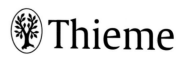

General and Visceral Surgery Review

Nicolas T. Schwarz, MD
Associate Professor
Friedrich Ebert Hospital
Surgical Clinic
Neumünster
Germany

Karl-Heinz Reutter, MD
Stuttgart
Germany

With contributions by
Hinrich Brunn, Ronald J. Elfeldt, Michael Fuchs,
Jan M. Mayer, Ingo L. Schmalbach, Nicolas T. Schwarz,
Alexander Selch, Burkhard Thiel, Michael Voelz

185 illustrations

Thieme
Stuttgart · New York

Library of Congress Cataloging-in-Publication Data

Allgemein- und Viszeralchirurgie. English.
  General and visceral surgery review/[edited by] Nicolas T. Schwarz, Karl-Heinz Reutter; with contributions by Hinrich Brunn ... [et al.]; [translator, Geraldine O'Sullivan; illustrators, P. Gusta ... et al.].
    p.; cm.
  Originally published in German as: Allgemein- und Viszeralchirurgie. 6th ed. 2009.
    ISBN 978-3-13-154311-0 (pbk.: alk. paper) 1. Operations, Surgical–Handbooks, manuals, etc. 2. Viscera–Surgery–Handbooks, manuals, etc. I. Schwarz, Nicolas T. II. Reutter, Karl-Heinz. III. Brunn, Hinrich. IV. Title.
    [DNLM: 1. Surgical Procedures, Operative–methods–Handbooks. 2. Viscera–surgery–Handbooks. WO 39]
    RD32.A56513 2011
    617'.9–dc23

                                          2011015799

This book is an authorized translation of the 6th German edition published and copyrighted 2009 by Georg Thieme Verlag, Stuttgart. Title of the German edition: Allgemein- und Viszeralchirurgie.

Translator: Geraldine O'Sullivan, Dublin, Republic of Ireland

Illustrators: P. Gusta, Champigny sur Marne, France; J. and K. Hormann, Stuttgart, Germany; Christiane and Dr. Michael von Solodkoff, Neckargemünd, Germany

© 2012 Georg Thieme Verlag,
Rüdigerstrasse 14, 70469 Stuttgart, Germany
http://www.thieme.de
Thieme New York, 333 Seventh Avenue,
http://www.thieme.com

Cover design: Thieme Publishing Group
Typesetting by Druckhaus Götz, Ludwigsburg, Germany
Printed in China by Everbest Printing Co. Ltd.

Important note: Medicine is an ever-changing science undergoing continual development. Research and clinical experience are continually expanding our knowledge, in particular our knowledge of proper treatment and drug therapy. Insofar as this book mentions any dosage or application, readers may rest assured that the authors, editors, and publishers have made every effort to ensure that such references are in accordance with **the state of knowledge at the time of production of the book.**

Nevertheless, this does not involve, imply, or express any guarantee or responsibility on the part of the publishers in respect to any dosage instructions and forms of applications stated in the book. **Every user is requested to examine carefully** the manufacturers' leaflets accompanying each drug and to check, if necessary in consultation with a physician or specialist, whether the dosage schedules mentioned therein or the contraindications stated by the manufacturers differ from the statements made in the present book. Such examination is particularly important with drugs that are either rarely used or have been newly released on the market. Every dosage schedule or every form of application used is entirely at the user's own risk and responsibility. The authors and publishers request every user to report to the publishers any discrepancies or inaccuracies noticed. If errors in this work are found after publication, errata will be posted at www.thieme.com on the product description page.

Some of the product names, patents, and registered designs referred to in this book are in fact registered trademarks or proprietary names even though specific reference to this fact is not always made in the text. Therefore, the appearance of a name without designation as proprietary is not to be construed as a representation by the publisher that it is in the public domain.

ISBN: 978-3-13-154311-0   1 2 3 4 5 6

List of Contributors

Hinrich Brunn, MD
Friedrich Ebert Hospital
Surgical Clinic
Department of Vascular Surgery
Neumünster
Germany

Ronald J. Elfeldt, MD
Associate Professor
Friedrich Ebert Hospital
Surgical Clinic
Department of Thoracic Surgery
Neumünster
Germany

Michael Fuchs, MD
Associate Professor
Friedrich Ebert Hospital
Trauma and Orthopedic Clinic, Sports Trauma Clinic
Neumünster
Germany

Jan M. Mayer, MD
Friedrich Ebert Hospital
Surgical Clinic
Neumünster
Germany

Ingo L. Schmalbach, MD
Friedrich Ebert Hospital
Surgical Clinic
Neumünster
Germany

Nicolas T. Schwarz, MD
Associate Professor
Friedrich Ebert Hospital
Surgical Clinic
Neumünster
Germany

Alexander Selch, MD
Friedrich Ebert Hospital
Surgical Clinic
Department of Vascular Surgery
Neumünster
Germany

Burkhard Thiel, MD
Friedrich Ebert Hospital
Surgical Clinic
Neumünster
Germany

Michael Voelz, MD
Friedrich Ebert Hospital
Surgical Clinic
Neumünster
Germany

Preface

General and Visceral Surgery Review was originally published in German in 1996 as a revision aid for surgery in general. Since then, as the individual surgical subspecialties continue to develop, and today's medical training is built around the "Common Trunk" (as it is called in Germany), with subsequent specialist training, it has been necessary to continually update and adapt the higher-training content according to the various surgical specialties. *General and Visceral Surgery Review* was published in its sixth German-language edition in 2009.

Karl-Heinz Reutter, MD, created *General and Visceral Surgery Review* and continued it through five successful editions in the German language. I am not only happy to take over the task of editor from him for further German language editions, I am also highly delighted to be able to present the first English-language edition.

The purpose of this textbook is higher training and examination preparation in general and visceral surgery. We have made every effort to include up-to-date information and to present this information in a concise and succinct format, thus enabling colleagues to acquire the necessary theoretical knowledge in the shortest possible time.

This book is designed to place emphasis on core statements, and includes suggestions for further reading to help consolidate what has been learned. Contributions were provided by surgeons actively working in this field. By calling on their own practical experiences they have produced an ideal learning tool suited to the current requirements of higher training and examination preparation.

Nicolas T. Schwarz   *Neumünster, Germany*

Acknowledgements

I thank my colleague K.-H. Reutter, MD, for giving me the opportunity to take over the editorship of this book. My special thanks also go to my medical colleagues in the Departments of Surgery and Trauma Surgery in Neumünster. We owe the production of this new edition to their enthusiasm for general and visceral surgery and to their constant thirst for knowledge, coupled with the desire to pass on this interest and their love of the specialty to their many colleagues.

Contents

1 Perioperative Medicine

N.T. Schwarz

- A patient's postoperative recovery has multifactorial influences (**Fig. 1.1**). The perfect surgical technique on its own does not suffice. The patient's progress is influenced particularly by physiological and psychological factors. "Evidence-based medicine" casts new light on traditional perioperative measures to produce new treatment concepts, the aim of which is to preserve or restore patient autonomy and homeostasis.

- Perioperative course has multifactorial influences.

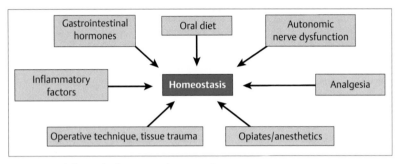

Fig. 1.1 Multifactorial influences on homeostasis.

■ Preoperative Phase

Risk Assessment

- The perioperative risk increases as the number of individual risk factors increases. Patients are classified prior to anesthesia according to the ASA (American Society of Anesthesiologists) classification (**Table 1.1**).
- In addition, a distinction can be made between patient-specific (**Table 1.2**) and operation-specific (**Table 1.3**) risks. Accordingly, preoperative investigations are necessary to assess the operative risk. In general, they are ordered when the results are likely to affect the management of the patient.
- Postoperative nausea and vomiting (PONV syndrome) are observed more
  - ► in females,
  - ► in nonsmokers,
  - ► with travel sickness,
  - ► with intraoperative opioid administration, and
  - ► with addition of nitrous oxide.
- PONV syndrome can be prevented effectively by various drugs (serotonin antagonists, dexamethasone, droperidol, propofol).

Table 1.1 ASA classification

Group	Description
I	Healthy, not taking any medication
II	Mild disease without functional limitation and need for medication
III	Disease requiring medication, mild limitation of activity
IV	Severe disease, permanent severe limitation of capacity
V	Moribund, life expectancy < 24 h
VI	Emergency surgery regardless of I–V

Source: ACC/AHA guideline update for perioperative cardiovascular evaluation for non-cardiac surgery. Circulation 2002:103:1257–1267.

Table 1.2 Patient risk factors

Low risk	Medium risk	High risk
• Advanced age • ECG abnormalities • Rhythms other than sinus rhythm • Low functional capacity • History of stroke • Poorly controlled hypertension	• Mild angina pectoris • Previous myocardial infarction • Compensated or early heart failure • Diabetes mellitus	• Unstable coronary syndrome • Decompensated heart failure • Severe arrhythmias

Source: ACC/AHA guideline update for perioperative cardiovascular evaluation for non-cardiac surgery. Circulation 2002:103:1257–1267.

Table 1.3 Operation risk factors

Low risk	Medium risk	High risk
• Endoscopic and superficial procedures • Cataract surgery • Breast surgery	• Carotid endarterectomy • Head and neck surgery • Intraperitoneal, intrathoracic and orthopedic procedures and prostate surgery	• Surgery on the aorta, other major vascular surgery and operations on peripheral vessels • Prolonged operations with major "volume shift" and/or blood loss

Source: ACC/AHA guideline update for perioperative cardiovascular evaluation for non-cardiac surgery. Circulation 2002:103:1257–1267.

Fasting

• Patients may generally drink low-fat liquids up to 2 hours preoperatively.

• Patients fast preoperatively to protect against aspiration. Aspiration of solid food can lead to vagal reactions, bradycardia, and asystole, and aspiration of liquids can also lead to pneumonia, respiratory insufficiency and, in extreme cases, to ARDS (adult respiratory distress syndrome). Adequate preoperative hydration is an important requirement for maintaining perioperative homeostasis.

- **Less than 6 hours preoperatively:** no high-fat liquids or solid foods
- **Up to 2 hours preoperatively:** clear fluids
- Deviations in the case of:
  - ► emergency surgery,
  - ► massive obesity,
  - ► gastric emptying disorder,
  - ► pyloric stenosis,
  - ► gastric atony,
  - ► esophageal stenosis and diverticula,
  - ► certain neurological diseases, and
  - ► apparent hypothyroidism.
- Prevention of stress-induced postoperative insulin resistance has been investigated in numerous studies. There is evidence that preoperative high-carbohydrate liquids, which are consumed up to 2 hours before the procedure, have a positive effect.

Patient-Informed Consent

- Apart from the legal requirement for patients to give informed consent, preoperative discussion of how patients can take an active part in their postoperative recovery is often positively motivating. Patients and relatives are given comprehensive information so that they are prepared as well as possible and can provide mutual support.

Bowel Preparation

- Orthograde bowel irrigation for bowel preparation before major abdominal surgery is obsolete. Like osmotically active irrigation fluids, they can lead to measurable electrolyte shifts and thus to fluid losses into the bowel lumen, which can be hazardous for patients with cardiovascular risks.
- In elective colorectal procedures using fast-track surgery, preparation with a laxative and an enema on the previous evening has proved to be sufficient.

- Orthograde bowel irrigation is virtually obsolete, and laxatives, enemas, or osmotically active solutions are used instead.

Premedication

- Apart from the anesthetic risk work-up and legal obligations, premedication serves to establish the perioperative anesthesiological treatment plan, particularly analgesia. The patient is given drug premedication for anxiolysis and sedation.

Pre- and Postoperative Anticoagulation

- The incidence of perioperative thrombosis in abdominal surgery averages 25% in studies. There are predisposing risk factors, which, together with the exposure factors (**Table 1.4**), define the individual's thrombosis risk (**Table 1.5**).

Table 1.4   Exposure factors

Low risk	Medium risk	High risk
• Minor or medium surgery with low trauma • Injuries without or with minor soft tissue damage • No additional or slight predisposing risk	• More prolonged surgery • Lower limb immobilization in a cast including a joint • Low thromboembolism risk due to operation or injury and additional predisposing thromboembolism risk	• Major surgery in the abdomen and pelvis for malignant or inflammatory disease • Polytrauma, severe injuries of the spine, pelvis and/or lower limb • Major surgery on the spine, pelvis, hip and knee • Major surgery in the chest, abdominal and/or pelvic body cavities • Medium risk due to operation or injury and additional predisposing risk • Patients with a history of thrombosis or pulmonary embolism

Source: AWMF (Working Group of German Specialist Scientific Medical Societies) guidelines: Inpatient and Outpatient Thromboembolism Prophylaxis in Surgery and Perioperative Medicine (April 24, 2003).
On the Internet: http://www.awmf-leitlinien.de/003-001.htm; revised February 28, 2009 [in German].

Table 1.5   Individual thrombosis risk

Thromboembolic complications	Low thromboembolism risk	Medium thromboembolism risk	High thromboembolism risk
Distal leg vein thrombosis	< 10%	10–40%	40–80%
Proximal leg vein thrombosis	< 1%	1–10%	10–30%
Fatal pulmonary embolism	< 0.1%	0.1–1%	≥ 1%

Source: AWMF guidelines: Inpatient and Outpatient Thromboembolism Prophylaxis in Surgery and Perioperative Medicine (April 24, 2003).
On the Internet: http://www.awmf-leitlinien.de/003-001.htm; revised February 28, 2009 [in German].

Predisposing Risk Factors
• Thrombophilia:
  ► History of venous thromboembolism
  ► Congenital or acquired thrombophilic defects of hemostasis (e.g., antiphospholipid syndrome, antithrombin, protein C or protein S deficiency, activated protein C resistance / factor V Leiden mutation, thrombophilic prothrombin polymorphism, etc.)
• Malignant disease
• Pregnancy and the postpartum period
• Advanced age (> 50 years; risk increases with age)

- Therapy with or block of sex hormones (including contraceptives and hormone replacement therapy)
- Chronic venous insufficiency
- Severe systemic infection
- Severe overweight (body mass index > 30)
- Heart failure: NYHA (New York Heart Association) grade III or IV
- Nephrotic syndrome
- Thrombosis prophylaxis consists of physical measures and, if necessary, medical thromboembolism prophylaxis.
- In patients with a low thrombosis risk, physical measures and early mobilization suffice, but in patients with a medium and higher thrombosis risk, medical thrombosis prophylaxis is usually indicated in addition.

Medical Thrombosis Prophylaxis
- In contrast to the common practice in North America, thrombosis prophylaxis in Europe is started on the evening before surgery, using unfractionated heparin (UFH) or low molecular weight heparin (LMWH).
- The duration of the medical thrombosis prophylaxis depends on predisposing risk factors, the degree of operative trauma, and postoperative immobilization. After major surgery for malignant disease in the abdomen, it lasts for an average of 4–5 weeks, but so far there are no binding recommendations.
- Current medications for thrombosis prophylaxis:
  - ► Heparins
    - – UFH
    - – LMWH
  - ► Danaparoid
  - ► Fondaparinux
  - ► Thrombin inhibitors
  - ► Hirudin
  - ► Vitamin K antagonists (coumarin)

- Perioperative thrombosis prophylaxis usually begins preoperatively.

■ Intraoperative Phase

- Most of the changes in recent years have been made in this phase.

Operation Technique

- Minimally invasive operation techniques have functional postoperative benefits compared with laparotomy, such as
  - ► less pain,
  - ► less postoperative intestinal atony,
  - ► altered postoperative immune response and inflammatory reaction, and
  - ► less postoperative pulmonary dysfunction.
- When laparotomy is performed, transverse incisions have proved to be superior compared with midline and paramedian laparotomy in respect of postoperative pain and pulmonary function. In general, they result in fewer incisional hernias.

Drains and Nasogastric Tubes

• Perioperative nasogastric tubes should remain in place for as short a time as possible.

• Experience has shown that anastomotic leaks and secondary hemorrhage are not identified despite intraperitoneal drains. This has also been confirmed in randomized controlled studies.
• The benefit of routine placement of a nasogastric tube has not been confirmed either. It does not prevent, but rather promotes, postoperative intestinal atony and may enable silent aspiration to occur.

Anesthesia

• Anesthesia and analgesia have an important influence on the postoperative course following general and visceral surgical procedures. The following are beneficial for these procedures:
  ► Rapidly controllable anesthetics
  ► Increase in the inspiratory oxygen concentration
  ► Normothermia
  ► Regional anesthesia methods (epidural anesthesia → analgesia and sympathetic block)
  ► Calculated intraoperative fluid replacement

Intraoperative Fluid Replacement

• Preoperative normovolemia is important for perioperative hemostasis.

• Maintenance of normovolemia and electrolyte balance is the most important goal. High infusion volumes were usual in the past to compensate assumed "third space" fluid losses. Avoidance of preoperative hypovolemia allows a restrictive fluid infusion regimen with complete electrolyte solution and colloid solution in a ratio of 2:1.
• Excessive infusion volumes can
  ► cause edema of the bowel wall;
  ► produce protracted postoperative intestinal motility dysfunction;
  ► have effects on cardiac function;
  ► cause pulmonary side effects; and
  ► lead to prolonged convalescence and hospitalization.

■ Postoperative Period

• Postoperative care is multidisciplinary.

• Postoperative care of patients is multidisciplinary. The postoperative period is characterized by analgesia, diet, mobilization, and discharge planning. The aim is freedom from pain while avoiding the use of systemic opioids. Where possible, mobilization should begin on the day of surgery.
• In meta-analyses of randomized studies, no advantage was found for postoperative fasting compared with early enteral feeding. In particular, anastomosis leak rates are not increased with early enteral feeding and there are fewer general infectious complications.

■ Fast-Track Surgery

Definition

- "Fast-track" implies an interdisciplinary and multimodal approach to improve and speed up convalescence and reduce postoperative complications, thus shortening hospitalization.
- Fast-track surgery comprises:
  - ► Preoperative patient informed consent
  - ► Atraumatic surgical technique
  - ► Reduction of stress
  - ► Elimination of pain, usually by regional anesthesia techniques (especially in the form of thoracic epidural anesthesia)
  - ► Optimized fluid and temperature management
  - ► Early enteral diet
  - ► Prevention of gastrointestinal atony and PONV
  - ► Rapid postoperative mobilization

- Fast-track surgery is evidence-based and is intended to reduce complications.

Therapeutic Approach for Colon Surgery

Preoperative
- Informed consent: discussion with the patient and relatives, planned discharge from the third postoperative day
- No bowel lavage, laxative if necessary
- Fasting: 6 hours for solids, 2 hours for liquids

Intraoperative
- Thoracic combined epidural anesthesia (EDA) and local anesthesia (LA)/opioids; coxibs IV, if necessary
- Laparoscopic surgery as far as possible, otherwise transverse or curved laparotomy
- Avoid drains as far as possible
- Remove gastric tube on extubation

Day of Surgery
- Transfer from recovery room to normal ward
- Limit postoperative infusion to 500 mL electrolyte solution
- Continuous thoracic EDA (LA/opioid), coxibs IV if necessary, avoid systemic opiates, morphine sulfate, 5 mg SC only if necessary
- Magnesium oxide or sodium picosulfate daily until first defecation
- Tea (maximum 100 mL), 2 portions of yogurt
- Early mobilization

First Postoperative Day
- Continuous EDA (LA/opioid), oral coxibs, avoidance of systemic opiates; morphine sulfate 10 mg orally, only if necessary
- Magnesium oxide or sodium picosulfate daily until first defecation
- Basic hospital diet, drinking volume > 1500 mL, mobilization out of bed for at least 8 hours or at least twice daily
- Removal of any drains and bladder catheter

Second Postoperative Day
- Removal of epidural and central venous catheters, oral coxibs, avoidance of systemic opiates; morphine sulfate 10 mg orally only if necessary
- Magnesium oxide or sodium picosulfate daily until first defecation, basic hospital diet, drinking volume > 1500 mL
- Full mobilization (retiring to bed only for an afternoon nap and at night)

Third Postoperative Day
- As second postoperative day
- Discuss discharge with patient and relatives, information sheet for post-hospital course (to return immediately if any problems)
- Dietary advice

From Fourth Postoperative Day
- As second postoperative day
- Final discussion with patient and relatives
- Discharge by agreement

Post-Hospital Outpatient Review
- Removal of sutures
- Discussion of histological results; if necessary schedule adjuvant therapy

Further Reading

ACC/AHA guideline update for perioperative cardiovascular evaluation for non-cardiac surgery. Circulation 2002; 105: 1257–1267

Fearon KC et al. Enhanced recovery after surgery : a consensus review of clinical care for patients undergoing colonic resections. Clin Nutr 2005; 24: 466–477

Kehlet H et al. Care after colonic operation – is it evidence based? Results from a multinational survey in Europe and the Unites States. J Am Coll Surg 2006; 202: 45–54

National Collaborating Centre for Acute and Chronic Conditions. Venous thromboembolism: reducing the risk of venous thromboembolism (deep vein thrombosis and pulmonary embolism) in patients admitted to hospital. National Institute for Health and Clinical Excellence (NICE); 2010 Jan. 50 p. (Clinical guideline; no. 92). http://www.guideline.gov/content.aspx?id=24106&search=thrombosis (accessed May 2011)

Schwenk W et al. Wandel der perioperativen Therapie bei elektiven kolorektalen Resektionen in Deutschland 1991 und 2000/2001. Zentralbl Chir 2003; 128: 1086–1092

2 Thyroid

B. Thiel

■ Anatomy

Ontogenic Development

The thyroid develops in the embryo from the floor of the pharynx (foregut) from day 24, initially as the thyroglossal duct. The two lobes of the thyroid arise from this. From week 7 they lie in front of the trachea. The duct often persists as a pyramidal lobe superior to the thyroid gland.

Histology

Follicles consisting of epithelial cells are the central feature. These are arranged in a single layer and produce thyroglobulin, the precursor of the thyroid hormones, in the follicle. The thyroid is surrounded by a capsule of connective tissue (fibrous capsule); connective tissue septa originate from this and divide the organ into individual lobules. Each lobule consists of several follicles. In

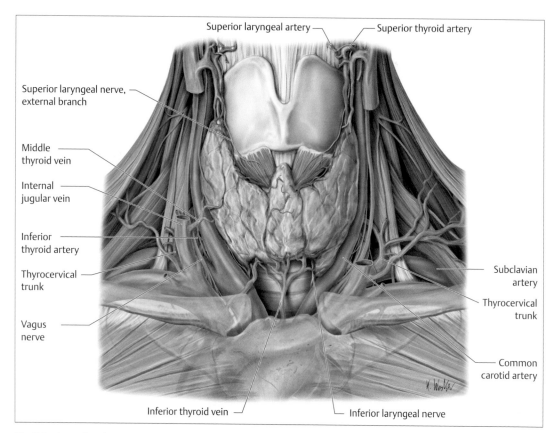

Fig. 2.1 Arterial and venous supply of the thyroid (from Thieme Atlas of Anatomy, Neck and Internal Organs, © Thieme 2006, Illustration by Karl Wesker).

mammals, the parafollicular C cells are located between the epithelial cells of the follicles and their basement membrane. Around the follicles are reticular fibers and a dense capillary network (blood and lymphatic capillaries).

Arteries (Fig. 2.1)

- Superior thyroid arteries
- Inferior thyroid arteries
- Thyroid ima artery

- **Superior thyroid arteries** from the external carotid artery
- **Inferior thyroid arteries** from the thyrocervical trunk (which arises from the subclavian artery)
- **Thyroid ima artery:** This unpaired artery is found in 10% of the population. It arises from the thyrocervical trunk or aortic arch and approaches the isthmus from below. Within the thyroid there are numerous anastomoses. The thyroid arteries are not end-arteries. There is good collateral circulation from extraglandular arteries, enabling all four thyroid arteries to be ligated without interfering with the nutrition of the gland.

Veins (Fig. 2.1)

- Unpaired thyroid plexus
- Middle thyroid vein
- Superior thyroid vein

- **Unpaired thyroid plexus** drains into the inferior thyroid vein and brachiocephalic vein (downward)
- **Middle thyroid vein** (the Kocher vein) drains into the internal jugular vein (laterally)
- **Superior thyroid vein** drains into the internal jugular vein (upward)

Nerves

- Superior laryngeal nerve
- Internal branch
- Recurrent laryngeal nerve
- **Warning:** recurrent laryngeal nerve and superior laryngeal nerve are at risk

- **Superior laryngeal nerve** from the inferior ganglion of the vagus nerve. The external branch innervates the cricothyroid muscle. It is at risk during ligature of vessels at the upper pole.

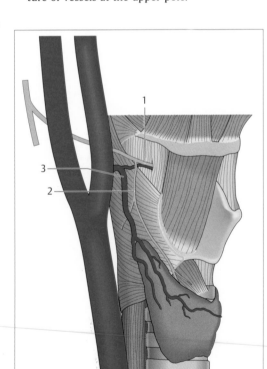

Fig. 2.2 The external branch of the superior laryngeal nerve runs close to the thyroid in ca. 15% of people and can be spared by ligating the vessels at the upper pole close to the capsule (from Frilling and Weber 2007, see p. 413).
1: Internal branch of superior laryngeal nerve
2: External branch of superior laryngeal nerve
3: Superior thyroid artery

- The **internal branch** contains mainly sensory fibers and supplies the mucosa of the epiglottis and larynx to below the glottis.
- The **recurrent laryngeal nerve** runs in the groove between the esophagus and trachea and crosses the inferior thyroid artery variably. It can run in front of, behind, and partially in front of and partially behind the branches of the thyroid artery. It is particularly at risk during ligature of the inferior thyroid artery. The motor branches of the recurrent nerve innervate the laryngeal muscles with the exception of the cricothyroid muscle. **Figure 2.2** shows the course of the nerves.

Surgically Relevant Groups of Lymph Nodes

- Four compartments are defined when the locoregional groups of lymph nodes and the anatomical boundaries are classified (**Table 2.1**). In the majority of differentiated thyroid carcinomas, lymph node metastases can be expected mainly in the central cervical (44%) and ipsilateral lateral cervical (34%) compartments (**Fig. 2.3**).

Table 2.1   Locoregional lymph nodes (LNs) and lymphatic drainage pathways

Three locoregional lymph node stations	Four surgically relevant compartments
Central cervical LN station	Central cervical compartment right and left (1a and 1b)
Lateral cervical LN station	Ipsilateral lateral cervical compartment (2) Contralateral lateral cervical compartment (3)
Upper mediastinal LN station	Mediastinal infrabrachiocephalic compartment right and left (4a and 4b)

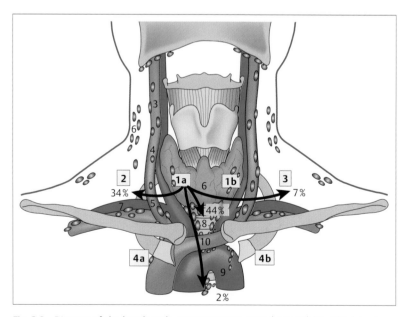

Fig. 2.3   Diagram of the lymph node compartments: central cervical (1a, 1b), lateral cervical (2, 3) and mediastinal (4a, 4b) with the percentages of the incidence of LN metastases (from Frilling and Weber 2007, see p. 413).

■ Physiology

- Hormones: thyroxine (T4), triiodothyronine (T3), and calcitonin
- Mode of action of T3 and T4: energy metabolism ↑
- Mode of action of calcitonin: calcium level ↓
- Feedback loop: TRH ↑ → TSH ↑ → T4 and T3 ↑ → TSH ↓ → TRH ↓

- The hormones produced by the thyroid gland are **thyroxine (T4), triiodothyronine (T3)**, and **calcitonin.** T3 and T4 are produced by the epithelial cells of the follicles. Thyroglobulin, their precursor, is released into the follicle cavity, where it takes up iodine (iodination) and divides to form the hormones thyroxine and triiodothyronine. The parafollicular C cells produce calcitonin.
- The thyroid hormones thyroxine and triiodothyronine act on nearly all the cells in the body and stimulate energy metabolism. They are necessary for growth and differentiation. Other effects include, for example, vasodilatation, a rise in body temperature, and a rise in blood pressure and pulse rate. Calcitonin reduces the calcium level in the blood and is thus an antagonist of parathyroid hormone (PTH), which regulates the extracellular calcium level.
- To regulate the degree of secretion of thyroid hormones, the body possesses a hormonal feedback control mechanism.
  - ► When there is a lack of thyroid hormones, the thyroid hormone level in the blood falls.
  - ► The hypothalamus releases more thyroliberin (TRH, thyroid releasing hormone).
  - ► TRH in turn causes the pituitary to release more thyrotropin (TSH, thyroid stimulating hormone) into the blood.
  - ► The TSH reaches the thyroid via the circulation. There it stimulates production of the thyroid hormones T3 and T4.
  - ► Negative feedback: high concentrations of T3 and T4 inhibit secretion of TSH and TRH.
  - ► T3 and T4 deficiency increases the secretion of TRH and TSH.
- The aim of this feedback control system is to keep the concentrations of free T3 and T4 constant. Persistent TSH secretion leads to hyperplasia of the thyroid (goiter).

■ General Epidemiology

- Up to two out of three Germans are affected, women and men equally.

- Studies have shown that in Europe one in three people has a pathologically altered thyroid as a result of iodine deficiency.
- Women and men are affected equally, and over the age of 45 years, one in two persons is affected in Germany.

■ General Diagnostic Approach

■ Clinical Examination

- Diagnosis starts with the medical history and physical examination (**Fig. 2.4**). The size and consistency of the thyroid and its movement on swallowing are palpated.
- In the history, attention is paid to the most varied symptoms, which are described below with the respective thyroid disorders.

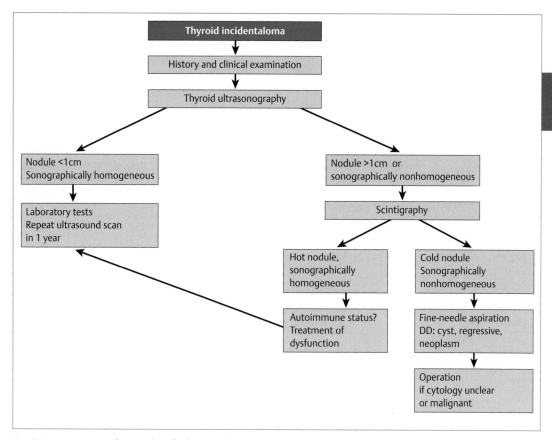

Fig. 2.4 Investigation of an incidentally discovered nodule (DD: differential diagnosis).

■ Laboratory Tests

Baseline Tests

- **Basal TSH:** normal range = 0.27–4.2 μIU/mL. Regulation of TSH secretion is sensitive and specific, even in borderline hypothyroidism or hyperthyroidism.
- A normal TSH level rules out overt hyperthyroidism and hypothyroidism.
- The most important parameters for monitoring treatment with T4 medication:
  - ► Normal TSH with replacement therapy (e.g., in hypothyroidism)
  - ► Low TSH with suppression therapy (e.g., in goiter)
  - ► Do not suppress TSH fully, as otherwise iodine uptake is not stimulated (iodine deficiency = stimulus to proliferation)
- fT_3 and fT_4 normal ranges: fT_3 = 3.4–7.2 pmol/L and fT_4 = 0.73–1.95 ng/dL. Thyroid hormones are biologically available and active only in the free form.

- Thyroid disease can be present despite a euthyroid metabolic state, for example, thyroid carcinoma or a compensated adenoma.

Special Tests

- **TRH test** ("TSH after TRH"): TSH level increases above the normal range 30 minutes after IV injection of TRH (positive test). Indication: borderline TSH levels.
  - ► Latent and overt hypothyroidism: excessive rise in TSH
  - ► Hyperthyroidism: no rise in TSH (negative test)

2

- **Specific antibodies** to thyroid tissue in autoimmune thyroiditis:
  - ► TRAB (anti-TSH receptor antibodies)
  - ► TAB (thyroglobulin antibodies)
  - ► TPO-MAB (TPO = thyroid peroxidase, a membrane-bound protein in the thyroid cells; MAB = microsomal antibodies)
- **Thyroglobulin:** normal range is < 75 µg/mL in healthy persons and < 3 µg/mL in post-thyroidectomy patients.
  - ► Normal levels are possible with small carcinomas.
  - ► Very high levels can be expected with metastases.
  - ► Normalization can be expected after successful treatment.
  - ► Normalization fails to occur if metastases are not removed.
  - ► Levels increase again in the event of recurrence.
- **Calcitonin:** normal range is up to 4.6 pg/mL in women and up to 11.5 pg/mL in men.

■ Diagnostic Imaging

Ultrasonography

Volumetry

- Ultrasonography is the mainstay of thyroid diagnostic imaging.

- **Determination of thyroid volume.** Approximate results are obtained by calculation: length × height × width (in cm) × 0.5 = volume in mL. The normal volume is 18 mL in adult women and 25 mL in men.

Assessment of the Echo Pattern

- Diffusely hypoechoic parenchyma can represent autoimmune disease but neither Graves disease nor Hashimoto thyroiditis can be deduced from this.

Assessment of Vascularization (Color-Coded Doppler or Duplex Ultrasonography)

- The perfusion pattern supplements the other findings and does not allow either assessment of function or reliable diagnosis of malignancy.

- Increased vascularization is often found in the active hyperthyroid stage of Graves disease. However, it is not pathognomonic as it also occurs in hypothyroidism with high TSH stimulation.
- Vascularization is diminished in thyroiditis with hypothyroidism (Hashimoto disease). The perfusion pattern at the margins (a possible benign finding) and in the center of the nodule (suspicious for malignancy) can assist in the differential diagnosis.

Focal Lesions and Nodules

An exact description of thyroid nodules includes the following information:
- Position
- Consistency such as: solid nodule, partially cystic, cysts
- Dimensions in three planes
- Echogenicity
  - ► Anechoic: cyst
  - ► Hypoechoic: adenoma, malignant tumor, hemorrhage
  - ► Hyperechoic: fibrosis, adenoma, calcification
- Margins
- Demarcation
- Calcification: macro- or microcalcification
- Perfusion at the margins (a possible benign finding) and in the center of the nodule (suspicious for malignancy)

Assessment of Cervical Lymph Nodes
- Lymph nodes > 1 cm and lymph nodes with virtually equal transverse and longitudinal diameter should be considered abnormal.

Parathyroid Glands
- The sensitivity of ultrasonography in detecting a parathyroid adenoma in primary or secondary hyperparathyroidism is about 50% and up to 85% in conjunction with a sestamibi scan.

Scintigraphy

- The radionuclide ^{99m}Tc pertechnetate is used almost exclusively. This is a pure gamma source with a short half-life (6 hours), which is taken up ("trapped") by the thyroid cells, like iodine. Since pertechnetate is not metabolized further, iodine isotopes are indicated in special situations, for example, to detect dystopic thyroid tissue.

Indications
- Investigation of suspected functional autonomy or Graves disease
- Investigation of palpable nodules or space-occupying lesions found on ultrasonography (suspected malignancy)
- Identification and localization of dystopic thyroid tissue
- Investigation for residual tissue or local recurrence of differentiated thyroid carcinoma

Interpretation of the Result
In scintigraphy, the uptake pattern is assessed with regard to
- areas of increased uptake (hot spots),
- areas of reduced uptake (cold spots), and
- ^{99m}Tc thyroidal uptake (TcTU),
taking into account the clinical symptoms, any previous treatment, the ultrasound result, and laboratory tests.

Cold Nodule on Scintigraphy
Possible causes of an area of low radionuclide uptake in the thyroid:
- Carcinoma
- Cyst
- Hemorrhage
- Follicular adenoma
- Regressive changes
- Focal inflammatory lesions

- Differential diagnosis is often possible with ultrasound imaging, but fine-needle biopsy is necessary when the acoustic pattern is hypoechoic or complex.

The reflection pattern on ultrasound scanning often allows differential diagnosis. However, when the acoustic pattern is hypoechoic or complex, a biopsy must always be obtained for cytology by fine-needle aspiration.

Hot Nodule on Scintigraphy
This is an area of increased uptake in the thyroid.
- Autonomic adenomas can often be identified on the scintigram only when the remainder of the thyroid shows no or slight uptake because of an oversupply of hormones (**Table 2.2**).

2

Table 2.2 T3 suppression and TSH stimulation to unmask an adenomatous nodule

Finding on palpation	Scintigraphy	Further investigation	Suspected diagnosis
Unilateral solitary nodule		T3 suppression	Compensated auto-nomic adenoma
Unilateral solitary nodule		TSH stimulation	Decompensated auto-nomic adenoma

- **Compensated autonomic adenoma:** in a nonsuppressed thyroid autonomic adenomas often do not stand out from the surrounding tissue.
- **Decompensated autonomic adenoma:** in the case of active adenomas, which often cause hyperthyroidism, endogenous suppression may already be present due to the hormones produced in the adenoma.

Assessment of functional activity subsequently is often possible only by repeating scintigraphy with exogenous TSH suppression (by giving the thyroid hormone T3 orally) or by TSH stimulation (**Table 2.2**), for instance, to unmask hot nodules or demonstrate disseminated autonomy.

Other Imaging Methods

- MRI and CT play a minor role in the routine diagnosis of thyroid disorders.

- An **MRI** or **CT** scan (without contrast) can be considered for assessing the surrounding soft tissues.
- Imaging can influence further management, especially in the case of large goiters or invasive thyroid carcinomas, for example, whether extensive resection is indicated if there is local metastasis.
- These imaging methods play a subordinate role in routine investigation of the thyroid.

■ **Invasive Diagnostics**

Fine-Needle Biopsy

- In the case of thyroid nodules, a narrowly circumscribed group of suspicious lesions should be selected for surgical diagnosis and/or treatment.
- The requirements for fine-needle biopsy (FNB) are that the physician performing it should be experienced in the technique and that the pathologist should be experienced in cytology; the percentage of nonassessable aspirates should be less than 10%.
- Thyroid ultrasonography (to distinguish cysts from focal lesions and assess echogenicity and margins) and thyroid scintigraphy should be performed beforehand.

Indications

- Suspected malignancy
- Presence of solitary, hypoechoic, cold, rapidly growing or poorly demarcated nodule
- Suspected subacute or chronic lymphocytic thyroiditis
- Solitary nodule when there is a history of percutaneous high-voltage radiation of the neck region
- Therapeutic FNB of large thyroid cysts producing signs of local compression or of acute purulent thyroiditis is possible.

- FNB is especially indicated if malignancy is suspected.

Interpretation of the Result

- The diagnostic certainty varies greatly among the different nodules; sensitivity is reported to be 70–100% and specificity 20–90%.
- In contrast to follicular neoplasm, it is often possible to draw a clear conclusion in papillary, medullary, and anaplastic carcinoma. This requires either further investigation or treatment and no further observation of a cold nodule.

- In the case of follicular neoplasm, it is not possible to distinguish between thyroid follicular carcinoma and a benign follicular adenoma from the cytology. A biopsy must be obtained for histological examination

■ General Treatment Approach

■ Indications

Absolute Indications for Surgery

- Large goiters causing mechanical obstruction (grade II–III; e.g., sensation of tightness, dyspnea, difficulty swallowing, venous congestion, tracheal stenosis, or tracheomalacia)
- Suspected malignancy
- To rule out carcinoma
- Treatment of carcinoma
- Solitary cold nodule
- Goiters with autonomous activity

Relative Indication for Surgery

- Cosmetic reasons in the case of grade I–II goiters

■ General Surgical Therapy

Tactical Considerations

- The aim of modern thyroid surgery is resection according to the results of investigations, preserving function where possible (**Fig. 2.5**). Diseased or functionally overactive thyroid tissue should be removed completely. Macroscopic assessment of the tissue by the surgeon is very important.
- Because of these tactical considerations, surgical management of thyroid disease has moved from subtotal bilateral resection of the goiter, which was performed frequently in the past, to hemithyroidectomy with subtotal resection of the contralateral side. The vessels at the upper pole are not ligated; tissue that is still normal is usually found here. This change in concept has resulted in the increasing importance of exposing the recurrent laryngeal nerve and the parathyroid glands, as surgery is now increasingly performed posterior to the fascia and close to the nerve. Inspection of both lobes of the thyroid is essential but complete mobilization of both lobes is not necessary when preoperative diagnosis of a unilateral abnormality was reliable.

- Operation tactics: resection according to results and preserving function, where possible

2

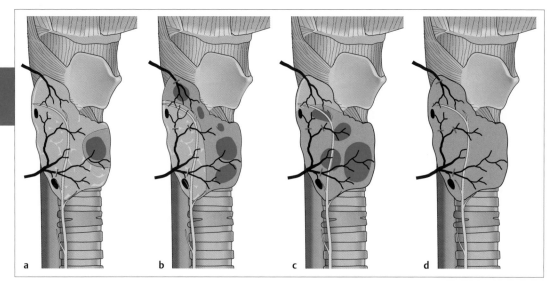

Fig. 2.5 a–d   Operation techniques according to morphology and with preservation of function.
a Enucleation
b Subtotal resection (conventional)
c Subtotal resection leaving the upper pole
d Lobectomy

- Surgery is performed under endotracheal anesthesia, ideally with tube electrodes to allow intraoperative neuromonitoring.
- The previously popular extreme hyperextension of the head has now been abandoned. Surgery is performed either with the upper body elevated 30° or supine with, at most, moderate extension of the cervical spine.

Operative Technique

- Access is through a transverse incision, one to two fingerbreadths above the sternal notch, if possible in a skin crease or after drawing the line of incision or marking it with a suture. Modern surgical methods (ligature using ultrasonic scissors or bipolar forceps) often allow the incision to be only 4–5 cm in length. If a complicated procedure is anticipated, a bigger incision should be planned beforehand as subsequent lateral extension of the incision leads to a poorer cosmetic result.
- Divide the subcutaneous fat and platysma with bipolar scissors. The anterior jugular veins can be spared to diminish any tendency to postoperative swelling.
- The strap muscles are split in the midline from the thyroid cartilage downward to the trachea.
- Dissection is in the midline down to the avascular layer on the capsule.
- **Preparation of one side:** Division of the infrahyoid neck muscles, which is often described in the literature, is necessary only in very rare cases. This can sometimes be unavoidable when the operation field cannot be seen in full (recurrent goiter, giant goiter).

- For further dissection, finding the "correct" plane between the outermost and inner thyroid capsule is very important to allow full anatomical and bloodless mobilization of the thyroid lobes.
- Lateral mobilization strictly close to the capsule with bipolar forceps gives lateral access to the upper pole. The upper pole of the thyroid is dissected with bipolar forceps or ultrasonic scissors. Dissection must be strictly close to the capsule so as not to irritate the superior laryngeal nerve.
- The upper pole vessels are managed with ultrasonic scissors, bipolar current (e.g., Ligashure), clips or ligatures.
- After dividing the middle thyroid vein, the upper pole can be increasingly dislocated forward with the lobe.
- Exposure of the capsular branches of the inferior thyroid artery and ligation close to the capsule.

Exposure of the Recurrent Laryngeal Nerve
- This is essential when dissecting close to the nerve, for example during hemithyroidectomy, thyroidectomy, resection of recurrent goiter, and enucleation of dorsal nodules. The occurrence of variations in the course of the nerve argues for intraoperative identification of the nerve. Loupes and neuromonitoring can be helpful.
- If the nerve cannot be exposed during dissection, it may be necessary to leave a posterior remnant of the thyroid capsule in situ. If complete resection is essential, for example because of diffuse autonomy or carcinoma, and the nerve cannot be exposed bilaterally, only one side should be resected initially. After checking vocal cord function in the awake patient, surgery can be performed on the other side in an early second stage. This procedure can be better explained to patients if the possibility of deciding on a two-stage operation has been discussed with them preoperatively.

  - No signal after hemithyroidectomy: two-stage surgery on the contralateral side

Dissection of the Parathyroid Glands
- In any more extensive dissection, the parathyroids must be demonstrated and preserved with their blood supply except when radical surgery necessitates their removal. When the recurrent nerve is exposed, the superior parathyroids are located slightly above where it crosses the inferior thyroid artery, and the inferior parathyroids are located anterior and inferior to this, and also in the cervical part of the thyrothymic ligament.
- Juxtacapsular dissection of the branches of the inferior thyroid artery prevents interference with the blood supply of the parathyroids. However, if perfusion is reduced at the end of the operation, the parathyroid in question should be excised, divided into three or four smaller pieces and reimplanted in a pocket of the sternocleidomastoid muscle.

  - If the perfusion of the parathyroids is impaired, dissect them out and reimplant them in muscle.

Ligation of the Vascular Supply
- The upper pole vessels are ligated in hemithyroidectomy, and in subtotal resection the upper pole vessels are spared on the contralateral side, since the upper pole is not reached through the paratracheal blood supply. The inferior pole vessels are managed close to the capsule, for example with bipolar forceps or ultrasonic scissors or ligatures.

2

Conclusion of Surgery

Removal of the thyroid is followed by:

- Meticulous hemostasis, with ligatures or clips when close to nerves and with bipolar forceps or diathermy when distant from nerves
- Final neuromonitoring of the recurrent nerves
- Suture of the strap neck muscles
- Suture of the subcutaneous tissue, especially the platysma

The needle should not pass too close to the skin surface to avoid skin puckering on the neck. Insertion of drains is not recommended if hemostasis has been meticulous. This does not prevent secondary hemorrhage due to slipping of a ligature but a drain interferes with patient comfort.

Intraoperative Neuromonitoring Procedure

- The neural structures at the paratracheal thyroid hilum can be better distinguished from other connective tissue or vascular structures by means of intraoperative neuromonitoring (IONM).
- Even the use of IONM does not provide 100 percent security. The rate of recurrent nerve paresis is not lower if intraoperative monitoring alone is relied on, but it allows safer and faster dissection when the anatomy is unclear.
- The use of IONM is increasingly regarded as a component of the operation tactics.

- Atraumatic leads, such as tube electrodes, are recommended for IONM.

- When intraoperative neuromonitoring was first used, the signal was conducted directly in the vocalis muscle through transligament electrodes (cricothyroid ligament). Tube electrodes, which allow atraumatic recording, are used today.

■ Special Surgical Therapy

Enucleation of a Nodule

Indications
- Small nodule with smooth margins
- No dysfunctional tissue in the remainder of the thyroid
- No evidence of malignancy, fine-needle aspiration beforehand, if necessary
- Histological diagnosis
- Cosmetically troublesome
- Enucleation can also be performed as a minimally invasive procedure (see below).

Operative Technique

- Small incision in the sternal notch
- Dissection down to the capsule of the side in question (see above)
- Enucleation of the nodule with bipolar forceps and meticulous hemostasis or resection with ultrasonic scissors
- Suture of capsule
- Subcutaneous suture
- Intracutaneous skin suture

Subtotal Resection

Indications
- Subtotal resection with bilateral reduction of thyroid volume is a rather rare procedure nowadays.
- It can still be employed for diffuse autonomy when there is normal posterior tissue bilaterally.

Operative Technique

The dissection is carried out as described above.
- During resection, the posterior capsule is not dissected free, but part of the thyroid around the nerves and parathyroids is left in situ.
- The latter also involves uncertainty as to whether the extent of the resection leaves the nerves and parathyroids unharmed.
- Establish the resection margin.
- Divide the thyroid tissue from lateral to medial.
- Hemostasis and suture of the residual thyroid capsule
- Skin suture

- **Caution:** nerve injury when suturing capsule

Hemithyroidectomy

Indications
- Large solitary nodule
- Diagnosis of suspected carcinoma (cold nodule)
- Papillary microcarcinoma

Operative Technique

- Unilateral dissection of the thyroid lobe (see above)
- Neuromonitoring
- Division of the isthmus with ligatures, bipolar forceps/scissors or ultrasonic scissors
- Resection of the thyroid lobe and exploration of the contralateral side
- Wound closure

Hemithyroidectomy with Subtotal Resection of the Contralateral Side (Dunhill Operation)

Indications
- Unilateral nodular goiter at the lower pole of the contralateral side
- Debulking of euthyroid goiter
- Reduction of functionally altered tissue in hyperthyroidism

In contrast to bilateral subtotal thyroid resection, this procedure involves removal of the thyroid lobe where most of the thyroid disease is located, with subtotal resection of the contralateral side according to the investigation results. The thyroid volume is not reduced schematically but the extent of resection is determined functionally. Healthy tissue is usually found at the upper pole, so that the upper pole of the less affected side can be left in situ.

2

Operative Technique

- Dissection with mobilization of the more affected lobe (see above)
- Neuromonitoring
- Sparing of the parathyroids
- Dissection across the trachea to the contralateral side
- Juxtacapsular management of the branches of the superior thyroid artery
- Determine the resection margins of the contralateral lobe
- Divide the thyroid tissue with bipolar current or ultrasonic dissector
- Spare the upper pole if possible, otherwise extend the surgery to thyroidectomy if the tissue of the upper pole is abnormal also
- Wound closure

Thyroidectomy

Indications
- Bilateral nodular goiter
- Bilateral giant goiter
- Carcinoma surgery when tumor is large
- Medullary carcinoma
- Differentiated carcinoma (apart from papillary microcarcinoma)
- Undifferentiated carcinoma
- Secure prevention of recurrence of Graves disease
- Thyrotoxic crisis
- Relative indications: thyroiditis or hyperthyroidism not controlled by conservative treatment

• Consider the possibility of two-stage surgery if the nerve is injured on one side

Thyroidectomy requires cautious dissection of both posterior thyroid capsules. Neuromonitoring is essential so that intraoperative injury on one side can be identified promptly and the surgical plan can be switched to two-stage resection.

Operative Technique

- Dissection of both thyroid lobes as an anatomic unit, that is, the specimen is not divided at the isthmus.
- Neuromonitoring
- Exposure of the parathyroids and, if necessary, reimplantation in a pocket of the left sternocleidomastoid muscle should perfusion be impaired
- Mark the specimen with sutures

■ Minimally Invasive Surgery Techniques

Minimally invasive techniques of thyroid surgery have been developed in recent years and the proportion of these operations in some centers is around 10%.

Purely Endoscopic Procedures
- Collar (Gagner/Hüscher/Ikeda/Kataoka)
- Prethoracic (Ishii/Kim/Shimizu/Yamashita)
- Axillary (Ikeda)

- Supra- or submandibular (Inabent III/Yamashita)
- Perimamillary (breast: Ohgami/Park/Shiamazu)

Open Video-Assisted Procedures
- Medial (Miccoli/Bellantone)
- Lateral (Henry)

Open Approach with Minimal Incision Length
- Medial (Ikeda)
- Lateral (Sackett)

Minimally Invasive Video-Assisted Thyroid Surgery

Minimally invasive video-assisted thyroid surgery (MIVAT) has become established as the most frequent technique; this does not always mean that thyroidectomy is performed.

Use of MIVAT depends on the correct indication (**Table 2.3**).

• MIVAT is the most common surgical technique.

Operative Technique

- Video unit at the patient's head
- If necessary, anesthetic equipment at the patient's feet, ventilation through an extension
- Surgeon on the right or left depending on findings, first assistant opposite, second assistant at the patient's head
- Small, 1–3-cm incision in sternal notch, size depending on findings
- Division of neck muscles in the midline
- Use of 5-mm camera, partly as "miner's lamp" in an open procedure with direct vision of the operation site or as an endoscopy camera at the upper pole
- Dissection of the thyroid capsule with a dissector/spatula
- Juxtacapsular management of the branches of the thyroid artery at the lower pole to mobilize the lobe
- Exposure of the parathyroids
- Dissection on the posterior capsule with exposure of the recurrent laryngeal nerve
- Dissection of the upper pole with dissector and microsurgical instruments, bipolar forceps
- Management of the upper pole vessels with clips, bipolar current or diathermy, for example with Ligashure precise
- Anterior dislocation of the mobilized thyroid lobe and division at the isthmus
- Exploration of the contralateral side
- Wound closure, absorbable intracutaneous skin suture

- MIVAT is still controversial today but has become more established because of increasing patient acceptance.
- The advantages cited are the cosmetic result, fewer postoperative symptoms, and the detailed view afforded by magnification. The disadvantages—such as longer operating times and the poorer overall view, and possibly greater risk of complications as a result—have not been confirmed in comparative studies.

2

• The criteria are relative and are currently being extended.

Table 2.3 Inclusion and exclusion criteria for MIVAT

Inclusion criteria	Exclusion criteria
• Nodules ≤ 3.5 cm • Goiter with a volume 25–30 mL • Small Graves goiter	• Multiple large nodules • Goiter with a volume > 40 mL • Thyroiditis • Thyroid carcinoma

Total Video-endoscopic Goiter Resection Via Axillo-Bilateral Breast Approach (ABBA)

Thyroid surgery from a submammary and axillary approach represents another minimally invasive technique. The ABBA technique for the first time provides a method of thyroid resection without a neck scar. This technique is employed in only a few centers.

Indication
• Patient's wish

Operative Technique

• Skin incision in the axilla and at the edge of the nipple
• Insertion of trocars
• Dissection with an ultrasonic dissector
• Procedure as in MIVAT
• Specimen removed through the axilla

• However, minimally invasive surgery is an alternative to conventional surgery in only 5–10% of all cases. All other patients will continue to undergo conventional surgery.

■ Postoperative Management

Routine Treatment
• Monitoring in the recovery room, analgesia

Routine Tests
• Ca^{2+} measurement on the first day, replacement only if the patient shows clinical signs or a very low level and when symptoms are anticipated
• ENT check on day 2 when the patient is still in hospital, otherwise as an outpatient
• Measure thyroid hormones in 4–6 weeks and initiate replacement according to basal TSH with benign goiter

■ Complications

Secondary Hemorrhage

Secondary hemorrhage occurs in the first 12–24 hours. It requires close monitoring when there are few signs. If dyspnea occurs with major swelling outside the operation tract, opening the wound to release the hematoma is a life-saving measure. After this, how to proceed further can be planned calmly. Surgical revision is then unavoidable.

Recurrent Nerve Injury

- Unilateral injury:
    - ► Usually without respiratory complication
    - ► Repeat ENT examination in 4 and 8 weeks.
    - ► Start speech therapy.
- When bilateral injury is suspected:
    - ► Monitoring in intensive care unit and early ENT examination
    - ► Intubation necessary if there is increasing stridor
    - ► Puncture tracheotomy with more prolonged ventilation
    - ► Further procedure with ENT treatment strategy

Hypoparathyroidism

The surgical procedures used frequently nowadays, such as thyroidectomy and hemithyroidectomy, more often lead to a postoperative drop in the serum calcium without clinical symptoms. When the parathyroids have been correctly exposed, this is due to trauma during mobilization. If reduced serum calcium levels are immediately replaced, resumption of parathyroid activity will be delayed so calcium replacement may be continued for longer than actually necessary. Therefore substitution of calcium is usually only done when clinical signs of hypocalcemia are observed.

- Asymptomatic postoperative hypocalcemia should not be directly replaced.

Symptoms of **hypocalcemia:**

- Tingling
- Muscle spasm
- Carpopedal spasm
- Risus sardonicus

Reduced serum calcium:

- Asymptomatic: monitor closely
- Symptomatic: monitor closely, give calcium IV immediately, up to 1 g t.i.d., early switch to oral calcium 2–8 g, measure parathyroid hormone level.
- In most cases, parathyroid insufficiency is reversible and symptomatic treatment with oral replacement is adequate. After 4 weeks, oral calcium therapy should normalize the calcium level; otherwise, permanent parathyroid insufficiency must be assumed.
- Long-term treatment: calcium with a vitamin D preparation:
    - ► Vitamin D3 (1,25-dihydroxycholecalciferol): 0.25–0.5 µg/d; dose adjustment according to laboratory results
    - ► Dihydrotachysterol: 0.5–1 mg/d

Despite the presence of hypocalcemia, so-called paradoxical calcifications can occur subsequently because of intermittent hyperphosphatemia depending on the amount of dietary phosphate; these are typically manifested as tetanic cataract or basal ganglia calcification.

Follow-up and Prevention of Recurrence of Benign Thyroid Conditions

Thyroid function must be monitored postoperatively. Prophylactic replacement therapy should be started only after the histology has been obtained so as not to delay the start of radioiodine therapy if carcinoma is found incidentally in the resected specimen. The need for and level of replacement after thyroid surgery have not been finally established but postoperative clinical prophylaxis is in accordance with the guidelines given in **Table 2.4.**

- Replacement therapy is undertaken only after histology has been obtained.

Table 2.4   Guidelines for replacement therapy after thyroid surgery

Operation	Guidelines
Thyroidectomy or near-total thyroidectomy	Standard dosage of 100–150 µg L-thyroxine Dose adjustment after 4–6 weeks when basal TSH is optimized
Hemithyroidectomy	No general replacement If uncertainty about the level of function of the residual thyroid tissue, replace with 50–75 µg L-thyroxine and iodide Short-term measurement of thyroid parameters, if levels reduced start replacement with 50–75 µg L-thyroxine and iodide Dose adjustment after 4–6 weeks when basal TSH is optimized
Enucleation	Prevention with iodide

■ Diseases of the Thyroid

Euthyroid Goiter

Epidemiology

- Euthyroid goiter is the commonest thyroid disorder (90% of all thyroid disorders), 10%–15% of the population is affected, women four times more often

- Thyroid enlargement with normal thyroid metabolism (euthyroid goiter) is the commonest thyroid disorder (90% of all thyroid disorders).
- 10%–15% of the population is affected, women four times more often than men.

Etiology

By far the most frequent cause of euthyroid goiter is a deficiency of dietary iodine. In areas far from the sea, drinking water contains too little iodine so that the daily intake is less than the required 150–200 mg. Because of this, thyroid hormone synthesis is reduced and the thyroid is stimulated via the feedback loop to grow more to increase thyroid hormone production.

Classification

The World Health Organization (WHO) classifies goiter into several grades, depending on its size (**Table 2.5**).

Table 2.5   WHO classification

Grade	Description
Grade 0a	No goiter
Grade 0b	Goiter palpable but not visible
Grade I	Goiter palpable and just visible with the head extended
Grade II	Visible goiter
Grade III	Large visible goiter

Symptoms

Euthyroid goiter is often an incidental finding. The patients do not exhibit any symptoms at the start of the disease but the following can occur as the thyroid enlarges:

- Sensation of tightness
- Difficulty swallowing
- Visible increase in neck size
- Dyspnea on exertion, stridor

Diagnostic Approach

- **Laboratory Tests:** TSH, fT_3 and fT_4 normal, no further laboratory tests needed when euthyroid
- **Ultrasonography:** size, analysis of nodules, follow-up of treatment
- **Scintigraphy:** not necessary with diffuse goiter, follow-up of nodular goiter
- **Aspiration Cytology:** optional with conservative treatment, obligatory with nodular goiter with a cold nodule

Treatment Approach

■ Indications

- Surgery after prolonged unsuccessful pharmacologic treatment (if possible not before the age of 16 years), mechanical obstruction, usually above grade III–IV

• Indication for surgery: failed treatment, mechanical complications, grade III

■ Conservative Treatment

- Diffuse goiter up to grade II: suppression of TSH stimulation with thyroid hormones, mainly T4 preparations, also in combination with iodide, ca. 100–250 µg L-thyroxine and 100–150 µg iodide

■ Surgical Treatment

- Standard resection leaving a defined remnant of the posterior part of the thyroid as performed in the past has now been abandoned in favor of a surgical procedure guided by function and morphology.
- The extent of the resection is determined by the local findings at operation; tissue that is functionally or cystically altered is resected.

Surgical Procedures
- Selective enucleation of a nodule from an otherwise normal thyroid for diagnosis and treatment
- Subtotal resection leaving normal thyroid tissue posteriorly or at the upper pole
- Hemithyroidectomy with predominantly unilateral change
- Hemithyroidectomy with contralateral resection if one lobe is predominantly affected and the contralateral lobe is only partially affected. Often, the upper pole is not involved so that the upper pole vessels and parathyroid can be left in situ
- Thyroidectomy if both lobes are enlarged and affected

• Extent of resection determined individually by morphology and function

Hyperthyroidism

Etiology

Commonest Causes

- Three different morphological forms of thyroid autonomy: unifocal, multifocal, disseminated
- Immunogenic hyperthyroidism (Graves disease)

Less Common Causes

- Preparations containing iodine
- Thyroiditis

Rare Causes

- TSH-producing pituitary adenoma
- Pituitary thyroid hormone resistance
- Hyperthyroidism with differentiated thyroid carcinoma

■ Thyroid Autonomy

In the thyroid, there are always areas, known as autonomic adenomas, which produce hormones uncoupled from the TSH feedback loop. They are classified into three morphological forms:

- Unifocal autonomy with a solitary thyroid nodule
- Multifocal autonomy with multiple nodules
- Disseminated form with autonomic cells distributed widely throughout the thyroid

The thyroid metabolic status must also be diagnosed so that treatment can be planned. A euthyroid state can be found with autonomy (nontoxic nodules) but hyperthyroidism can also develop (toxic nodules). Autonomic adenomas account for 15–50% of cases of hyperthyroid disease; the incidence is higher in regions of iodine deficiency and women are affected more often, especially after the age of 40 years.

Symptoms

- Nervousness, insomnia, restlessness
- Weight loss despite increased appetite
- Heat intolerance with increased sweating
- Increased defecation, possibly with diarrhea
- Hair loss
- Menstrual irregularities in women
- Muscle spasms

Diagnostic Approach

- **Laboratory Tests:** TSH level is reduced
- Nodule on **ultrasonography**
- Hot nodule on **scintigraphy,** if necessary unmasked by suppression scintigraphy (see **Table 2.2**)
- **Aspiration cytology** of cold areas on scintigraphy

- Thyroid autonomy and Graves disease are the most important causes of hyperthyroidism.

2

Treatment Approach

■ Indications

Small solitary adenomas without functional significance can be observed. If treatment is indicated, the choice is between surgery and radiotherapy. However, if the nodule alters, if it becomes bigger or the metabolic status alters, or if the remainder of the gland is abnormal, surgical treatment is recommended (see **Table 2.3**), as this also allows histology to be obtained.

Surgery is indicated particularly in:

- Hyperthyroidism
- Decompensated adenoma
- Large adenoma with mechanical symptoms
- Multinodular goiter with adenoma
- Cold spots
- Suspected carcinoma

- Every patient with an autonomic adenoma and hyperthyroidism must be rendered euthyroid.

■ Conservative Treatment

- Perchlorate

Or ideally

- Methimazole, 40–80 mg/d initially, then 10–20 mg/d
- Carbimazole, 40–80 mg/d initially, then 10–20 mg/d
- Combined with thyroid hormone replacement because of ALP (anterior lobe of pituitary) activation and risk of goiter enlargement
- Elective surgical treatment at intervals (when euthyroid state is achieved)
- Concomitant β-blockers and, if necessary, benzodiazepines to alleviate symptoms caused by increased sympathetic tone

■ Surgical Treatment

A summary of the surgical management of autonomic adenoma is presented in **Table 2.6**.

Table 2.6   Surgical management of autonomic adenoma

Type of autonomy	Procedure
Unifocal autonomy	• Resection of the solitary nodule with margin when the remaining tissue is normal • Hemithyroidectomy when the residual thyroid is of small volume or the thyroid lobe is nodular
Multifocal autonomy	• Hemithyroidectomy of the more involved lobe with subtotal resection of the contralateral side • Thyroidectomy when the entire thyroid is nodular
Disseminated autonomy	• Resection adapted to the tissue, e.g., hemithyroidectomy with subtotal resection of the contralateral side • Thyroidectomy in the case of complete autonomy or nodularity of the entire thyroid

Graves Disease, Immunogenic Hyperthyroidism

Definition

Graves disease or immunogenic hyperthyroidism is an autoimmune disease that causes overactivity and enlargement of the thyroid. In this disease, TRAB are produced, which attach to cell receptors and stimulate the cell to produce T3 and T4.

Etiology

The exact causes have not been determined. It is assumed to be multifactorial.
- A **genetic predisposition** obviously plays a large part as there is a higher incidence of autoimmune diseases in patients with certain HLA (human leukocyte antigen) subtypes over the course of their lives.
- Infections due to viruses and bacteria (e.g., *Yersinia*) are increasingly suspected.
- Psychological stress
- Triggering factors can also be immunostimulating drugs such as α-interferon or interleukin 2.
- Graves disease occurs rarely in pregnancy but often following pregnancy. Pregnancy is regarded as a confirmed precipitating factor of Graves disease. The reason is not known. The hormone changes during and after pregnancy probably play an important part.
- Excessive iodine intake

Symptoms

- Graves disease is characterized by a symptom triad.

The symptom complex results from the thyroid and extra-thyroid manifestations of Graves disease. The typical triad of symptoms consists of
- Goiter
- Tachycardia
- Exophthalmos

More specifically, the symptoms can be divided into three groups.

1) Symptoms of Overactivity
- Palpitations, tachycardia
- High blood pressure
- Nervousness, irritability, restlessness
- Muscle weakness, muscle pains
- Tremor of the hands
- Sleep disorders
- Sweating, moist warm skin
- Ravenous hunger and thirst
- Weight loss despite eating large amounts
- Headaches
- Diarrhea
- Menstrual cycle disorders (irregular or heavier bleeding, amenorrhea)
- Increased libido (decrease is also possible, though rarer)

2) Symptoms of Immunopathology
- Joint pains
- Muscle and back pain
- Flu-like symptoms
- Hair loss
- Pretibial edema

3) Symptoms of Endocrine Orbitopathy
Immunologically induced inflammation of the orbit with:
- Swelling of the retro-orbital muscles
- Exophthalmos
- Visual disturbances
- Eyelid retraction (Dalrymple sign)
- Lid lag on looking downward (Graefe sign)
- Dryness and infrequent blinking (Stellwag sign)
- Convergence weakness

Diagnostic Approach

- **Laboratory Tests:** levels of TSH reduced, fT3 and fT4 raised, TSH receptor antibodies raised
- **Ultrasonography:** diffusely diminished echogenicity, organ hypervascularized
- **Scintigraphy:** diffuse goiter with homogeneous uptake of radioactivity
- Radiographic imaging tends to be less important in diagnosing Graves disease

Treatment Approach

- There is no causal treatment and therapy is directed toward the symptoms.

- Treatment of cause is not possible, therapy is symptomatic only.

■ Indications

Conservative Treatment
- Patients with hyperthyroidism and a small thyroid without endocrine orbitopathy
- Preparation for ablative treatment methods
- Particularly in children and adolescents
- Patients with contraindications to radioiodine or surgical treatment (children and adolescents, more elderly patients)

If pharmacologic treatment is unsuccessful, ablative forms of therapy are employed.

Radioiodine Treatment
- Patients who fail to respond to antithyroid pharmacologic treatment after 1 year
- Patients with contraindications to surgical treatment
- Severe side-effects of the antithyroid drugs
- Patient wish
- Recurrence after surgical treatment
- **Contraindications:**
  - ► Children and adolescents
  - ► Pregnant women

► Large goiter with mechanical impairment
- **Advantage:**
  ► No injury to the recurrent nerve and parathyroids

Surgery
- Large goiters with local complications
- Recurrence after antithyroid treatment
- Poorly controlled hyperthyroidism
- Poor patient compliance
- History of thyrotoxic crisis
- Hyperthyroidism in pregnant women
- Nodular reorganization with cold nodules, suspected malignancy
- Severe orbitopathy
- **Contraindications:**
  ► Patients with increased operation risk
  ► Mild disease without a previous trial of pharmacologic treatment

■ Conservative Therapy

Pharmacologic Therapy
- Antithyroid drugs (see autonomic adenoma)
- Suppression of hormone overproduction
- Treatment of symptoms of hyperthyroidism, not causal therapy
- Treatment continued for 1 year, long-term results are not good.
- After 1 year a further rise in thyroid parameters occurs in 50% of patients.
- A further trial of antithyroid drug therapy is successful in only 20% of cases.

Radioiodine Treatment
- Using the radioactive isotope ^{131}iodine in capsule form
- The radioactive iodine is taken up mainly in the thyroid, where the β radiation causes death of thyroid cells. Since it takes some weeks before the onset of its action, it must be preceded and followed by antithyroid drug treatment.

■ Surgical Treatment

- The immune reaction is stopped by thyroidectomy

The aim of surgery is to abolish the hyperthyroidism by stopping the immune reaction, eliminating local mechanical problems and providing the best possible prevention of recurrence. Extensive reduction or complete removal of thyroid tissue is necessary.
- **Near-total thyroidectomy, hemithyroidectomy with subtotal resection of the contralateral side.** The residual thyroid tissue at the upper pole is kept below 2–4 mL. However, since patients are always given thyroid replacement, complete removal of the thyroid is recommended today.
- Thyroidectomy is the safest way to prevent recurrence and stop the immune reaction.

■ Treatment of Endocrine Orbitopathy

- When the disease follows a three-stage course, treatment should as far as possible begin in the first active phase to achieve a better inactive end stage.
- Euthyroidism through antithyroid drugs, radioiodine treatment, surgery
- High-dose steroid treatment
- Decompression surgery or orbital radiation with optic nerve decompression

Thyrotoxic Crisis

Etiology

Thyrotoxic crisis is usually triggered by multiple endogenous and exogenous mechanisms in the presence of untreated or undiagnosed thyroid autonomy or Graves autoimmune hyperthyroidism (**Table 2.7**).

- The most important triggers of thyrotoxic crisis are infections and iodine exposure.

2

Table 2.7 Endogenous and exogenous triggering mechanisms

Endogenous	Exogenous
• Metabolic disturbance • Acute cardiovascular event • Pregnancy • Emotional stress • Mania	• Infection • Iodine exposure • Discontinuation of antithyroid drugs • Surgical procedures • Acute trauma • Radioiodine therapy

Classification

A system for staging thyrotoxic crisis is shown in **Table 2.8**.

Table 2.8 Stages of thyrotoxic crisis

Stage I	Stage II	Stage III
	In addition:	In addition:
• Tachycardia > 150 beats/min • Cardiac arrhythmias • Hypertension • Hyperthermia • Red face, dehydration • Muscle weakness, tremor • Restlessness, agitation	• Disordered level of consciousness • Confusion, psychosis, stupor • Somnolence	• Coma

Stages I, II, and III: a < 50 years, b > 50 years.

Diagnostic Approach

- Diagnosis is based exclusively on clinical findings.
- There are no laboratory parameters that allow overt hyperthyroidism to be distinguished from thyrotoxic crisis.

- Cardinal symptoms of thyrotoxic crisis: hyperthyroidism with fever, unexplained tachycardia, and agitation

Treatment Approach

- Start immediately in an intensive care unit
- Treatment of the trigger mechanism (infection etc.)
- Blockage of peripheral thyroid hormone action (anti-adrenergic blockade)
- Antithyroid treatment
- Treatment of systemic complications, supportive measures
- If stabilization does not occur in 12–24 hours, emergency thyroidectomy is indicated.

Prognosis

An early interdisciplinary decision on emergency thyroidectomy made by endocrinologist, anesthesiologist, and surgeon is crucial. Mortality rates of 0–10% are cited with early surgery, and a mortality rate of 28% is reported in stage III.

Thyroiditis

- Rare diseases of the thyroid
- Possible classification according to course and etiology into:
  - ► Acute (bacterial)
  - ► Subacute (de Quervain)
  - ► Chronic (Hashimoto)
- This classification does not include other forms of thyroiditis so a classification into **painful** and **painless** forms is employed (**Table 2.9**).

Table 2.9 Forms of thyroiditis

Painful forms	Painless forms
• Subacute thyroiditis (de Quervain) • Acute purulent thyroiditis • Radiation thyroiditis	• Hashimoto thyroiditis • Postpartum thyroiditis • Silent thyroiditis • Drug-induced • Riedel fibrous thyroiditis

■ Painful Thyroiditis

Subacute Thyroiditis (de Quervain)

Etiology
- Unclear, often preceded by a history of upper respiratory tract infection indicating viral origin
- A genetic predisposition (e.g., HLA-B35) is also suspected

Symptoms
- General malaise
- Muscle pains
- Subfebrile temperatures
- Diffuse neck pain

Diagnostic Approach

• Diminished nuclide uptake, in contrast to Graves disease

- **Laboratory tests:** transient hyperthyroidism, leads to permanent hypothyroidism in 5% of cases, ESR is raised, no antibodies are detected
- **Ultrasonography:** nonhomogeneous appearance
- **Scintigraphy:** diminished nuclide uptake (in contrast to Graves disease where nuclide uptake is increased)
- **Fine-needle aspiration:** granulomatous inflammation with giant cells

Treatment Approach
- Nonsteroidal anti-inflammatory drugs, high-dose corticosteroid therapy

Acute Purulent Thyroiditis

Etiology
- Usually bacterial infections, local or hematogenous or lymphatogenous

Symptoms
- Pain predominantly unilateral
- Fever
- Tenderness in the neck
- Skin erythema

Diagnostic Approach
- **Laboratory tests:** C-reactive protein level and leukocytes raised
- **Ultrasonography:** possibly abscess

Treatment Approach
- Immediate antibiotics, anti-inflammatories, surgical intervention if an abscess forms to stop extension of the inflammation (e.g., mediastinitis)

- Bacterial infection, immediate antibiotics

Radiation Thyroiditis

Etiology
- Following radioiodine capsule treatment, an inflammatory reaction can occur in 1% of patients after 5–10 days; also after percutaneous radiotherapy.

Symptoms
- Similar to subacute thyroiditis

Treatment Approach
- Local measures (icepack)
- Anti-inflammatory drugs
- Corticosteroids

■ Painless Thyroiditis

Chronic Lymphocytic Thyroiditis (Hashimoto Disease)

Epidemiology
- This form of thyroiditis is the commonest inflammatory thyroid disease and affects women much more than men.

- Commonest inflammatory thyroid disease

Etiology
- The central feature in pathogenesis is infiltration with cytotoxic T-lymphocytes. A high iodine intake or smoking may be trigger mechanisms.

Symptoms
- Usually without local symptoms, depends on the metabolic status

Diagnostic Approach
- **Laboratory tests:** hyperthyroidism initially; in the hypothyroid phase, lifelong replacement may be necessary
- **Scintigraphy:** diminished radionuclide uptake
- **Ultrasonography:** diminished echogenicity

• Increased incidence of thyroid lymphoma and thyroid papillary carcinoma

Treatment Approach
• Depends on current metabolic status; in the hypothyroid phase, lifelong replacement may be necessary
• Hashimoto thyroiditis is associated with an increased incidence of thyroid lymphoma and thyroid papillary carcinoma, so patients should be regularly monitored clinically and by ultrasonography. Nodule formation warrants close monitoring and, if necessary, fine-needle aspiration or histological diagnosis.

Postpartum Thyroiditis and Silent Thyroiditis

Epidemiology
• The course of postpartum thyroiditis resembles Hashimoto thyroiditis and occurs in mothers ca. 2–8 months after delivery. Metabolism normalizes after a year in 80% of patients but 30–50% of them may develop underactivity in the longer term, which must be monitored and detected. If the patients are found to have thyroid autoantibodies, postpartum thyroiditis can recur in 70% of patients with a subsequent pregnancy.
• "Silent thyroiditis" is a special form, with hyperthyroidism of brief duration, followed by hypothyroidism and subsequent normalization. Anti-TPO antibodies can be found in this case also.

Symptoms
• Depends on the metabolic status

Treatment Approach
• Symptomatic, as in Hashimoto thyroiditis

Drug-Induced Thyroiditis

Etiology
• Some drugs can cause destructive thyroiditis with an alternating metabolic state: amiodarone, lithium, thalidomide, interleukin, α-interferon, and lenalidomide

Treatment Approach
• Symptomatic

Fibrous Thyroiditis (Riedel Disease)

Etiology
• Unclear, manifestation of systemic fibrosis
• Can extend beyond the capsule to adjacent tissue and lead to local symptoms

Symptoms
• Increasing sensation of tightness, difficulty swallowing

Treatment Approach
• Nonsteroidal anti-inflammatory drugs, high-dose corticosteroid therapy
• In the case of localized symptoms or suspected malignancy, surgery may become necessary, up to and including thyroidectomy.

Thyroid Carcinoma

The majority of operations involve benign thyroid disease but the number of patients with thyroid malignancy is increasing steadily. This results on the one hand from better diagnostics but also from the increasing willingness to operate on nodular lesions. A large number of cases are often only identified postoperatively on histology, necessitating a second operation. This disease has a good survival rate because of surgery and the possibility of radioiodine therapy.

• Good survival rate with surgery and radioiodine therapy

Epidemiology

- About 44670 new cases and 1690 deaths annually in the United States
- 0.2–0.3% of deaths due to cancer are attributable to thyroid carcinoma
- Incidence is 3.1 in men and 6.3 in women, and the incidence is increasing worldwide in all age groups
- Average disease age is 55 years with a peak between the 6th and 7th decades
- Rare in childhood, but then usually grows aggressively
- The majority of thyroid carcinomas arise from the follicular cells (up to 90%) or parafollicular calcitonin-producing C cells (3–5%).
- There are marked geographical differences:
  - ▸ in regions with a good iodine supply, 80% of cases are thyroid papillary carcinoma and 14% follicular carcinoma;
  - ▸ in regions poorly supplied with iodine, the papillary forms are found in 66% of cases and follicular forms are increasingly found in up to 27% of cases.

Etiology

- Ionizing radiation
- Especially radiation during childhood
- Percutaneous radiotherapy of cervical disease

Classification

It is becoming increasingly apparent that local lymph node metastases have a low negative predictive value for long-term survival. However, the presence of distant metastases significantly reduces survival rates. The cellular origin of the individual carcinoma is important for prognosis (**Table 2.10**).

■ Forms of Carcinoma

Thyroid Carcinoma Originating from Follicular Cells
Carcinomas originating from follicular cells are divided into three groups according to the new WHO classification:

- **Differentiated carcinomas** (very good prognosis)
  - ▸ Metastasis of papillary carcinoma is predominantly lymphatogenous to the cervical and mediastinal lymph nodes. Lymph node metastases increase significantly when the primary tumor is greater than 3 cm in size.
  - ▸ Metastasis of follicular carcinomas is predominantly hematogenous. However, lymph node metastases are also found in 10%–20% of patients.
  - ▸ Good overall prognosis with a 10-year survival rate of 75%–90%.
- **Poorly differentiated carcinomas** (poor prognosis)
  - ▸ Classified between differentiated and anaplastic carcinomas
  - ▸ Associated even initially with hematogenous metastasis.
  - ▸ This results in a much poorer 10-year survival rate of only 25%–35%.

Metastasis
- Papillary cancer: lymphatogenous
- Follicular cancer: hematogenous

• TNM classification

Table 2.10   TNM classification

Stage		Description
pT1	a	< 1 cm, limited to the thyroid, not penetrating the capsule
	b	1–2 cm, limited to the thyroid, not penetrating the capsule
pT2		> 2–4 cm, limited to the thyroid
pT3	a	> 4 cm, limited to the thyroid
	b	Any tumor with minimal spread outside the thyroid, penetration of the capsule
pT4	a	Subcutaneous spread, infiltration of larynx, trachea, esophagus and/or recurrent laryngeal nerve
	b	Penetration of the prevertebral fascia, mediastinal vessels and/or carotid artery
		Undifferentiated thyroid carcinomas only:
	a	Limited to the thyroid
	b	Spread beyond the thyroid capsule
pN1	a	Cervical lymph node metastases (central)
	b	Unilateral, bilateral, contralateral or mediastinal lymph node metastases

- **Undifferentiated** (anaplastic) **carcinomas** (very poor prognosis)
  - ► Incidence less than 10% of all thyroid cancers
  - ► Occurrence after the 5th decade
  - ► No thyroglobulin detectable in the tumor
  - ► Poorest prognosis with a survival rate of less than 12 months after diagnosis.

Thyroid Carcinomas Arising from Parafollicular C Cells

C-cell carcinomas
- Sporadic form: 75%
- Familial form: 25%

- C-cell carcinomas are medullary thyroid carcinomas originating from parafollicular C cells. The sporadic form accounts for 75% and the familial form for 25% of cases.

Classification of Familial Medullary Carcinoma (C-cell Carcinoma)
- Autosomal dominant inheritance
- Nearly 100% penetrance with multiple endocrine neoplasia type II (MEN II) as the only malignant component of the syndrome (**Table 2.11**).

Table 2.11   Forms of medullary thyroid carcinoma in multiple endocrine neoplasia type II syndrome

MEN type IIa	MEN type IIb	Third manifestation
• Familial medullary carcinoma	• Familial medullary carcinoma	• Only familial medullary carcinoma occurs clinically
• Bilateral pheochromocytoma	• Bilateral pheochromocytoma	
• Hyperplasia or adenoma of the parathyroids	• Intestinal ganglioneuromatosis	
	• Marfanoid habitus	

Genetic Changes

The cause of the MEN II syndrome is a genetic mutation in the RET proto-oncogene. In ca. 98% of all cases of MEN II, a point mutation can be detected in this RET proto-oncogene. These mutations are associated with close genotype–phenotype correlation so that patients with MEN II syndromes can increasingly be provided with customized treatment.

Symptoms

- Nonspecific symptoms
- Clinically relevant symptoms such as dyspnea, recurrent laryngeal nerve paresis, and dysphagia occur mainly at advanced stages
- Sudden vocal cord paralysis with hoarseness: this must be regarded as a sign of malignant disease

- Fine-needle aspiration with every suspicious thyroid

Diagnostic Approach (Fig. 2.6)

Thyroid carcinoma is often diagnosed only at operation for a nodular thyroid swelling. The diagnosis is often made from fine-needle aspiration of a cold area or after removal of enlarged cervical lymph nodes. Fast-growing, hard, and nonmobile solitary nodules are suspicious.

■ History and Clinical Examination

- Rate of nodule growth, familial incidence, general symptoms
- Mobility of the nodule, abnormal lymph nodes, hoarseness, nodule consistency
- **Laryngoscopy:** examination of vocal cord function by an ENT specialist.

■ Laboratory Tests

- No specific tumor marker for carcinomas of follicular cell origin
- fT_3, fT_4, TSH, parathyroid hormone
- Diagnosis of medullary thyroid carcinoma is immunohistochemical, based on detection of calcitonin. Measurement of calcitonin should be considered when investigating abnormal thyroid nodules.

■ Diagnostic Imaging

- **Ultrasonography:** hypoechoic nodule, irregular margins, increased vascular supply and microcalcifications
- **Scintigraphy:** area of reduced or absent radionuclide uptake
- **Chest X-ray** (lung metastases)

■ Invasive Tests

- **Fine-needle aspiration:** Every thyroid nodule that appears suspicious on imaging or is suspected clinically to be malignant should be investigated by fine-needle aspiration. If the result is suspicious and requires further investigation or follicular neoplasia is suggested, histological diagnosis is essential. Follicular neoplasia can indicate both adenoma and follicular thyroid carcinoma. Evidence of carcinoma extending beyond the capsule or with follicular invasion can be adduced only by histological examination.

- Fine-needle aspiration with every suspicious thyroid nodule or clinical suspicion of malignancy

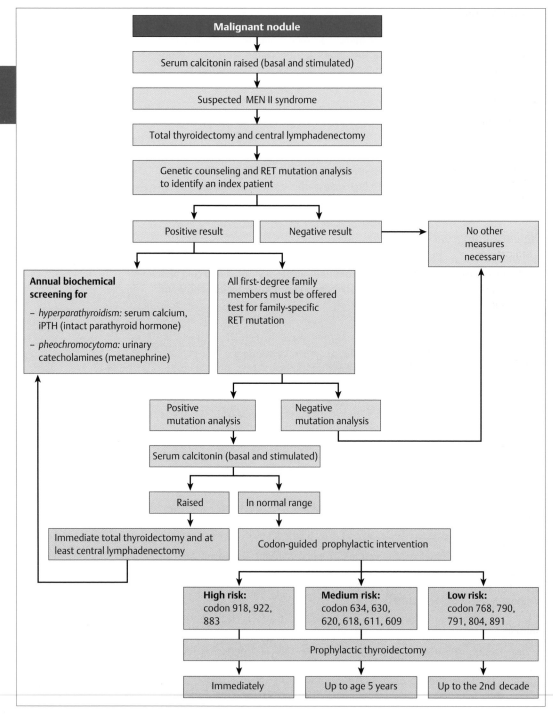

Fig. 2.6 Diagnostic procedures for medullary thyroid carcinoma.

Fine-needle aspiration assists the surgeon
- in choosing the operation strategy: preserving function or radical surgery, planning with or without frozen section;
- in planning the timing: urgent or elective; and
- in confirming the diagnosis.

■ Genetic Analysis

When a patient has medullary carcinoma, it is important to establish whether this is a sporadic or hereditary form. On further investigation, 5% of patients prove to have unrecognized MEN IIa or belong to familial medullary thyroid carcinoma families. In MEN type IIb, a family history has often not yet been obtained in 50% of patients. This is why genetic testing for RET mutations should be performed in all patients with medullary thyroid carcinoma.

- With medullary carcinoma, think of genetic analysis to filter out familial forms.

2

Therapeutic Approach

■ Indications

- When the diagnosis of thyroid carcinoma is confirmed, thyroidectomy and lymph node dissection in the central compartment are performed in accordance with the guidelines in surgery (**Table 2.12**).
- When carcinoma is suspected, the first step is complete removal of the thyroid lobe containing the nodule as hemithyroidectomy. If carcinoma is confirmed, the operation is completed by hemithyroidectomy of the contralateral side and lymphadenectomy in the central compartment.
- Thyroidectomy and hemithyroidectomy with removal of lymph nodes should, as a rule, be carried out en-bloc, and also when neighboring organs, for example the neck muscles, are infiltrated.

Table 2.12   Treatment of thyroid carcinoma types

	Hemithy-roidectomy	Thyroidec-tomy	Functional neck dissection	Functional neck dissection	Radio-iodine therapy	Suppression therapy with T4	Radio-therapy
Microcar-cinoma	+	–	–	–	–	–	–
Papillary carcino-ma T2–4	–	+	Central	Lateral, uni-lateral if ap-plicable	+	+	Palliative
Follicular carcino-ma	–	+	Central	Lateral, uni-lateral if ap-plicable	+	+	Palliative
Undiffer-entiated carcino-ma	–	+	Central		–	– (+)	Palliative
MEN II	–	+	Central	Lateral, bilat-erally	–	–	Palliative
Sporadic	–	+	Central	Lateral, bilat-erally	–	–	Palliative

2

Specific Indications

Solitary Differentiated Microcarcinoma: Papillary Carcinoma T1 N0 M0
- A large proportion of thyroid carcinomas are represented by solitary differentiated microcarcinoma, which is diagnosed by chance on partial thyroid resection. When there is no evidence of lymph node metastases and when complete tumor removal is confirmed histologically, further resection is not necessary and it is not followed by radioiodine therapy.
- In the case of all other thyroid carcinomas diagnosed incidentally on postoperative histology, whether because of vascular or capsule invasion, size or cell origin, further resection is required. This can be performed within 24–48 hours after the primary procedure during the first hospitalization, or 6–8 weeks later. Even when patients desire early surgery on receiving the diagnosis, as they often do, completion surgery after 4–6 weeks is acceptable for oncological reasons. The local tissue structure is then better for re-operation.
- If a differentiated thyroid carcinoma extending beyond the gland is present, multivisceral resection is justified if the tumor can be removed as an R0 resection, as a good prognosis can be achieved by this means.

Indications with Thyroid Carcinoma Arising from Parafollicular C Cells

Sporadic Medullary Carcinoma
- Regardless of the size of the primary tumor, thyroidectomy with lymph node dissection in the central and both lateral cervical compartments is indicated.

Clinically Manifest Hereditary Thyroid Carcinoma

- In familial medullary thyroid carcinoma, treatment is guided by the risk profile.

- Here, too, the standard procedure is thyroidectomy with lymphadenectomy in all three cervical compartments.
- Apparently normal genetic carriers of MEN II or familial medullary thyroid carcinoma represent a special case. The procedure should be adapted to the calcitonin level and the presence of a RET mutation.
  - ► If abnormal basal and pentagastrin-stimulated calcitonin levels are found, thyroidectomy with lymphadenectomy should be performed, regardless of age and the type of mutation.
  - ► If the stimulated calcitonin level is still in the normal range, the timing of surgery is guided by the severity of the RET mutation.
  - ► If there is a high-risk profile, surgery should be performed within the first months of life.
  - ► With a medium-risk profile, surgery should be performed by the age of 5 years.
  - ► When the risk profile is low, thyroidectomy can be postponed until the 2nd decade.

Indications with Poorly Differentiated or Undifferentiated Thyroid Carcinoma

- When the carcinoma is still limited to the thyroid, the surgical treatment of poorly differentiated or undifferentiated thyroid carcinoma corresponds to the treatment of more differentiated carcinomas. Patients should also receive adjuvant percutaneous radiotherapy.
- When growth extends beyond the gland, the patient undergoes further multimodal oncological treatment following histological confirmation of the diagnosis.

2

■ Surgical Treatment

Operative Technique
- For general steps, see pp. 17–25.
- Additional lymph node dissection:
    - ► Central cervical compartment medial to the jugular vein bilaterally
    - ► Ipsilateral lateral cervical and contralateral lateral cervical compartment lateral to the jugular vein bilaterally
    - ► Mediastinal infrabrachiocephalic compartment retrosternally (see **Table 2.1**)
- With papillary and differentiated follicular thyroid carcinoma < 1 cm in size, lymph node metastases are found predominantly in the central cervical (44%) and ipsilateral lateral cervical compartments (34%), so lymphadenectomy includes resection of the cervico-central and ipsilateral cervico-lateral compartments.
- For all other carcinomas and higher stages, lymphadenectomy of all four compartments should be performed.

■ Postoperative Management

- Following thyroidectomy because of differentiated thyroid carcinoma, radio-iodine therapy is given after 4–6 weeks to ablate any thyroid tissue still present.
- Post-treatment scintigraphy can also provide information on definitive tumor staging as differentiated thyroid carcinoma metastases are visible. Following successful ablation, levothyroxine replacement is started, optimized according to the basal TSH value.
- A raised TSH level is increasingly obtained by means of short-term exogenous recombinant human TSH (rh-TSH) while maintaining the replacement dose so that radioiodine therapy can be started after 4–6 weeks.
- Chemotherapy and percutaneous radiotherapy are palliative treatments for differentiated carcinomas not responding to [131]iodine or in R1 situations.

Prognosis

Thyroid carcinoma has a good prognosis in general. The influencing factors are the tumor stage and the patient's age, along with the cellular origin of the carcinoma.

- Prognosis is generally good.

Ten-Year Survival Rate
- 93% for papillary carcinoma
- 85% for follicular carcinoma
- 75% for C-cell carcinoma
- 14% for anaplastic carcinoma

Further Reading

Aschebrook-Kilfoy B, Ward MH, Sabra MM, Devesa SS. Thyroid cancer incidence patterns in the United States by histologic type, 1992–2006. Thyroid February 2011: 125–134

Gemsenjaeger E. Atlas of Thyroid Surgery: Principles, Practice, and Clinical Cases. Stuttgart: Thieme; 2008

Wartofsky L, Van Nostrand D, eds. Thyroid Cancer: A Comprehensive Guide to Clinical Management. Heidelberg, Berlin: Springer; 2006

3 Parathyroid

B. Thiel

■ Anatomy

- < 3 parathyroids in 3% of individuals
- > 4 parathyroids in 13%– 37% of individuals

- The parathyroid glands, usually four in number, are situated between the investing fascia and fibrous capsule of the thyroid (**Fig. 3.1** and **Table 3.1**).

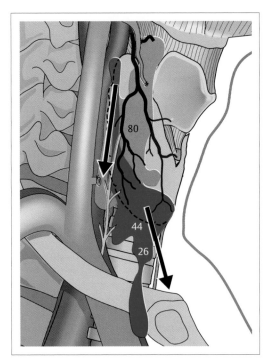

Fig. 3.1 Location of the parathyroids: superior gland above and posterior to the crossing of the nerve and artery in 80%, inferior gland inferior and anterior in 44%, in the thymus compartment in 26%. Arrow: direction of parathyroid dislocation, inferior gland toward the thymus.

Table 3.1 Typical position of the parathyroids

Superior parathyroids	Inferior parathyroids
• On the back of the upper and middle part of the thyroid, superior and posterior to the site where the recurrent laryngeal nerve crosses the inferior thyroid artery (in 80%) • Atypical position rather seldom: inferior position in 4%, retropharyngeal or retroesophageal in 1% and within the thyroid in only 0.2%	• Rather variable, usually inferior and anterior to the site where the nerve and artery cross (in 44%) • Often also in the upper part of the thymus, ca. 26% in the cervical part and 2% in the mediastinal part of the thyrothymic ligament

- Fewer than three parathyroids may be found in 3% of the population and more than four in 13%–37%.
- The glands produce parathyroid hormone (parathormone, PTH), which regulates calcium and phosphate metabolism, together with vitamin D3 and calcitonin from the thyroid.

■ Physiology

Normal Levels
- Serum parathormone: 12–72 ng/L or 1.5–6.0 pmol/L
- Calcitonin: in adults less than 10 ng/dL (equivalent to 2.8 pmol/L)
- Calcium: 2.15–2.75 mmol/L in serum, 4.02–4.99 mmol/L in 24-hour urine
- Phosphate: 0.84–1.45 mmol/L in serum

Action of Parathormone: Negative Feedback Regulation
- Hypocalcemia and deficiency of 1,25-dihydroxy vitamin D3 promote secretion of parathormone.
- Parathormone elevates the serum calcium level by:
  - ► Increasing bone breakdown by releasing calcium phosphate
  - ► Increasing calcium absorption from the small intestine
  - ► Increasing reabsorption in the kidneys by increasing phosphate excretion
- Vitamin D is required for this.
- If the calcium or vitamin D concentration in the blood is too high, parathormone secretion in the parathyroids is inhibited.
- Calcitonin reduces the calcium level in the blood by:
  - ► Inhibiting calcium release from bone
  - ► Increasing calcium excretion in the kidney

■ Primary Hyperparathyroidism

Definition

- Continuous hypersecretion of parathormone
- In primary hyperparathyroidism (pHPT), the cause of the hypersecretion is in the parathyroids themselves.

Epidemiology

- Four cases per 100 000 population
- Third commonest endocrine disease after thyroid disease and diabetes mellitus
- Women are affected more than men in the ratio 3 : 1.

• Third commonest endocrine disease

Etiology

Causes and Their Frequency
- Solitary adenoma: 80%–85%
- Hyperplasia of multiple glands: 10%–15%
- Double adenoma: 5%
- Carcinoma: < 1%

3

In multigland hyperplasia or double adenoma, a hereditary syndrome may be present in up to 25% of cases, so the diagnosis must be followed by further investigations to rule out multiple endocrine neoplasia (MEN) syndrome type I or type IIA (see also **Table 2.11**).

Parathyroid hyperplasia associated with MEN plus pHPT:

- Type I: tumors of the pancreas, usually insulinomas, pituitary tumors, parathyroid hyperplasia present in 90% of cases
- Type IIA: bilateral pheochromocytoma, thyroid medullary carcinoma, parathyroid hyperplasia present in 50% of cases

Symptoms

Functional Disorders Caused by Hypercalcemia

- pHPT symptoms: "stones, bones, and abdominal groans"

- **Renal manifestation:**
  - ► Nephrolithiasis in up to 40% of cases: nephrocalcinosis with renal failure, renal water loss with polyuria, dehydration
- **Bony manifestation:**
  - ► Bone resorption ranging from characteristic changes in the subperiosteal zones on the radial side of the digital phalanges to generalized osteitis fibrosa cystica (rare nowadays)
- **Gastrointestinal manifestations:**
  - ► Anorexia, weight loss, vomiting
  - ► Constipation, meteorism
  - ► Duodenal and gastric ulcers and pancreatitis are associated rather rarely
- **Neuromuscular manifestations:**
  - ► Muscle weakness
  - ► Neurological changes with fatigue, lethargy
  - ► Cognitive disturbances

Diagnostic Approach

■ Laboratory Tests (Table 3.2)

- Serum levels: calcium ↑, phosphate ↓, parathormone ↑
- Urine levels: calcium ↑, phosphate ↑
- Constellation remains the same after repeat tests: diagnosis of pHPT is very reliable.
- 24-hour urine calcium measurement: in the rare familial hypocalciuric hypercalcemia, the level is low-normal with high serum calcium levels.

Table 3.2 Typical calcium and phosphate levels in the different forms of hyperparathyroidism

Form	Serum level		Urine level	
	Calcium	Phosphate	Calcium	Phosphate
Primary	High	Low	High	Low
Secondary	Low/Normal		High	Low
Tertiary	High	High	High	Low
Acute	High		High	
Reference range	2.15–2.6 mmol/L	0.83–1.67 mmol/L	2.5–10 mmol/24 h	23–48 mmol/24 h

■ Diagnostic Imaging

- pHPT is diagnosed from the laboratory parameters, imaging methods are used for localization.
- Prior localization is important for a focused procedure, especially when minimally invasive techniques are used.

Ultrasonography
- Localization of an enlarged parathyroid gland
- Establishes whether a double adenoma or multigland disease is present
- Possibility of fine-needle aspiration for clear identification of the adenoma and localization (an elegant method of localization in the minimally invasive procedure in experienced hands)

Scintigraphy
- **^{99m}Tc sestamibi scintigraphy:** There is increased and prolonged ^{99m}Tc sestamibi accumulation in tissues high in mitochondria, such as hyperplastic or adenomatous parathyroids.

Other Imaging Methods
CT and MRI are not methods of first choice but may be used for:
- Localization when the position is unclear after ultrasound and scintigraphy
- Preoperative imaging of the anatomy after surgery on the neck
- Persisting pHPT or recurrent pHPT
- Localization of an ectopic parathyroid gland

Despite these possibilities for localization, none of these methods is capable of clearly identifying or ruling out multigland disease.

- None of these imaging methods is capable of clearly identifying or ruling out multigland disease.

■ Differential Diagnosis

- Malignancy
- pHPT
- Vitamin D intoxication
- Sarcoidosis
- Immobilization
- Hyperthyroidism
- Addisonian crisis
- Drug effect (lithium, thiazides)
- Milk-alkali syndrome
- Familial hypocalciuric hypercalcemia

Treatment Approach

■ Indication

- Surgery in principle for symptomatic pHPT
- Hypercalcemia confirmed by at least three measurements on different days and measurement of parathormone
- Early indication for operative therapy even in asymptomatic pHPT, as the supposedly mild symptoms often become obvious after successful operation
- Longer-term hypercalcemia is associated with increased morbidity and mortality.
- Reoperation: if the hyperparathyroidism persists

- Surgery in principle for symptomatic pHPT

■ Surgical Treatment

General Tactical Surgical Considerations
- The aim is complete removal of tissue producing too much parathormone, while leaving a residue of normal parathyroid tissue to normalize the serum calcium level.
- In pHPT this is usually achieved by adenoma removal; persistence of hyperparathyroidism is avoided by rapid intraoperative tests to measure parathormone and frozen section examination.
- When preoperative localization is not clear and the intraoperative parathormone level is raised, further exploration is necessary.
- The uncertainty of missing diffuse hyperplasia or a second adenoma is always present but can be justified by the possibility of an early second operation.

Preoperative pHPT Checklist
- History, clinical examination
- Laboratory tests: serum calcium, parathormone, calcitonin, phosphate, creatinine, urea; optional: fT3, fT4, TSH
- Ultrasonography of the neck, optional: fine-needle aspiration cytology
- ^{99m}Tc sestamibi scintigraphy
- Laryngoscopy: ENT check of vocal cord neural function
- Before reoperation: operation report, repeat ^{99m}Tc sestamibi scintigraphy, CT or MRI

Standard Operation: Bilateral Cervical Exploration

- Every parathyroid surgeon should master bilateral exploration.

- Increasingly in the background nowadays due to advancing localization tests and intraoperative tests such as parathormone and frozen section diagnosis
- This operation technique is still necessary when the localization tests are unclear or the intraoperative parathormone level does not fall adequately.

Operative Technique

- Position as for thyroid surgery with the head only slightly reclined.
- Access through a transverse incision made one to two fingerbreadths above the sternal notch, if possible in a skin crease or after drawing a line on the awake patient.
- Start the exploration at the site of supposed localization.
- Expose the recurrent laryngeal nerve and inferior thyroid artery; in bilateral resection, the nerve should be exposed before resection.
- The parathyroids are usually located in the fat behind the thyroid; by careful dissection of the fat, they become apparent because of their different consistency and color (somewhat darker and brownish; hence, a bloodless field is essential for identification).
- The exploration starts from above, as the upper parathyroids are usually located above and posterior to the site where the recurrent laryngeal nerve and inferior thyroid artery cross.
- The position of the lower parathyroids is variable; they are often inferior and anterior to the site where the nerve and artery cross, and also in the upper part of the thymus.
- Expose the four parathyroids. The enlarged one is removed and examined by frozen section; if the diagnosis of adenoma is confirmed and if the parathormone level has fallen adequately, the operation is concluded.

- If three or more parathyroids are enlarged, three and a half glands should be resected if familial hyperparathyroidism or MEN syndrome was ruled out beforehand. Part of the least conspicuous gland is left in situ; another possibility is complete removal of the parathyroids and reimplantation in a pocket of the sternocleidomastoid muscle or forearm muscle.

- Cryopreservation of part of a parathyroid allows operative treatment of permanent hypoparathyroidism 6 months postoperatively.

Procedure When an Enlarged Parathyroid Is Not Found

- A definite diagnosis is essential, ruling out familial hyperparathyroidism or MEN syndrome, so that multigland hyperplasia or an unfound adenoma can be assumed at operation.
- If the parathormone level persists and isolated enlargement of one gland cannot be identified, proceed as shown in **Fig. 3.2**.

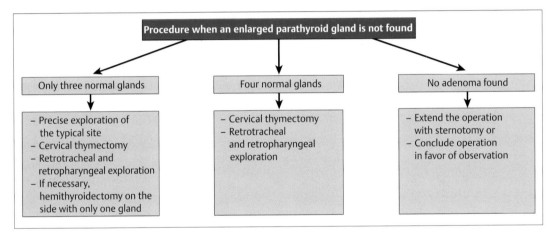

Fig. 3.2   Procedure when an enlarged parathyroid gland is not found.

Dystopic Parathyroid Glands

- In 15% of patients dystopic parathyroid glands may be present in the thyrothymic ligament, within the thyroid, or as undescended glands at the origin of the superior thyroid artery and along the carotid sheath.
- Intramediastinal parathyroids can be reached via sternotomy or minimally invasive video-assisted mediastinoscopy or thoracoscopy—for example, as far as the lower border of the thymus or in the aortopulmonary window.

Operative Procedures Focused on Localization

- **MIVAP:** minimally invasive video-assisted parathyroidectomy through a 2-cm incision at the sternal notch assisted by the 30° optic
- **OMIP:** open minimally invasive parathyroidectomy through an incision ca. 3 cm in length over the localized adenoma; surgery under local anesthesia may be possible in a favorable case
- **ELPA:** endoscopic parathyroidectomy through a lateral approach with dissection in the space behind the thyroid; three trocars are inserted, similar to the ABBA technique of thyroidectomy (p. 24)

Reoperation

Indications
- Repeated confirmed diagnosis of pHPT
- Marked hypercalcemia (> 2.9 mmol/L)
- Specific disease symptoms in milder forms

Necessity
- Persistence of the pHPT, defined by persistently high calcium levels post-operatively or by a further rise within 6 months after temporary normocalcemia
- Due to recurrence characterized by postoperative normocalcemia with a rise only after at least 6 months

Causes of Persistence or Recurrence with Subsequent Reoperation
- Inadequate exploration of the neck at the first operation
- Failure to identify disease in multiple glands
- An excessive number of parathyroid glands
- Ectopic location

Investigations
- Repeat tests for pHPT
- CT or MRI to assist localization and demonstrate the anatomy after previous surgery

Timing
- As soon as possible or before the second week, and again only after the sixth week because of unfavorable adhesions

Operative Procedure
- Repeat exploration through the existing access except in the case of a mediastinal adenoma.
- Carry out bilateral neck exploration if localization has not been confirmed, to allow a focused procedure.
- If adhesions are present, dissect posterior to the strap neck muscles and anterior to the sternocleidomastoid muscle in the retropharyngeal space to circumvent adhesions.
- Nerve exposure is obligatory; intraoperative neuromonitoring with exposure of the vagus nerve and recurrent laryngeal nerve
- Intraoperative parathormone measurement

■ Postoperative Management

- Close monitoring of postoperative calcium
- Examine for clinical signs of hypocalcemia
- No replacement necessary in most cases when focused operation technique for pHPT
- Normalization of calcium level in 2–4 days
- After marked hyperparathyroidism, deficiency states can occur due to increased recalcification, necessitating IV calcium replacement.
- Measure parathormone before discharge.
- Check vocal cords before discharge.

■ Complications

- Low mortality (0.1%–1%)
- Rate of recurrent nerve paresis below 1% after primary surgery, up to 10% after reoperation
- Postoperative hypocalcemia in 2%, up to 10% after surgery for multigland hyperplasia
- Persistent HPT or recurrent HPT

Postoperative Problems
- **Immediate postoperative hypocalcemia:**
  - ► Initially calcium replacement IV as needed
  - ► Later, up to 1–2 g q.i.d. orally
  - ► Magnesium and phosphate if necessary
- **Permanent hypocalcemia:**
  - ► Autotransplantation of cryopreserved parathyroid tissue
  - ► Long-term replacement with calcium 0.5–1.5 g daily p.o. and vitamin D3 20 000 to 100 000 IU/d, dihydrotachysterol 0.5–1.5 mg/d or 1,25-dihydroxy vitamin D3 0.25–2 mg/d
  - ► Early reoperation in the case of persistent HPT or recurrent HPT

■ Secondary Hyperparathyroidism

Definition

- Compensatory increase in parathyroid hormone secretion in hypocalcemia
- In secondary hyperparathyroidism (sHPT), the cause of the increased secretion is outside the parathyroid, due in 90% of cases to endocrine and exocrine dysfunction of the kidney.

Epidemiology

- More than 90% of cases are diagnosed in patients with chronic renal failure requiring dialysis.
- sHPT is rarely due to other, underlying diseases.
- Only 2%–5% of patients with sHPT require surgery.

Etiology

Renal sHPT
- Renal failure with an increase of the phosphate level and inhibition of renal calcitriol production
- Followed by hypocalcemia with compensatory hyperplasia of the parathyroids and stimulation of parathyroid hormone production

Extrarenal sHPT
- Deficiency of calcium and/or calcitriol, for geographic or regional reasons
- Malabsorption syndrome (sprue, Crohn disease)
- Hepatic cirrhosis, cholestasis
- Vitamin D resistance, hypomagnesemia

• 90% due to renal disease

3

• 90% due to renal disease

■ Tertiary Hyperparathyroidism

Definition

- sHPT becomes autonomous

- Originally secondary hyperparathyroidism becomes autonomous.

Etiology

- Develops after prolonged sHPT.
- Hyperplastic parathyroids develop to compensate.
- These initially demonstrate overcompensation with calcium mobilization from bone and overproduction of parathormone.
- Also occurs after treatment of the cause, that is, after renal transplantation.
- sHPT becomes autonomous and so becomes tertiary hyperparathyroidism.

Treatment Approach

■ Surgical Treatment

- Indication under the same conditions as given for clinically obvious pHPT

Surgical Approach
- Bilateral exploration
- Resection of three and a half parathyroids
- Autotransplantation of part of the least abnormal parathyroid in the forearm

■ Postoperative Management

- As for sHPT

■ Parathyroid Carcinoma

Epidemiology

- Extremely rare, occurs in 0.5% of cases
- Women affected more often than men (3 : 1)
- Peak incidence is between the ages of 50 and 60 years

Symptoms

- Symptoms as in pHPT

Diagnostic Approach

- Occurs very rarely
- Usually diagnosed at operation

- Extremely high serum calcium and parathormone levels
- Rarely diagnosed preoperatively, more often intraoperatively when there is infiltration of the surrounding tissue and frozen section is performed

Treatment Approach

■ Surgical Treatment

- Parathyroidectomy with hemithyroidectomy on the affected side
- If necessary, en-bloc resection of infiltrated soft tissues
- Systematic lymphadenectomy

■ Postoperative Management

- As after parathyroidectomy without autotransplantation and with replacement of calcium and vitamin D3.
- External radiotherapy and chemotherapy are employed mainly for palliation

■ Hypoparathyroidism

Etiology

- Usually iatrogenic after thyroid or parathyroid surgery, idiopathic

Congenital
- Parathyroid aplasia, isolated or as part of a syndrome (Di George syndrome)
- Pseudohypoparathyroidism types Ia, Ib, II (end-organ resistance to parathormone)
- Gene mutations in the calcium receptor of the end-organs

Acquired
- Usually iatrogenic after thyroid or parathyroid surgery or after radiotherapy
- Functional after hypomagnesemia, neonatal
- Autoimmune disorder in isolation or as part of syndromes (polyendocrine autoimmune syndrome)

Symptoms

- Tetany, seizures
- Glottic spasm
- Visceral spasm
- Skin and nail defects
- Chvostek and Trousseau sign positive

- The functional consequences are reversible but the structural consequences can be influenced only slightly by treatment.

Functional Consequences
- CNS: tetanic syndrome, anxiety states, psychosis
- Eye: papilledema
- Kidney: hypercalciuria, hypophosphaturia
- Skin: paresthesias
- Heart: prolonged QT interval, cardiomyopathy

Structural Consequences
- CNS: basal ganglia calcification (Fahr disease)
- Eye: cataract
- Kidney: nephrocalcinosis
- Skin: subcutaneous calcification
- Bone: hyperostosis, growth disorders

Diagnostic Approach

- Laboratory tests: parathormone, calcium, magnesium reduced, phosphate raised

Treatment Approach

- In an acute tetanic episode, 10 mL of 10% calcium gluconate solution IV 1.5–2 mL/min
- Long-term therapy: oral calcium 0.5–2 g/d, vitamin D to increase calcium absorption from the intestine

Further Reading

Chan AK, Duh QY, Katz MH, Siperstein AE, Clark OH. Clinical manifestations of primary hyperparathyroidism before and after parathyroidectomy. A case-control study. Ann Surg 1995; 222(3): 402–414

Oertli D, Udelsman R, eds. Surgery of the Thyroid and Parathyroid Glands. New York: Saunders; 2010

Yano Y, Nagehama M, Sugino K, Ito K, Ito K. Long-term changes in parathyroid function after subtotal thyroidectomy for Graves' disease. World Journal of Surgery 2008; 32: 2612–2616

4 Thorax (Pleura, Lung)

R.J. Elfeldt

■ Anatomy

- The **thorax** consists of the bony thorax, the muscles, the two pleural cavities with the lungs, and the mediastinum between them containing the esophagus, heart, vessels, and nerves.
- The anterior, lateral, and posterior boundaries of the thorax are formed by the rib cage, the medial boundary by the spine and mediastinum, the inferior boundary by the diaphragm, and the superior boundary by the upper thoracic inlet.
- The **lungs** are covered by the visceral (pulmonary) pleura. The hilum of the lung—where it is entered by the main bronchus, vessels and nerves—is not covered by the serous covering as the visceral pleura here becomes the parietal pleura, which lines the inside of the chest wall.
- The **pleural cavity** between the layers of the pleura is a capillary potential space in the normal state. It has a negative pressure of -5 cm H_2O in expiration, which falls to -10 cm H_2O on deep inspiration.

■ Pleural Effusion

Definition

- Increased accumulation of fluid in the pleural space is called a pleural effusion. Depending on the protein content and specific gravity of the effusion, a distinction is made between a **transudate** and an **exudate**.
- **Transudate:** protein content < 3 g/100 mL and specific gravity < 1015, usually due to congestion, for example, in heart failure or as a result of dys- or hyperproteinemia
- **Exudate:** protein content > 3 g/100 mL and specific gravity > 1015, usually of inflammatory origin, for example, pneumonia, or neoplastic (e.g., pleural carcinomatosis)

- Increased accumulation of fluid in the pleural space
- Classified as transudate or exudate

Etiology

- The equilibrium between absorption and secretion in the pleura is maintained by the extensive lymphatic vessels, the capillary network, and the thin serosa of the two layers of the pleura. Outflow obstructions of the vascular system, lymphatic pathways, or excessively low oncotic pressure due to dysproteinemia or increased permeability of the serosa are possible causes of pleural effusion.

4

Symptoms

- Symptoms range from pain to dyspnea and shortness of breath.

- The symptoms of an effusion depend on its severity and its pressure on the right atrium. They range from mild pain with concomitant pleuritis to dyspnea and shortness of breath with compression of the lung due to large volumes of fluid.

Diagnostic Approach

■ Clinical Examination

- Dullness to percussion
- Diminished breath sounds

- There is a dull note on percussion with diminished breath sounds on auscultation.

■ Diagnostic Imaging

- The **p.a. radiograph** shows **shadowing** at the lateral thoracic wall with effusions of more than 400 mL; smaller volumes (over 100 mL of fluid) can be identified on the lateral decubitus film.
- A pleural effusion cannot only be diagnosed by **ultrasonography** but the optimal site for aspiration can be marked. In addition, incipient loculation of the effusion can be shown
- Even the smallest effusions can be shown by **thoracic CT. Measurements of the density** provide evidence regarding the nature of the effusion (serous, bloody, purulent, etc.). Early **loculation** of the effusion can also be shown.

Treatment Approach

- Pleural aspiration or chest drain
- For malignant effusions, pleurodesis is a possibility.

■ Surgical Treatment

Pleural Aspiration
- Pleural aspiration is indicated for greater effusion volumes and corresponding symptoms (dyspnea), to achieve immediate **relief.** It is also occasionally indicated for purely diagnostic purposes to clarify the nature of an unclear pleural effusion.
- The obtained aspirate must be tested for protein content, leukocyte count, lipase and amylase, LDH, bacteria (including *Mycobacterium tuberculosis*), fungi and malignant cells. When lymphocytes predominate in the effusion, fungal infection must be included in the differential diagnosis along with tuberculosis. If malignant cells are found in the aspirate, this indicates **pleural carcinomatosis,** that is, advanced malignancy.
- Strict **asepsis** and an assistant are essential for aspiration. The patient sits leaning forward slightly (with an assistant supporting the patient forward). The site of aspiration is determined according to the previous diagnosis (e.g., by percussion or ultrasound). This is usually in the **7th or 8th intercostal space** (ICS) in the seated patient. The aspiration is performed in the **posterior axillary line:**
  - ► Injection of local anesthetic (ask about allergic reactions)
  - ► Enter the pleural space at the **upper border of the rib** (vessels and nerves are at the lower border).
- For diagnostic and therapeutic aspiration, **syringes with a three-way stopcock** have proved effective; these allow airtight aspiration of the effusion. To avoid pneumothorax, the puncture can be made with a Veress needle.

Chest Drainage
- This is indicated when subsequent leakage of the effusion can be expected or the effusion accompanies a more prolonged disease (e.g., acute pancreatitis with sepsis). It is inserted with the patient lying down, if necessary on his/her side.
- The **site of puncture** depends on the cause of the symptoms:
  - ► In the 4th ICS in the posterior axillary line in the posterior direction for hemothorax or pleural effusion
  - ► Ventrally in the 2nd ICS in the midclavicular line for pneumothorax (**caution:** subclavian vessels, mammary artery)

Operative Technique

- After local anesthesia of the skin, subcutaneous tissue, and intercostal muscles, the skin is incised and the trocar with attached drain tube is advanced upward, initially subcutaneously parallel to the chest wall over the width of at least one ICS, to produce an airtight tunnel.
- After reaching the ICS to be punctured, the tip must point almost vertically toward the chest wall and the trocar is passed under the intercostal muscles.
- After passing through the intercostal muscles and parietal pleura, the drain is advanced in the desired direction and fixed in this position by a skin suture (**Fig. 4.1**).
- The tube is connected to an underwater seal and aspirated with suction of $-20\,cm\,H_2O$. The drain system must be airtight so that no pneumothorax can develop.
- The more viscous and high in protein that the pleural effusion is (hemothorax, pleural empyema), the larger should be the tube diameter so that it does not become occluded by precipitated fibrin.

Pleurodesis
- Generally indicated in **malignant pleural effusions.** The aim is to produce adhesions between the two layers of pleura by inducing an inflammatory reaction.
- The pleurodesing agent (e.g., talcum) is dissolved in normal saline (e.g., 2 g talcum in 50 mL NaCl). A **local anesthetic** is added to obtain local anesthesia of the pleura. This mixture is instilled through the chest tube after drainage of the pleural cavity.
- The tube is clamped for **1 hour** and the patient is turned through 90 degrees every **15 minutes** so that the pleural surfaces are moistened evenly. The tube can then be reopened. Depending on further effusion production (more than 100 mL/24 h), the treatment can be repeated after 24 hours.

After each puncture, drainage, or pleurodesis, a **chest x-ray** is taken to check the position of the tube and reduction of the effusion. Incorrectly positioned or insufficiently draining tubes are often the cause of adhesions (loculations) and therefore of later complications.

4

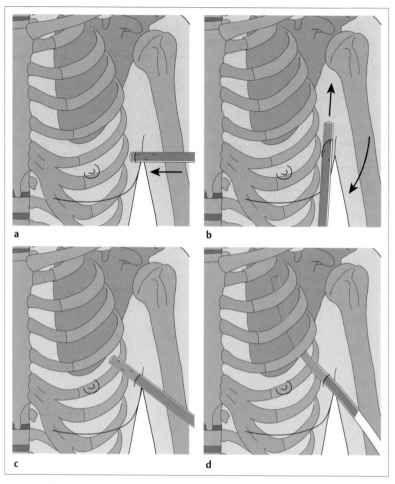

Fig. 4.1 a–d   Steps in placing a chest drain.
a After injecting local anesthetic and making a skin incision, the chest drain is first advanced perpendicularly to the chest wall.
b After reaching the ribs, the drain is angled through 90° and advanced subcutaneously, parallel to the chest wall.
c After reaching the next higher intercostal space, the intercostal muscles are punctured.
d After puncturing the chest wall, the drain is advanced into the thoracic cavity.

■ Complications

- Typical complications with chest drains are infections, injuries of the inter-costal vessels with more severe bleeding, or injuries of the intercostal nerves. **Incorrect puncture** and **incorrect positions** can also occur:
  - ► Subcutaneous position in obese patients without drainage
  - ► Intrapulmonary position with fistulation of the suction or bleeding
  - ► Intra-abdominal position with injury of the liver, spleen, or diaphragm
  - ► Mediastinal position with injury of the heart or great vessels.

■ Pleural Empyema

Definition

- Pleural empyema (synonym: pyothorax) is a collection of pus in the pleural cavity.

• Collection of pus in the pleural cavity

Etiology

- The most common causes are **extension of inflammatory processes** in the thorax (e.g., pneumonia, bronchiectasis, mediastinitis, or lung abscesses).
- Empyema can also develop with **intra-abdominal bacterial infections,** such as subphrenic or subhepatic abscesses, esophageal rupture, and hematogenous spread to the pleural cavity.
- **Postoperative** pleural empyema can occur as a wound infection following surgery on the lung or mediastinum (esophageal resection, partial lung resection).
- **Posttraumatic** pleural empyema is rare. If the pleural abscess penetrates the chest wall, this is called empyema necessitatis (or perforating empyema). In pleural empyema due to trauma, direct contamination of the chest wound is the cause.

4

Classification

Three stages of empyema are distinguished:
1. Exudative phase
2. Fibrinopurulent phase
3. Fibrosing/scarring phase

Symptoms

- Typical signs are dyspnea with breathing-related pain, leukocytosis, high **fever**, and **severe malaise**. Encapsulated processes may have few symptoms.

• Dyspnea with breathing-related pain
• Leukocytosis
• High fever
• Severe malaise

Diagnostic Approach

- **Shadowing** is seen on the a.p. **chest x-ray**.
- The extent and the presence of any loculation of the empyema can be established on **thoracic CT**.

Treatment Approach

■ Indications

- Stage 1: irrigation only
- Stage 2: lysis or video-assisted thoracoscopic (VAT) debridement
- Stage 3: decortication or resection of the empyema sac

Antibiotic treatment is essential after determining the resistance and **draining** the empyema. Further treatment of the empyema depends on the stage.

Symptoms

- Petechial hemorrhages in Perthes syndrome

- As with chest contusion, there is breathing-related pain and shallow breathing on the affected side. In Perthes syndrome, **petechial hemorrhages** occur in the upper half of the body and in the eye (retina, vitreous).

Diagnostic Approach

- A **chest radiograph in two planes** is essential and if rib fractures are suspected (marked localized tenderness), specific x-rays of the ribs or bony hemithorax must be obtained. **Repeat radiographs** after a delay of some hours often show the entire extent of the lung injury.
- As with all other chest injuries, a **thoracic CT** is always possible as this allows contusions of the lung in particular to be identified sooner than with a conventional chest x-ray.

Treatment Approach

- Admission to hospital, analgesic treatment, and intensive respiratory therapy are necessary to prevent pneumonia. In severe cases with **respiratory insufficiency, intubation** and **intensive care treatment** are necessary. If **pneumonia** occurs as a result of lung contusion, antibiotic treatment, in line with microbiology test results, is required.

Rib Fractures

Definition

- Rib fractures can occur as isolated fractures, multiple rib fractures, or flail segments.

- A distinction is made between fractures of the **upper** and **lower ribs**.
- **Multiple rib fractures** (at least three ribs on one side are fractured)
- **Flail segment** (when a rib is broken in two places); separation fractures are fractures at the costocartilage junction.

Etiology

- **Direct** and also **indirect force** on the chest wall. The severity of the injury ranges from an uncomplicated fracture of one rib, without any significant disturbance of the mechanics of breathing, to multiple rib fractures with an **unstable thorax** and **respiratory insufficiency,** necessitating **immediate intubation.**

Symptoms

- Breathing-related pain
- Dragging respiratory movements
- Paradoxical respiration

- The signs of rib fractures are breathing-related pain and dragging respiratory movements on the affected side. Characteristically, marked tenderness is found over the fracture, possibly with crepitation.
- An unstable chest wall with **paradoxical respiration** results from multiple rib fractures and can be caused by flail segments. Inspiratory indrawing and outward movements on expiration on the affected side of the chest are typical. **Respiratory insufficiency** develops due to the movement of air between the two lungs with inadequate gas exchange (dead-space ventilation).

Diagnostic Approach

- As with all chest injuries, a **chest radiograph** in two planes must be obtained initially with an x-ray photo of the bony **hemithorax** with the central beam through the area of maximum pain.
- Depending on the pattern of injury, concomitant injuries must be sought or further radiographs should be taken.
  - ► Fractures of the **upper ribs** (ribs 1–3) are caused by considerable force as the shoulder girdle protects the upper chest region like a bulwark. Concomitant trauma such as brachial **plexus injury, vascular injury,** or **ruptures of the tracheobronchial space** must be ruled out. **Angiography** is indicated when the pulse is absent in the upper limb, if hemothorax occurs, or there are motor or sensory deficits in the hand.
  - ► With fractures of the **lower ribs, intra-abdominal** (liver, spleen) or **retroperitoneal organs** (kidneys) can also be injured because of the absence of the stabilizing action of the sternum. **Ultrasonography of the abdomen** and examination of the **urine sediment** are primary investigations. The tests should be repeated after a few hours so that delayed complications (e.g., two-stage rupture of the spleen) can be identified promptly.

4

Treatment Approach

- Simple rib fractures are treated with analgesia. If there are multiple rib fractures, in-patient monitoring with repeat radiographs is essential. If hemo- or pneumothorax occurs, a chest drain must be inserted.
- If the **chest wall is unstable** (extensive multiple rib fractures) with respiratory insufficiency, the patient must be intubated and ventilated with PEEP (positive end-expiratory pressure). Whether treatment with internal splinting can be continued or whether surgical stabilization of the ribs is necessary can be decided later. Mechanical ventilation is usually the treatment of choice. Stabilization of the chest wall by internal fixation is performed only rarely.

■ Complications

- The most common complications of rib fractures are hemothorax, pneumothorax, and lung contusion. Intra-abdominal or retroperitoneal injuries should also be considered. Patients must be hospitalized for analgesia and monitoring. If any of the aforementioned concomitant injuries occur (vascular tear, splenic, liver or renal injury), surgical treatment is indicated.

- Hemothorax
- Pneumothorax
- Lung contusion

Fracture of the Sternum

Etiology

- **Direct trauma to the sternum** is usually the cause of this injury (typical road-traffic injury), in which the sternum is deformed backward; it can cause **cardiac contusion.** The injury is usually a transverse fracture between the body of the sternum and the manubrium.

Symptoms

- There is severe tenderness over the fracture and breathing-related pain at the same time. Sternal fractures are often accompanied by rib fractures and cartilage tears.

Diagnostic Approach

- Cardiac contusion must be ruled out.

- A **chest x-ray with a lateral view** of the sternum is essential.
- If the result is unclear, **ultrasonography** or **conventional tomography** of the sternum can be performed as this may show the fracture line.
- **ECG** and **measurement of the cardiac enzymes** (CK-MB, GOT, LDH) are required urgently to rule out **cardiac contusion.** The time course of the enzyme pattern is important, and **echocardiography** can be performed in addition.

Treatment Approach

- Patients with a sternal fracture require **in-patient monitoring.** In the absence of complications, analgesia is sufficient treatment.

■ Complications

- If there is cardiac contusion, **cardiac arrhythmias** with corresponding hemodynamic changes can occur.

Lung Contusion

Definition

- Lung contusion is damage of the lung parenchyma as a result of force.

Etiology

- Hemorrhage within the lung parenchyma

- After both blunt and sharp chest injuries with transmission of force to the lung, the lung parenchyma becomes **interspersed with blood.**
- Changes in permeability at the same time cause interstitial alveolar **edema** with microatelectasis. These changes can lead to an intrapulmonary **right-to-left shunt** with consequent **arterial hypoxia** (respiratory insufficiency).

Classification

- If the lung injury is apparent only on x-ray, this is a simple lung contusion but if the arterial oxygen saturation is below normal, this is a lung contusion with respiratory insufficiency.

Symptoms

- The symptoms depend on the extent of the lung injury and are often masked by the concomitant injuries (rib fractures, pneumothorax), which often predominate symptomatically.
- Since lung contusions only develop after a certain interval, they can be initially "silent" clinically and radiologically.

Diagnostic Approach

- The **chest x-ray** can be normal initially but usually the full extent of the contusion can be seen, even on the first chest radiograph. The x-ray appearance ranges from diffuse, soft, demarcated, small opacities to extensive infiltrates or opacification of entire lung lobes.
- **Repeat radiographs** of the lung are important for diagnosing lung contusion.
- The same applies for **arterial blood gas analysis,** as this is the only way to promptly identify the right time for intervention.

Treatment Approach

- Active and intensive **respiratory therapy** of lung contusion without respiratory insufficiency.
- Adequate **analgesia** is more important if there are concomitant injuries (e.g., rib fractures).
- If there is respiratory insufficiency, **mechanical ventilation** with PEEP is the treatment of choice.

- Early intubation and ventilation for respiratory insufficiency

4

■ Complications

- The patients often develop **pneumonia.**
- Progression to **shock lung** or **acute respiratory distress syndrome (ARDS)** is possible.

■ Chest Trauma: Penetrating Chest Injuries

Traumatic Pneumothorax

Definition

- In a traumatic pneumothorax, air gets into the pleural cavity because of injury.

Etiology

- **Perforating injuries** of the chest wall and **blunt chest trauma** with injury of the lung can both cause pneumothorax.
- When the leak is in the **visceral pleura,** this is an **internal pneumothorax** and when the leak is in the **parietal pleura,** this is an **external pneumothorax.** An external pneumothorax occurs after stab, gunshot and impaling injuries and an internal pneumothorax after rib fractures or blunt chest trauma with injury of the lung. The defect can close spontaneously, remain patent or act like a check valve that allows air to pass through only during inspiration.

Classification

Closed Pneumothorax
- No connection with the outside air
- Depending on the location, this can be an **internal** or **external** closed pneumothorax.

- The lung can be more or less **collapsed** and therefore **atelectatic,** depending on the duration and size of the opening.
- **Perfusion** continues but oxygenation is absent, at least partially, and venous blood is admixed in this lung (**right-to-left shunt**).
- The lung volume is reduced by 50% if the lung surface is ca. 3 cm distant from the chest wall.

Open Pneumothorax
- Persisting communication between the pleural cavity and the outer air; it can be present as an initial pneumothorax in the form of a lung injury.
- The lung usually collapses completely. In addition, the affected lung cannot follow the respiratory excursions of the chest wall so that **"pendelluft"** develops with defective gas exchange.
- Because of the movements of the healthy side, the **mediastinum can move** (mediastinal flutter) with kinking of the inferior vena cava and impaired venous return to the heart. This leads to **cardiocirculatory insufficiency.**

Tension Pneumothorax

- Positive pressure in the pleural cavity with mediastinal shift to the healthy side.

- Valve mechanism in which air is sucked into the affected pleural cavity during inspiration. The defect closes during expiration and the inspired air cannot escape.
- This produces **positive pressure** in the pleural cavity with **mediastinal shift** to the healthy side. This results in compression of the heart with impairment of venous flow.

Symptoms

- Tension pneumothorax is an acute life-threatening condition.

- In simple pneumothorax, **dyspnea** occurs with **breathing-related pain** on the affected side.
- In open pneumothorax, there is respiratory insufficiency in addition because of the **extensive lung collapse.**
- In tension pneumothorax, the clinical signs of venous obstruction are increasing **cyanosis, tachycardia** and **venous congestion.** Overall, this results in a **life-threatening condition** due to respiratory and circulatory insufficiency.

Diagnostic Approach

- The physical signs of simple pneumothorax are diminished or absent **breath sounds** and a **hyperresonant percussion note.**
- The absence of lung markings on **x-ray** is characteristic. Depending on the extent of lung collapse, a distinction is made between an **apical pneumothorax** over the lung apex, a **simple pneumothorax** with a 1–2 cm lateral space and a **total collapse** of the lung. In tension pneumothorax, mediastinal shift to the healthy side is found in addition.

Treatment Approach

- Immediate decompression of the positive pressure in tension pneumothorax by insertion of a chest drain

- The spontaneous course of apical or simple pneumothorax can be observed clinically and radiologically as small volumes of air are reabsorbed.
- When there is an extensive pneumothorax, the negative pressure in the pleural space must be restored by a **drain with suction** to preserve the

lung. With a pure pneumothorax, this is placed in the 2nd ICS in the mid-clavicular line as the air moves upward (in the supine patient). A narrow tube can be used, which is attached to suction of $-20\,\mathrm{cm\,H_2O}$. After insertion of the chest drain and aspiration, an x-ray to check the position and outcome is essential. In the case of an external open pneumothorax with a chest wall injury, a loose airtight dressing that is permeable to air must first be applied. (**Caution:** valve mechanism.) After a chest drain is inserted, the wound can be closed and suction is attached to the drain.

- The life-threatening condition of pneumothorax requires **immediate decompression** of the pleural cavity by inserting a chest drain (4th ICS, posterior axillary line). In an emergency, the 2nd ICS can be **aspirated** with a stout cannula. The cannula should be covered with a fingerstall that acts like a pressure relief valve (Tiegel cannula). A chest drain is inserted subsequently.
- The patient must not be ventilated until the tension pneumothorax is relieved and a chest drain is inserted. Once the breathing mechanism has been restored, the cause of the condition can be treated.

4

Hemothorax

Definition

- Hemorrhage into the pleural cavity is called hemothorax.

Etiology

- A hemothorax results from injuries of the lung, pleura, and chest wall. The causes can include: puncture wounds (pleural aspiration, central venous routes); injuries of the tracheobronchial system; rib fractures; aortic rupture and, in rare cases, spontaneous rupture of lung cysts or lung tumors.

• Result of lung, pleura, and chest wall injury

Symptoms

- Patients complain of **dyspnea** and **breathing-related pain.** On examination, the **breath sounds are reduced** and there is **percussion dullness;** depending on the severity of the bleeding, there may be a drop in **hemoglobin** and **symptoms of shock**.

Diagnostic Approach

- The chest radiograph shows a homogeneous reduction in transparency on the affected side. In erect views, fluid can be seen only when the volume exceeds 400–500 mL.
- A supplementary thoracic CT can show the quantity of blood better.

• Thoracic CT can show the quantity of blood better.

Treatment Approach

- A **chest drain** must be inserted to decompress the pleural cavity and monitor the volume of bleeding. Complete evacuation of the pleural cavity prevents fibrosis with later lung fistulation.
- **Surgical treatment** is indicated with persistent bleeding of more than 100 mL/h for several hours.

Chylothorax

Definition

- This is a collection of chyle in the pleural space.

Etiology

- Results from injury of the thoracic duct or cisterna chyli

- Chylothorax is nearly always the result of injury of the thoracic duct or cisterna chyli after trauma.
- However, chylothorax is more often caused by **iatrogenic injuries** during thoracic surgery, for example, esophageal resection or operations on the aorta.
- Other rare causes are **obstructions of lymph drainage** due to tumors or inflammation (e.g., tuberculosis).
- A congenital anomaly is a rare cause, which is always associated with chyloperitoneum (chyle in the abdomen).

Symptoms

- The symptoms, as with any pleural effusion, are **dullness to percussion** and **diminished breath sounds**. If the volume of chyle is large, the patient is **dyspneic**.

Diagnostic Approach

- **Aspiration** of cloudy fluid with a fat content of 0.4%–4%, a protein content of up to 30% and containing lymphocytes is diagnostic.

Treatment Approach

- Treatment is initially conservative, with insertion of a chest drain and observation of the spontaneous course with a **low-fat diet** to reduce chyle production.
- If chyle production does not cease, **surgical ligature of the thoracic duct** is indicated.

Tracheal and Bronchial Injuries

Definition

- Tracheal and bronchial injuries are usually the result of very severe blunt thoracic trauma, particularly in children (elastic chest wall).

- Ruptures of the tracheobronchial system are usually the result of very severe blunt thoracic trauma, particularly in children with an elastic chest wall.

Symptoms

- Since tracheal and bronchial injuries seldom occur in isolation, nearly all of the symptoms of possible chest injuries are found. Hemothorax, pneumothorax, atelectasis, and cutaneous or mediastinal emphysema result from bronchial rupture. Particularly in the case of pneumothorax that cannot be abolished despite adequate drainage, bronchial injuries should be sought.

Diagnostic Approach

- Radiographic findings as in explosion injury
- **Bronchoscopy** is important to establish the extent and location of the injuries before surgery

Treatment Approach

- The affected side of the chest is first **drained.** If there is a tear of the bronchus or trachea, the **defect is sutured,** an avulsion is **re-anastomosed,** and with more minor tracheal injuries, especially in the region of the membranous wall, endoscopic insertion of a **coated tracheal stent** may be sufficient.

Further Reading

Boffa DJ, Sands MJ, Rice TW et al. A critical evaluation of a percutaneous diagnostic and treatment strategy for chylothorax after thoracic surgery. Eur J Cardiothorac Surg 2008; 33: 435–439

Hill S, Edmisten T, Holtzman G, Wright A. The occult pneumothorax: an increasing diagnostic entity in trauma. Am Surg 1999; 65: 254–258

Roberts JR, Hedges JR. Clinical Procedures in Emergency Medicine: Expert Consult–Online and Print (Roberts, Clinical Procedures in Emergency Medicine). 5th ed. Philadelphia, USA; Saunders: 2009

Schmidt U, Stalp M, Gerich T, Blauth M, Maull KI, Tscherne H. Chest tube decompression of blunt chest injuries by physicians in the field: effectiveness and complications. J Trauma 1998; 44: 1115

4

5 Mediastinum

R.J. Elfeldt

■ Anatomy

- Anterior mediastinum
- Middle mediastinum
- Posterior mediastinum
- Superior mediastinum

- The boundaries of the mediastinum are formed by the thoracic spine (behind), the sternum (in front), the diaphragm (below) and the two lungs at the sides.
- Above, it is connected with the connective tissue spaces of the neck, which are continuous with the fascia of the mediastinum. This explains the spread of collar inflammation to the mediastinum (descending sepsis).
- The mediastinum is divided into the anterior mediastinum located between the pericardium and the posterior surface of the sternum, the middle mediastinum, which is filled mainly by the heart, the posterior mediastinum, which is between the posterior pericardium and the spine, and the superior mediastinum, which is above the level of the sternal angle.
- The mediastinum contains all the organs of the thoracic cavity apart from the lungs (**Fig. 5.1** and **Table 5.1**).

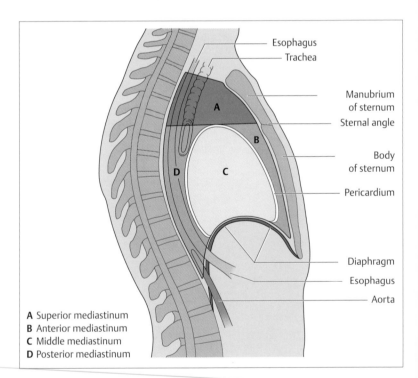

A Superior mediastinum
B Anterior mediastinum
C Middle mediastinum
D Posterior mediastinum

Fig. 5.1 Diagram of the division of the mediastinum in midline sagittal section.

Table 5.1   Contents of the mediastinum

Location	Contents
Anterior mediastinum	• Loose connective tissue between sternum and pericardium • Lymphatic vessels • Minor blood vessels
Middle mediastinum	• Heart and pericardium • Ascending aorta • Terminal segments of the superior vena cava and azygos vein • Pulmonary trunk with its branches • Pulmonary veins • Phrenic nerves with pericardiophrenic vessels
Posterior mediastinum	• Esophagus with vagus nerves (vagal trunks) • Descending aorta with its branches • Thoracic duct • Azygos and hemiazygos veins • Sympathetic trunk and greater and lesser splanchnic nerves
Superior mediastinum	• Arch of the aorta, brachiocephalic artery, initial part of the left common carotid artery, and left subclavian artery • Superior vena cava (upper part), brachiocephalic vein • Thymus • Vagus nerve, left recurrent laryngeal nerve, cardiac and phrenic nerves (upper segments) • Trachea • Esophagus • Thoracic duct (upper segment)

5

■ Mediastinoscopy

- Mediastinoscopy allows direct inspection of the paratracheal, subcarinal, and bilateral tracheobronchial mediastinum.

Indications
- Establishing operability of malignant bronchial tumors when mediastinal lymph node metastases are suspected on radiography (staging).
- Confirmation of the diagnosis when systemic disease with mediastinal involvement is suspected (e.g., malignant lymphoma, sarcoidosis, etc.).
- The indication should be highly restricted on account of the risk of injury when there is upper venous congestion, a large goiter, or a history of previous mediastinoscopy or radiotherapy.

Contraindications
- Acute inflammatory mediastinal or pulmonary processes are contraindications to mediastinoscopy (bacterial contamination).

- Collar mediastinoscopy: assessment of the paratracheal, subcarinal, and bilateral tracheobronchial space
- Anterior mediastinoscopy: retrosternal space

Collar Mediastinoscopy

Operative Technique

- Make a transverse skin incision 2 cm above the sternal notch under general anesthesia.
- The pretracheal fascia is then dissected and opened and the anterior wall of the trachea is dissected bluntly with a finger.
- After introducing the mediastinoscope, further blunt dissection is performed with a dissecting swab.
- The pre- and paratracheal space as far as both main bronchi can be evaluated in this way.

Anterior Mediastinoscopy

Operative Technique

- Allows diagnostic exploration of the anterior mediastinum, which is not accessible with collar mediastinoscopy.
- The examination is performed through a horizontal incision made lateral to the sternum at the level of the second or third costal cartilage.
- The cartilaginous part of the corresponding rib is resected and the internal thoracic artery and vein are identified, ligated, and divided.
- The parietal pleura is then pushed laterally, so that the anterior mediastinum can be opened.

Complications
- Injuries of the trachea and main bronchi, vascular injuries (aortic arch, right brachiocephalic trunk, left carotid artery), so always **be prepared to carry out sternotomy or thoracotomy** when performing mediastinoscopy.
- Recurrent nerve paresis and pneumothorax
- Esophageal perforation can also occur when the esophagus is atypically displaced.

■ Subcutaneous Emphysema

- Collection of air in the subcutaneous tissue and muscle due to injury

- **Definition:** Subcutaneous emphysema is a collection of air in the subcutaneous tissue and muscle due to injury.
- **Etiology:** There is a communication due to trauma between air-containing organs and the subcutaneous region. It often occurs with bronchial or tracheal injuries.
- **Symptoms:** Crepitus (a crunching sensation) is felt on palpation of the involved areas.
- **Diagnostic approach:** Typical **streaky lucencies** are seen on x-ray photos.
- **Treatment approach:**
  ► If the **injury is minor,** treatment of the subcutaneous emphysema is not necessary as the air will be absorbed.
  ► If a **lung fistula** is the cause, a **drain** should be inserted.

■ Mediastinal Emphysema

- Collection of air in the mediastinum as a result of injury to central air-containing organs such as the trachea, bronchi, and esophagus

- **Definition:** This refers to a collection of air in the mediastinum as a result of injury.
- **Etiology:** Air passes into the mediastinum due to a traumatic opening in the mediastinal pleura. Typical injuries are **esophageal perforation** and **bronchial or tracheal rupture.**
- **Symptoms:** There is usually **subcutaneous emphysema**, with **dyspnea** and **venous congestion** when severe (**Fig. 5.2**). Mediastinitis can occur as a result of the injury.
- **Treatment approach:**
  ► Minor injuries can be observed (subsequent reduction of the mediastinal emphysema). If mediastinitis develops, **antibiotic treatment** and **drainage** by jugular mediastinostomy are necessary.

5

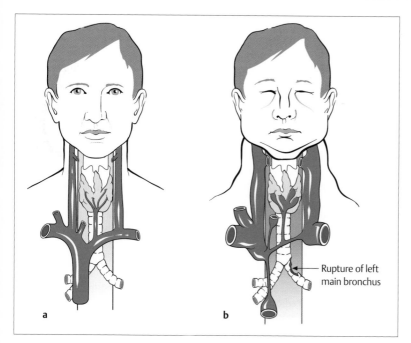

Rupture of left
main bronchus

Fig. 5.2 a, b   Mediastinal emphysema and its clinical consequences.
a Normal.
b The development of mediastinal emphysema leads to excess pressure in the mediastinum
with compression of the veins located in the mediastinum (superior vena cava, left brachiocephalic vein) and resulting congestion.

▸ Major injuries are managed with operative closure of the leak and/or
  insertion of a chest drain, depending on the cause (esophageal perforation, pneumothorax).
▸ For minor tracheal injuries, endoscopic placement of a **coated tracheal
  stent** is often sufficient.

■ Mediastinitis

Definition

• This is an inflammatory process in the mediastinum, spread of which is
  favored by the loose fatty connective tissue and prominent lymphatic system
  of the mediastinum. A distinction is made between **acute mediastinitis** and
  chronic mediastinitis.

• Acute and chronic mediastinitis

Etiology

• **Acute mediastinitis** most often arises directly from **perforation** of the **trachea** or **esophagus** by: a tumor or ulcer, during endoscopy, due to foreign
  body ingestion, blunt trauma, after violent choking or vomiting (known as
  Boerhaave syndrome), or **leakage** from **an esophageal anastomosis**. Moreover, it can be caused by spread of inflammatory purulent processes from

neighboring areas (pleural empyema, lung abscess), or by lymphatogenous or hematogenous spread in measles, pleuritis, pneumonia, or scarlet fever (very rare).

- **Chronic mediastinitis** occurs most frequently as a result of **tuberculosis**, syphilis or **actinomycosis**. However, **penetrating foreign bodies** (e.g., shrapnel) can also cause chronic mediastinitis, even after many years.

Symptoms

- In **acute mediastinitis**, there is usually considerable impairment of the patient's general condition with fever, chills, tachycardia, dry tongue, hiccup, retrosternal pain, and possibly also subcutaneous emphysema in the neck and face.
- In **chronic mediastinitis**, there is more likely to be retrosternal pain, possibly with compression of the trachea, esophagus, or great vessels.

Diagnostic Approach

- Diagnostic imaging: a widened mediastinum and pneumomediastinum can be seen on **chest radiographs in two planes**.
- If esophageal perforation or a leaking anastomosis is suspected, **contrast radiography** (using water-soluble contrast agent only) and **esophagoscopy** can confirm the diagnosis.
- **Bronchoscopy** must be performed if tracheal or **bronchial rupture** is suspected.
- In addition, the diagnosis can be confirmed by **CT**.

Treatment Approach

Acute Mediastinitis

- **Surgical decompression** and **drainage**, as collar, abdominal, or transpleural mediastinostomy, depending on the location of the focus
- Perforation of the esophagus or tracheobronchial system is managed either surgically (thoracotomy, primary oversewing, transpleural drainage) or **endoscopically** by means of a tube bridging the perforation.
- In addition, the patient is given high-dose **antibiotics** and is monitored in the intensive care unit. When the mediastinitis is severe, mortality is still high today.

Chronic Mediastinitis

- The treatment is guided by the cause (foreign body removal, tuberculostatic drugs, antibiotics, etc.).

Further Reading

Berger H. Mediastinal emphysema. Harmlose Kuriosität oder Notfall? Pneumologe 2006; 3: 216–223
Tamura Y, Takahama M, Kushibe K, Taniguchi S. Ectopic pancreas in the anterior mediastinum. Jpn J Thorac Cardioavasc Surg 2005; 53: 498–501
Van Schil PE, De Waele M. A second mediastinoscopy: how to decide and how to do it? Eur J of Cardiothorac Surg 2008; 33: 703–706

6 Diaphragm

I.L. Schmalbach

■ Anatomy

- The diaphragm forms the double, dome-shaped fibromuscular layer that separates the thorax from the abdomen.
- It consists of striated muscle and is the most important respiratory muscle in mammals (75% of breathing work at rest).

• Most important respiratory muscle

Origins of the Muscle Groups
- Lumbar part, costal part, sternal part
- Ligament of Treitz = suspensory muscle of the duodenum: originates from the right medial crus of the lumbar part of the diaphragm
- The muscle groups are connected through the central tendon in the apex of the domes: right leaf (over the liver), left leaf (over the gastric fundus), and central leaf (covered by the pericardium).

• Three muscle groups with central tendon, phrenic nerve (C4), phrenic and pericardiophrenic arteries, phrenic veins

Innervation
- Afferent and efferent innervation by the right and left phrenic nerves (mainly C4), peripheral afferents accompany the intercostal nerves.

6

Arteries
- Right and left inferior phrenic arteries, arising from the aorta after it passes through the aortic hiatus: posterior, central, and lateral diaphragm. Right and left pericardiophrenic arteries (central diaphragm) and right and left musculophrenic arteries (anterior diaphragm), both arising from the internal thoracic artery, which in turn originates from the subclavian artery.

Veins
- Venous drainage is through the inferior phrenic veins, suprarenal veins, and renal veins into the inferior vena cava.

Physiological Openings (and Thus Weak Points) (See Fig. 6.1)
- Aortic hiatus (at the level of T12): aorta, thoracic duct, thoracic splanchnic nerves, azygos vein (right), and hemiazygos vein (left), each lateral to the medial crus of the lumbar part
- Esophageal hiatus (at the level of T10): esophagus, vagus nerves, esophageal branches of the left gastric arteries and inferior phrenic artery, lymphatic vessels (hiatal hernia is an axial or paraesophageal hernia)
- Caval opening: inferior vena cava

• Weak points: aortic hiatus, esophageal hiatus, caval opening

Other Anatomical (Connective Tissue) Weak Points
- Right sternocostal triangle (Morgagni hernia)
- Left sternocostal triangle (Larrey hernia)
- Lumbocostal triangle (Bochdalek hernia)
- Central tendon (pleuroperitoneal hernia)

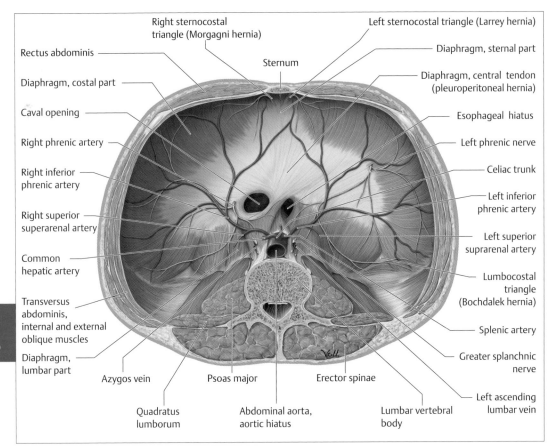

Fig. 6.1   Anatomy of the diaphragm. Inferior view with parietal peritoneum removed. The veins (not shown here) accompany the arteries. (From Thieme Atlas of Anatomy, Neck and Internal Organs, © Thieme 2006; illustration by M. Voll.)

■ Diaphragmatic Hernias

Definition

- Diaphragmatic hernias represent a displacement (complete or partial) of abdominal organs into the thorax through a defect in the diaphragm, with corresponding compression effects and potential incarceration.
- They occur at physiological openings or anatomical weak points (see above) and can be congenital, acquired, or traumatic.

Classification

- Hiatal hernias (90% of diaphragmatic hernias) are axial or paraesophageal hernias, hernias of the anatomical weak points, traumatic hernias

- Hiatal hernias (through the esophageal hiatus, the most frequent form accounting for 90%) in two variants:
  - ▶ Axial sliding hernia (**Fig. 6.2**): the cardia slides into the thorax along the esophageal axis over the distal esophagus

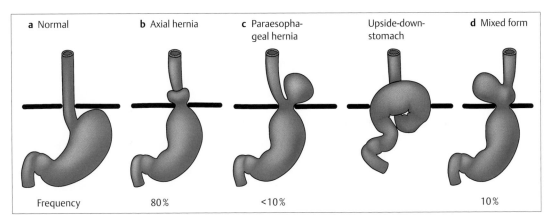

a Normal	b Axial hernia	c Paraesopha-geal hernia	Upside-down-stomach	d Mixed form
Frequency	80%	<10%		10%

Fig. 6.2 a–d Portrayal of types and frequency of occurrence of hiatus hernia.

- ► Paraesophageal hernia (**Fig. 6.2**): the cardia is fixed, and parts of the stomach (usually the fundus) slide through the hiatus beside the esophagus and past the cardia into the thorax; an extreme variant is the upside-down or thoracic stomach
- Mixed forms consisting of an axial and paraesophageal hernia (**Fig. 6.2**)
- Morgagni, Larrey, and Bochdalek hernias and pleuroperitoneal hernias (see above)
    - ► Bochdalek hernia nearly always occurs on the left as the right lumbocostal triangle is covered by the liver. The Morgagni hernia is 10 times commoner than the Larrey hernia as the left sternocostal triangle is sealed off by the heart and pericardium.
- Traumatic hernias: unilateral or bilateral with abdominothoracic compression or perforating trauma

Symptoms

- Depending on their location and size or volume and the nature of the content displaced into the thorax, all hernias can be asymptomatic, have nonspecific symptoms, or have or develop acute or hyperacute symptoms.
- Cardiopulmonary symptoms: dyspnea/tachypnea with atelectasis, pleural effusion, pleurisy, pleural empyema, pneumonia, tachycardia, cardiac arrhythmias
- Gastrointestinal symptoms: bloating, belching, vomiting, gastroesophageal reflux, possibly with bleeding erosions (anemia) and ulceration or Barrett metaplasia (hiatal hernia), esophageal stenosis with regurgitation, acute or subacute ileus, organ ischemia, acute abdomen due to strangulation with gangrene
- Retrosternal pressure or pain, nonspecific pressure in the upper abdomen or lower thorax

- Cardiopulmonary symptoms: dyspnea, cardiac arrhythmias
- Gastrointestinal symptoms: bloating, reflux, ileus, acute abdomen

6

Diagnostic Approach

■ Clinical and Laboratory Examination

- Auscultation and percussion: bowel sounds heard over the thorax, tympanitic percussion note or dullness in the thorax, iron deficiency anemia with chronic bleeding, leukocytosis, raised C-reactive protein, fever

■ Diagnostic Imaging

- Ultrasonography: interrupted diaphragm line, bowel loops, stomach and lung in proximity, pleural effusion, pathological subphrenic fluid collection
- Chest x-ray: elevated diaphragm, mediastinal shift and widening, intrathoracic gastric or intestinal structures with consequent lung atelectasis, pleural effusion, fluid level, irregularity of the diaphragm domes with abnormal mobility
- Contrast radiography (GI series): contrast-filled stomach/intestine above the diaphragm, pathological gastroesophageal reflux (hiatal hernia), delayed passage of contrast
- Cross-sectional diagnostic imaging (CT, MRI): differential diagnosis to exclude other space-occupying processes, more precise determination of location, size and contents of the hernia, relationship to neighboring organs, concomitant injuries in the case of traumatic hernias

■ Invasive Investigations

- Endoscopy (hiatus hernias): direct vision into the hernia, identification of co-existing gastroesophageal reflux disease; if reflux disease also: 24-hour pH monitoring, sphincter manometry

Treatment Approach

■ Indications

Indication for Surgery of Hiatal Hernias

- Most asymptomatic diaphragmatic hernias do not require surgical treatment.
- Axial hernias with grade III–IV reflux according to Savary and Miller
- Volume reflux
- Failure of proton pump inhibitor (PPI) therapy
- All paraesophageal hernias because of the risk of incarceration and lack of alternative forms of treatment

Indication for Surgery of Hernias of the Anatomical Weak Points

- Any definite symptoms
- Relative indication if few or no symptoms
- Repair prior to planned pregnancy to avoid complications

Traumatic Hernias

- The timing and nature of management depend on the overall pattern of injuries.

■ Conservative Treatment

- Conservative treatment only if asymptomatic
- PPIs; classically in hiatal hernias with reflux
- Weight reduction (reduction of intra-abdominal pressure)
- Abstention from alcohol and nicotine (reduction of acid production)

■ Surgical Treatment
Hiatal Hernias

Operative Technique

- Laparoscopic access
- Reduction of the hernia contents into the abdomen
- Resection of the hernial sac if appropriate
- Narrowing of the hiatus ring by nonabsorbable interrupted sutures of the crura of the diaphragm posterior to the esophagus as posterior hiatus repair
- Fixation of the gastric fundus to the diaphragm (fundophrenicopexy) to reconstruct the angle of His
- If signs of reflux disease, Nissen fundoplication (360°) or Toupet hemifundoplication (270°; see Chapter 8)
- Open surgical approach necessary in rare cases, thoracic approach indicated even more rarely

- Laparoscopy with reduction, hiatoplasty, fundophrenicopexy, and fundoplication/hemifundoplication

Hernias of the Anatomical Weak Points

Operative Technique

- Abdominal access, usually laparoscopic, possibly additional thoracic access with large hernias, thoracic access alone more rarely
- Reduction of the hernia contents
- Attempt resection of the hernial sac
- If necessary, (partial) resection of incarcerated hernia contents (e.g., intestine, stomach)
- Closure of the hernial gap in the diaphragm by direct suture (tightening or doubling) is possible in most cases; otherwise, implantation of a nonabsorbable mesh or lyophilized dura
- In children, no alloplastic material as far as possible because growth is not complete

- Surgery indicated when patient complains of symptoms
- **Caution:** children who are still growing

6

Traumatic Hernias

- Occur mainly in patients with multiple injuries/polytrauma, so life-threatening injuries are treated first.
- Recent ruptures: thoracic or abdominal access (open), or both if appropriate depending on concomitant injuries. Operative tactics otherwise as with hernias of the anatomical weak sites.
- Old ruptures: if adhesions with the lung/pleura are anticipated, open thoracic access is preferable. Otherwise laparoscopic access also. Operative tactics otherwise as with hernias of the anatomical weak sites.

■ Rare Disorders of the Diaphragm

Diaphragm Duplication
- Unclear etiology
- Very rare
- Congenital

- Always unilateral (usually on the right in the interlobar gap between the middle and lower lobes)
- Surgical indication: only with pronounced symptoms (respiratory disorders, recurrent pneumonia)

Diaphragmatic Relaxation (Synonyms: Eventration, Megadiaphragm)
- Congenital incidence (1 : 8500) or acquired (phrenic nerve irritation due to inflammation, tumor, trauma)
- Variable extent, and symptoms depend on this
- Surgical indication: only if overt clinical features
- Operative procedure: tightening or folding/doubling of the diaphragm, open abdominal access

Cysts
- Congenital (e.g., bronchogenic cysts) or acquired (e.g., posttraumatic)
- Clinical features and necessity of treatment depend on location and size

Tumors
- Primary tumors of the diaphragm are very rare, secondary metastatic involvement (stomach, lung, liver) is more frequent
- Necessity of treatment depends on symptoms and underlying disease

Functional Disorders
- For example, postoperative hiccup due to phrenic nerve irritation after laparoscopy or as a symptom of a subphrenic abscess, pleurisy, or pericarditis

Further Reading

Hartnett KS. Congenital diaphragmatic hernia: advanced physiology and care concepts. Adv Neonatal Care 2008; 8(2): 107–115

Scharff JR, Naunheim KS. Traumatic diaphragmatic injuries. Thorac Surg Clin 2007; 17 (1): 81–85

Schumpelick V. Atlas of General Surgery. Stuttgart: Thieme; 2009

6

7 Hernias

J.M. Mayer

Definition

- Hernial sac: bulging of the parietal peritoneum
- Hernial orifice: opening for the hernial sac and its contents (musculoaponeurotic gap in the abdominal wall or pelvis)
- Hernia contents: most frequently greater omentum or loops of small bowel but nearly any abdominal viscus possible
- Hernial covering: layers of abdominal wall pushed away by the hernial sac

Epidemiology

- Hernia is the most common disorder in surgery; 10%–15% of general surgical procedures are hernia operations.
- Men are affected much more often than women.
- There are three peaks in the **age range** at which hernias are manifested:
  - Children under 5 years: usually inguinal hernias in boys
  - Between 20 and 30 years: increased physical exertion
  - Between 50 and 70 years: incipient connective tissue weakness

- Most common disorder in surgery
- Older men affected in particular

Etiology

7

- Various factors cause hernias to develop:
  - Increase in intra-abdominal pressure: obesity, ascites, constipation
  - Connective tissue weakness: collagen disorders, pregnancy, previous surgery, age
  - Persistent vaginal process (processus vaginalis) of the peritoneum: in inguinal hernias
- Hernias usually occur in areas of preformed anatomical gaps in a muscle aponeurosis.

- The causes are connective tissue weakness and increased intra-abdominal pressure.
- Hernias occur in areas of preformed anatomical gaps in a muscle aponeurosis.

Classification

■ According to Their Relation to the Abdominal Wall

External Hernias (Fig. 7.1)
- Inguinal hernia:
  - Direct = medial to the epigastric vessels
  - Indirect = lateral to the epigastric vessels
- Femoral hernia
- Umbilical hernia
- Paraumbilical hernia
- Epigastric hernia
- Incisional hernia
- Spigelian hernia (abdominal wall hernia in the area of the linea semilunaris)

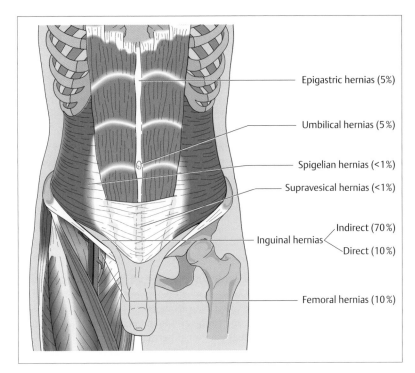

Fig. 7.1 External hernias and their frequency.

7

Internal Hernias
- Treitz hernia (the most frequent form of internal hernia at ca. 53% of cases): paraduodenal hernias at the duodenojejunal flexure
- Paracecal hernias: in the superior, inferior, or retrocecal recess
- In the foramen of Winslow
- In the sigmoid mesocolon
- In the mesentery (**caution:** open postoperative mesenteric defect)
- In a postoperative defect in the pelvic peritoneum
- Paravesical hernia

- **Note:** Always close the mesenteric defect in abdominal operations

■ According to Their Clinical Aspects

- **Reducible hernia:** Hernial sac and hernial contents can be pushed back easily into the abdominal cavity; often asymptomatic
- **Irreducible hernia:** Fixed hernial sac and hernial contents but without impaired perfusion, clinically identifiable as a persistent bulge
- **Incarcerated hernia:** Suddenly occurring, extremely painful bulge that cannot be reduced; associated with acute or subacute ileus; incarceration often leads to strangulation or even necrosis; absolute indication for surgery
- **Sliding hernia:** Hernial sac consists of partially fixed retroperitoneal structures (e.g., bladder, sigmoid) and should be reduced surgically
- **Symptomatic hernia:** Hernia as a symptom of another disease (e.g., ascites, peritoneal carcinomatosis)

- Incarcerated hernia: absolute indication for surgery

■ Inguinal Hernias

Anatomy of the Inguinal Canal (Fig. 7.2)

- Opening for the spermatic cord in men and the round ligament in women and thus a site of less resistance, especially in men
- Starts at the deep inguinal ring lateral to the epigastric vessels and runs in a medial and downward direction through the abdominal wall, to end at the superficial inguinal ring lateral to the pubic tubercle
- Anterior wall: aponeurosis of the external oblique muscle
- Posterior wall: transverse fascia and parietal peritoneum
- Upper boundary: lower border of the internal oblique and transverse abdominal muscles
- Lower boundary: inguinal ligament

• Inguinal canal: place of lesser resistance

Epidemiology

- Hernia operations are the most frequently performed general surgical procedures in Europe and the United States, with about 800 000 operations performed annually.
- Men are affected four to six times more often than women.
- The incidence is 2%–4% in men and 0.3% in women.
- Infants and children:
  - ► Hernias are nearly always indirect, with few exceptions.
  - ► The hernial sac is formed by a persistent patent processus vaginalis.
  - ► Boys are affected about eight times more often than girls.
  - ► About 40% of these hernias occur in infancy and 80% have become apparent by the age of 3 years.

• In adults, 70% of hernias are indirect and 30% are direct.
• In infants and children, hernias are usually indirect.

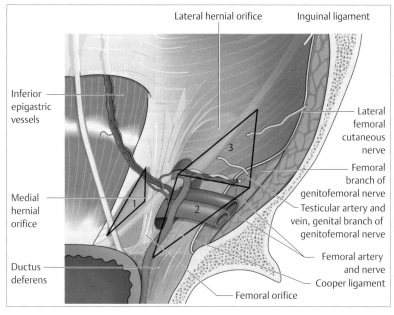

Fig. 7.2 Inguinal canal (1: Hesselbach triangle, 2: Triangle of doom, 3: Triangle of pain).

■ Conservative Treatment

Reduction of Acutely Incarcerated Hernia

- **Caution:** en bloc reduction
- Unsuccessful reduction: emergency surgery

- Analgosedation
- The edema is compressed bimanually with constant pressure and the hernial contents are massaged toward the hernial orifice (**caution:** reduction en bloc, in which the constricting ring is moved into the abdomen with the incarceration but persists).
- If closed reduction is successful, the patient must be monitored in hospital because of the risk of irreversible bowel damage.
- After unsuccessful reduction for more than 10 minutes, emergency surgery is indicated.

■ Surgical Treatment

- Meticulous hemostasis
- In older women, rule out a femoral hernia.
- In men, do not constrict the internal inguinal ring too much.

- Meticulous hemostasis is important.
- Use of a local anesthetic is recommended.
- In older women, rule out a femoral hernia by opening the transversalis fascia.
- In men, do not constrict the internal inguinal ring too much (should admit the little finger, Hegar size 11).
- In women, the internal inguinal ring can be closed firmly around the round ligament.

Bassini Herniotomy

- **Principle:** Stabilization of the posterior wall by suturing the transversalis fascia and the two inner abdominal muscles to the inguinal ligament (not tension-free) (**Fig. 7.3**)

Operative Technique

- Perform a groin incision, splitting the external oblique aponeurosis in the direction of its fibers.
- Protect the ilioinguinal nerve.
- Expose and retract the spermatic cord above the pubic tubercle.
- Identify the hernial sac as a direct or indirect hernia.
- **Lateral hernias:** Dissect the hernial sac down to its base, open it, and reduce the sac contents if necessary (**caution:** sliding hernia). Close the hernial sac close to its base by a transfixion ligature or internal purse-string suture and excise it. Open the transversalis fascia.
- **Medial hernias:** Expose and open the transversalis fascia and resect the attenuated parts of it.
- Closure is with interrupted sutures (polypropylene, e.g., Prolene 0) by suturing the internal oblique, transversis abdominis and superior lip of the transversalis fascia to the inferior lip of the transversalis fascia and inguinal ligament (**caution:** do not constrict the internal inguinal ring too much (should admit the little finger, Hegar size 11).
- Continuous suture of the external oblique aponeurosis, skin closure.

7

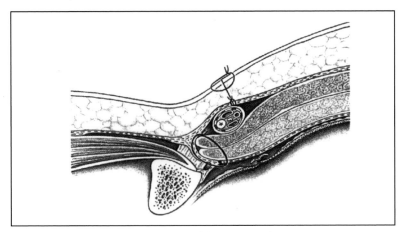

Fig. 7.3 Bassini herniotomy (from Schumpelick 2000, p. 413).

Shouldice Herniotomy

- **Principle:** Stabilization of the posterior wall by duplication of the transversalis fascia (not tension-free) (**Fig. 7.4**)

Operative Technique

- Perform a groin incision, splitting the external oblique aponeurosis in the direction of its fibers.
- Protect the ilioinguinal nerve.
- Expose and retract the spermatic cord above the pubic tubercle.
- Identify the hernial sac as a direct or indirect hernia.
- **Lateral hernias:** Dissect the hernial sac down to its base, open it, and reduce the sac contents if necessary (**caution:** sliding hernia). Close the hernial sac close to its base by a transfixion ligature or internal purse-string suture and excise it. Open the transversalis fascia.
- **Medial hernias:** Expose and open the transversalis fascia and resect the attenuated parts of it.
- Double-row duplication of the transversalis fascia by a continuous suture (polypropylene, e.g., Prolene 2–0), starting at the pubic tubercle (**caution:** vascular injuries, "corona mortis": vascular anastomosis between the epigastric artery and obturator artery).
- Tighten the internal inguinal ring to admit no more than the little finger (Hegar size 11) ensuring normal perfusion of the cord.
- Continuous suture (polypropylene, e.g., Prolene 2–0) of the muscles (transversus abdominis and internal oblique) to the inguinal ligament in two rows, beginning at the internal inguinal ring (usually only one row of sutures is possible because of the high tension).
- Continuous suture of the external oblique aponeurosis, skin closure

7

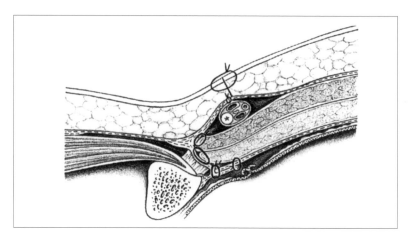

Fig. 7.4   Shouldice herniotomy (from Schumpelick 2000, p. 424).

Lichtenstein Herniotomy

- **Principle:** Tension-free reinforcement of the posterior wall and reconstruction of the internal inguinal ring by insertion of a mesh (**Fig. 7.5**)

Operative Technique

- Perform a groin incision, splitting the external oblique aponeurosis in the direction of its fibers.
- Protect the ilioinguinal nerve.
- Expose and retract the spermatic cord above the pubic tubercle.
- Identify the hernial sac as a direct or indirect hernia.
- **Lateral hernias:** Excise the hernial sac in the usual way.
- **Medial hernias:** Reduce the hernial sac without opening it, tighten the transversalis fascia by a continuous suture to correct the hernia.
- Insert a light, partially absorbable mesh (ca. 10 × 12 cm), which is cut to size (**caution:** if mesh is too small there is an increased risk of recurrence, mesh shrinkage). Important: ensure a tension-free mesh insertion.
- Suture fixation of the mesh (polypropylene, e.g., Prolene 2–0), initially with an interrupted suture on the pubic tubercle, followed by continuous suture (polypropylene, e.g., Prolene 2–0) to the inguinal ligament, starting at the pubic tubercle and continuing ca. 2 cm beyond the internal inguinal ring.
- Insertion of the spermatic cord into the previously made opening in the mesh.
- Fixation of the mesh (polypropylene, e.g., Prolene 2–0) to the internal oblique by loose interrupted sutures (**caution:** injury of the iliohypogastric nerve).
- Closure of the opening in the mesh by an interrupted suture between the superior lip of the mesh and the inguinal ligament, and reconstruction of the internal inguinal ring (**caution:** do not tighten the internal inguinal ring too much, should admit the little finger: Hegar size 11).
- Continuous suture of the external oblique aponeurosis, skin closure.

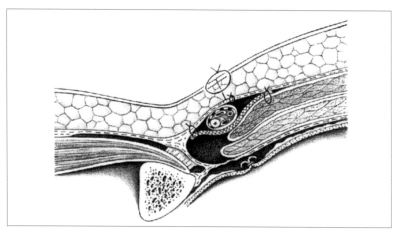

Fig. 7.5 Lichtenstein herniotomy (from Schumpelick 2000, p. 424).

Transabdominal Preperitoneal Hernia Repair—TAPP

- **Principle:** Tension-free reinforcement of the posterior wall by insertion of a preperitoneal mesh (**Fig. 7.6**)

Operative Technique

- Create the pneumoperitoneum.
- Make a curved incision of the peritoneum above the hernial orifice, from the anterior superior iliac spine to the medial umbilical fold.
- Dissect the peritoneum off the transversalis fascia, protecting the epigastric vessels and ductus deferens until the psoas muscle appears posteriorly.
- Expose the inguinal ligament and the pectineal ligament.
- Dissect the hernial sac of an indirect hernia from the inguinal canal, remove any preperitoneal lipoma present with direct hernias.
- Insert and position a light, partially absorbable mesh (size 10 × 15 cm), with suture or clip fixation of the mesh to the pectineal ligament, so that all three hernial orifices are covered (**caution:** never use sutures or clips in the triangle of doom or pain).
- Peritoneal closure by clips or suture.

- Never use sutures or clips in the triangle of doom or pain

7

- **Advantages:**
  - ► Laparoscopic assessment of the entire intraperitoneal space is possible, so incidental findings (adhesions, cysts) can be removed and biopsies can be taken
  - ► Good anatomical view during dissection
  - ► Nerve injuries are less frequent, so postoperative pain syndromes occur less often
  - ► Bilateral treatment possible
- **Disadvantages:**
  - ► Risk of major complications
  - ► Higher costs
  - ► More time-consuming

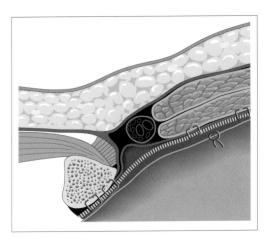

Fig. 7.6 Transabdominal hernia repair

Total Extraperitoneal Hernia Repair—TEP

- **Principle:** Tension-free reinforcement of the posterior wall by insertion of a preperitoneal mesh

Operative Technique

- Subumbilical insufflation of CO_2 into the preperitoneal space, if necessary creating the space using a transparent balloon (not absolutely necessary)
- Exposure of the epigastric vessels, ductus deferens, and hernial sac
- Hernial sac pushed back into the abdominal cavity
- Insertion of a light, partially absorbable mesh into the same position as in TAPP with minimal or no fixation

- **Advantages:**
  - ➤ Mesh implant is only inserted; there are no complications due to clip fixation.
  - ➤ There are no intraperitoneal complications, which are possible with the transperitoneal access.
- **Disadvantages:**
  - ➤ Poorer anatomical overview
  - ➤ Possible dislocation of the mesh, which is not fixed by clips, with risk of recurrence
  - ➤ Temporary subcutaneous emphysema (scrotum), usually can be expressed during surgery
  - ➤ More frequent postoperative seroma or hematoma
  - ➤ Higher costs
  - ➤ More time-consuming

Other Procedures

- Marcy/Ogilvie tightening of the internal inguinal ring
- Zimmermann tightening of the internal inguinal ring using the external oblique aponeurosis also

- Extensive abdominal wall reinforcement with bilateral cover of all hernial orifices by implanting a preperitoneal mesh through a midline lower abdominal laparotomy (Stoppa method)

Herniotomy in Infants and Children

- Always an indirect hernia through a patent processus vaginalis

---

Operative Technique

- Mobilization, suture ligature, and excision of the hernial sac at the internal inguinal ring. When the hernial sac extends beyond the external inguinal ring, only the part within the inguinal canal is excised.
- Tighten the inguinal canal without displacing the spermatic cord.
  - ► **Czerny:** tightening of the external oblique aponeurosis at the external inguinal ring without opening the external oblique aponeurosis
  - ► **Grob:** suture of the inferior border of the internal oblique to the inguinal ligament over the spermatic cord after opening the external oblique aponeurosis

---

■ Complications

Perioperative Complications

- Seroma/hematoma
- Infection
- Injury of the epigastric vessels or femoral vessels
- Femoral vein thrombosis, pulmonary embolism
- Injury of bowel or bladder (especially with sliding hernias)
- Spermatic cord injury
- Testicular atrophy
- Pain syndromes (due to nerve injury, among other things)
- Mesh intolerance
- Major complications with TAPP (intra-abdominal bleeding, bowel injury, adhesions, fistulas)

Late Complications

- Recurrence
- Infertility
- Chronic pain

Chronic Pain
- **Definition:** persisting pain 2–3 months after operation when healing process and scarring are complete
- **Incidence:** up to 30% (large number unreported)
- **Risk factors:**
  - ► Intraoperative nerve injury
  - ► Heavy mesh
  - ► Surgery for recurrence
  - ► High preoperative pain sensitivity
  - ► Young men
  - ► Genetic predisposition

- Incidence up to 30% (large number unreported)
- Neuropathic in 50% of cases

7

- **Classification:**
  - ► Neuropathic pain (50% of cases):
    - – Caused by nerve injury, compression, or traction (constricting sutures or clips, scars/meshes, neuromas)
    - – Mechanism: complex peripheral and central nerve dysregulation ("Sudeck disease of the groin")
    - – Causalgia-type pain, associated with hypo- or hyperesthesia
  - ► Non-neuropathic pain (25% of cases):
    - – Very heterogeneous causes, for example, dislocated mesh, periostitis due to deep sutures to the pubic tubercle
    - – Treatment: mesh removal, suture removal
  - ► Painful spermatic cord (25% of cases):
    - – Diffuse painfulness
    - – Sometimes with erectile and ejaculatory disorders
    - – Greater incidence in young men
    - – Genesis and treatment unclear
- **Treatment of neuropathic pain (step-by-step plan):**
  - ► Nonsteroidal anti-inflammatory drugs
  - ► Injection of local anesthetics
  - ► Surgical nerve removal ("triple neurectomy") as a last resort:
    - – Always resect all three inguinal nerves (reason: anastomoses between the nerves).
    - – Resect as long a segment as possible.
    - – Bury the proximal nerve end in muscle.
    - – No electric coagulation of the nerve ends
- **Prevention:**
  - ► No dissection of nerves (visual sparing), leave the cremaster fibers
  - ► Resection of long segment of nerve after injury
  - ► Use of light mesh
  - ► Use of a local anesthetic
  - ► No clips in the triangles of doom and pain
  - ► Lower risk of nerve injury with endoscopic procedures

Prognosis

- Lower recurrence rates with mesh methods compared with suture methods

- It is difficult to draw conclusions about recurrence rates after hernia operations in view of the many different individual studies.
- Meta-analysis of the EU Hernia Trialists Collaboration (2000) which evaluated 42 prospective randomized studies revealed significant advantage for mesh procedures compared with suture methods (2% versus 5%).
- With suture methods, a high cumulative risk of recurrence must also be expected.
- There is no significant difference with regard to recurrence when endoscopic and open mesh methods are compared (2.2% versus 1.7%).

■ Femoral Hernias

Definition

- Passage of a peritoneal hernial sac through the narrow femoral ring medial to the femoral vein

Symptoms

- Usually a painful bulge below the inguinal ligament (incarceration frequent)

Diagnostic Approach

- See inguinal hernias.

Treatment Approach

■ Indication

- Because of the narrow hernial orifice, incarceration occurs frequently, which is an emergency and an **absolute indication** for surgery.
- 50% of men and 10% of women with a femoral hernia have an inguinal hernia at the same time, so revision of the inguinal canal is always indicated in men.
- In elderly women, a femoral hernia often becomes apparent due to incarceration: during surgery of an inguinal hernia, a femoral hernia should therefore always be ruled out by opening the transversalis fascia.

- Emergency and an absolute indication for surgery because of the narrow hernial orifice and frequency of incarceration
- Men: always revision of the inguinal canal
- Elderly women: at inguinal hernia surgery always rule out a femoral hernia

■ Surgical Treatment

7

Operative Technique

- Access: low groin skin incision parallel to the inguinal ligament so that crural and inguinal dissection is possible
- Crural exposure of the hernial sac after splitting the fascia lata, retracting the femoral vein laterally
- Dissection of the hernial sac on all sides until the parietal peritoneum is visible
- Open the hernial sac, reduce the contents, place a transfixion ligature close to the base and excise the sac
- In the case of incarceration, extend the hernial orifice if necessary by nicking the lacunar or inguinal ligament medially. After opening the hernial sac, resect a segment of small bowel if necessary (**caution:** never carry out blind reduction).

- Never carry out blind reduction.

Shouldice Herniotomy

Operative Technique

- Exposure of the femoral ring after opening the transversalis fascia over the inguinal access
- Continuous suture of the pectineal ligament to the inguinal ligament (**caution:** constriction of the femoral vein)
- After exposing the hernial orifice from the crural aspect (through the same skin incision), continuous suture of the inguinal ligament to the pectineal fascia
- Manage the inguinal canal in the typical Shouldice manner (p. 90, **Fig. 7.4**).

Lotheissen/McVay Herniotomy (Fig. 7.7)

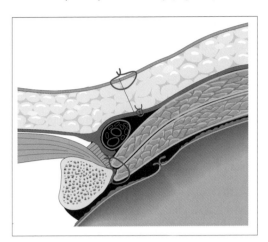

Fig. 7.7 Lotheissen/McVay herniotomy

Operative Technique

- Exposure of the femoral ring after opening the transversalis fascia over the inguinal access
- Closure by means of interrupted sutures, attaching the internal oblique, transverse abdominal muscle, and cranial lip of the transversalis fascia to the pectineal fascia and the inferior lip of the transversalis fascia
- The last lateral suture passes through the adventitia of the femoral vein (**caution:** thrombosis due to constriction, bleeding).

Other Methods

- Closure of the hernial gap from the inguinal aspect by interrupted sutures (polypropylene, e.g., Prolene 0) between the inguinal ligament and pectineal ligament/ileopubic tract (Moschkowitz operation)

■ Incisional Hernias

Anatomy of the Abdominal Wall

- The muscles and tendons of the abdominal wall form an extraordinarily adaptable bracing system, which extends between the ribs, xiphoid, lumbar vertebrae, and pelvis.
- The abdominal wall opposes the back muscles, acts during respiration and trunk movements, and adapts flexibly to the level of filling of the abdominal organs.

Definition

- Acquired fascial defect with a peritoneal hernial sac

- Acquired fascial defect, usually due to secondary dehiscence of the fascia
- Typical structure with a peritoneal hernial sac
- This situation must be distinguished from a burst abdomen, which is an early postoperative wound rupture without a peritoneal covering.

Epidemiology

- Incidence is 2%–11%, up to 15% according to more recent studies.
- In the United States 2.7 million laparotomies per year, in Germany 700 000 laparotomies per year: in total 100 000 incisional hernias in Germany and 400 000 incisional hernias in the United States.
- The greatest risk of developing an incisional hernia is after **median laparotomy** (10%–15%).
- Risk factors contributing to the development of incisional hernias are listed in **Table 7.3.**

- Greatest risk after midline laparotomy (10%–15%)

Pathogenesis

- The integrity of the complex system of the abdominal wall is disturbed by operations on the abdomen, which can result in **loss of stability**.
- Another cause is a **disorder of collagen metabolism,** resulting in diminished scar stability; in this connection, disorders of collagen biosynthesis, diminished collagen stability and altered fibroblast activity have been demonstrated.
- Incisional hernias initially occur more frequently postoperatively, which can be explained by surgical errors.
- There is then a subsequent steady increase in the rate of recurrence; these late recurrences are not a result of surgical technique but are a biological phenomenon ("biological recurrence"), which can be influenced very little by the surgeon and which are due to disorders of collagen metabolism.
- Late biological recurrences occur with both suture and mesh repair, but manifest later after mesh repair.

- Early postoperative occurrence due to surgical errors
- Late occurrence due to disorders of collagen metabolism: "biological recurrence"

Symptoms

- Complaints range from complete absence of symptoms to complete incapacity for work because of pain or limitation of physical capacity.
- As the fascial defect increases in size there is displacement forward of intestinal organs from the abdominal cavity into the hernial sac (loss of "right of residence").

- Symptoms are very varied, often asymptomatic.
- With very large hernias the hernial contents lose their "right of residence."

7

Table 7.3   **Risk factors for the development of incisional hernias**

Demographic	Patient factors	Intraoperative	Postoperative
• Age (> 45 years) • Male sex	• Obesity (BMI > 25) • Ascites • Malnutrition • COPD • Consuming diseases • Diabetes mellitus • Renal failure • Collagen metabolism disorders • Anemia • Smoking • Chemotherapy • Steroids	• Emergency operation • Recurrence procedure • Surgeon's experience • Suture technique • Suture material	• Wound infection

BMI: body mass index, COPD: chronic obstructive pulmonary disease.

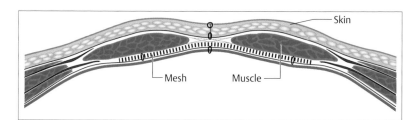

Fig. 7.9   Sublay technique

- **Disadvantage:**
  - ► Time-consuming dissection

Onlay Technique (Fig. 7.10)

Operative Technique

- Implantation on the muscle fascia (subcutaneous)
- Adequate mesh overlap on all sides (at least 5 cm)

- **Advantages:**
  - ► Less invasive
  - ► Shorter operation time
- **Disadvantages:**
  - ► Absence of mesh abutment
  - ► Major tissue trauma (risk of infection, seromas more frequent)
  - ► Adequate overlapping of bony structures not possible

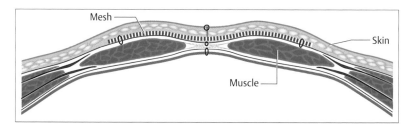

Fig. 7.10   Onlay technique

Intraperitoneal Technique—IPOM (Fig. 7.11)

Operative Technique

- Access to the abdominal cavity through minilaparotomy
- Division of adhesions
- Measurement of the hernial opening
- Mesh implantation (correct alignment, overlap of at least 5 cm on all sides, fixation with sutures or staples after pressure reduction)
- Licensed composite meshes: ePTFE, PP/PE (see **Table 7.4**) with collagen coating (on intestinal side)

- **Advantages:**
  - ► Low trauma
  - ► Low infection risk
  - ► Mesh can also be placed behind bone (sternum, symphysis)

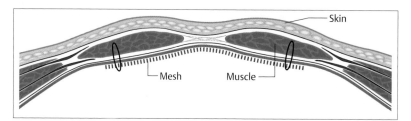

Fig. 7.11 Intraperitoneal technique (IPOM)

- **Disadvantages:**
  - ➤ Risk of major complications (e.g., bowel injury, adhesions, fistulas)
  - ➤ Cannot be used if there are extensive intra-abdominal adhesions
  - ➤ Expensive

Bridging
- If the fascial defect cannot be closed on account of its size and if there is adequate soft-tissue cover by skin and subcutaneous fat, the defect can be bridged by a mesh; the mesh then represents a substitute for the abdominal wall (**Fig. 7.12**).

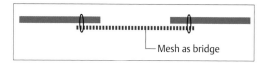

Fig. 7.12 Bridging

7

Operative Technique

- **Retromuscular** mesh implantation (equivalent to the sublay technique)
  - ➤ Peritoneal mesh covering essential
  - ➤ Difficult dissection lateral to the linea semilunaris with risk of injuring the neurovascular bundles that radiate inward from the lateral aspect
- **Intraperitoneal** mesh implantation
  - ➤ Use of composite meshes
  - ➤ Suitable for large defects as simple fixation is possible even lateral to the linea semilunaris

---

Other Methods

Double-Door Technique

Operative Technique

- Closure of peritoneum and inner borders of the rectus sheath is effected with a continuous suture.
- For reinforcement, the two anterior layers of the rectus sheath are incised laterally throughout their length and dissected off the muscle in a medial direction.
- The two layers of fascia obtained thus are joined in the midline by interrupted sutures.
- If necessary the muscle defect can be covered with a Lyodura flap.

Ramirez Component Separation (Fig. 7.13)

- Closure of fascial defects with a diameter of up to 20 cm in the midline by separation of the muscle components of the abdominal wall
- Recurrence rate is ca. 10%
- Technically demanding method

Operative Technique

- The external oblique aponeurosis bilaterally is split lateral to the linea semilunaris in a longitudinal direction so that the external and internal oblique can be separated.
- The rectus sheath bilaterally is split in a longitudinal direction starting from the midline.
- By medializing the two posterior layers of the rectus sheath, closure in the midline can be achieved.

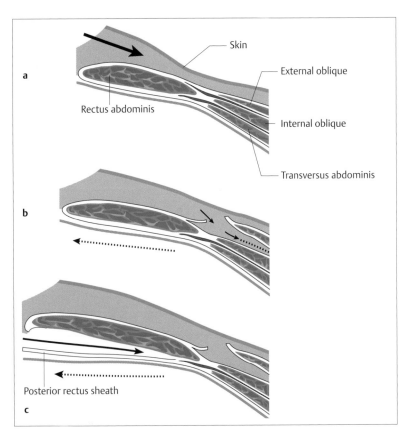

Fig. 7.13 a–c   Ramirez component separation
a Subcutaneous dissection as far as the lateral edge of the rectus abdominis.
b Incision of the external oblique fascia over its entire length.
c Incision of the rectus sheath and elevation of the muscle from the posterior layer over its entire length.

Loewe and Rehn Skin Graft

Operative Technique

- The skin flap is obtained from the excess skin of the hernial sac.
- It is then cleaned with alcohol and all of the subcutaneous tissue is removed.
- The flap is perforated in numerous places.
- After peritoneal closure and dissection of the free fascial margin, the skin flap is fixed to the fascia with strong interrupted sutures, with the epidermis side facing toward the peritoneum.
- An overlap of at least 2–3 cm should be ensured.
- The implant should finally be stretched like a drum.

Prognosis

- Direct comparison of the different methods by randomization is not permissible because of the heterogeneous characteristics of incisional hernias.
- The majority of study data has been obtained retrospectively and is difficult to compare.
- The longer patients are followed up, the greater the recurrence rate will be, which can be explained by biological late recurrences.
- Very high recurrence rates were apparent in different studies with suture methods (25%–46%), so this method is no longer important in the management of incisional hernias.
- Suture repair may be considered only in the case of very small defects such as trocar hernias.
- Mayo–Dick fascial duplication is obsolete nowadays; even higher recurrence rates are apparent with this method in studies than with the other suture methods.
- Mesh methods are the standard procedure today for managing incisional hernias.
- The recurrence rate after mesh repair is significantly lower than after suture repair; however, the complication rate is significantly higher after mesh implantation.
- The lowest recurrence rates were seen with sublay and IPOM techniques (1%–7%), while the onlay method has recurrence rates between 4% and 14%.

- Mesh method is standard, with sublay and IPOM techniques being the best.
- Very high recurrence rates with suture methods, permissible only for small defects (e.g., trocar hernia)
- Biological late recurrences cannot be avoided with all methods.

■ Umbilical Hernia

- The hernial orifice is the umbilical ring.
- Incidence is ca. 5%.
- If postnatal scarring does not occur, an umbilical hernia develops.
- Surgery is not usually indicated before the age of 2 years, as there is a very great tendency to spontaneous regression and the risk of incarceration is minimal in childhood.
- Obesity and ascites are predisposing factors.

- High tendency to spontaneous regression in infants, minimal risk of incarceration

Treatment Approach

Operative Technique

- Semicircular inferior periumbilical incision (Spizzi) in the case of small defects or semicircular lateral periumbilical incision (Drachter)
- Sharp dissection of the umbilicus (**caution:** skin injury, if necessary leaving the roof of the hernial sac on the umbilicus)
- After dealing with the hernial sac, transverse closure of the hernial defect with continuous or interrupted sutures
- Mesh implantation using the sublay technique for hernial defects > 3 cm
- Refixation of the umbilicus to the fascia

- With extremely large hernias, omentectomy may be necessary (inform the patient!).

■ Epigastric Hernia

- Often an incarcerated pre-peritoneal lipoma

- Supraumbilical in the linea alba with an incidence of ca. 5%
- Often appears as a small painful irreducible bulge
- Often consists of an incarcerated preperitoneal lipoma

Treatment Approach

Operative Technique

- Transverse skin incision
- After dealing with the hernial sac, transverse closure of the hernial defect with continuous or interrupted sutures
- Mesh implantation using the sublay technique for hernial defects > 3 cm

■ Internal Hernias

- Often an incidental finding

- Often an incidental finding at laparotomy or becomes apparent due to symptoms of intestinal obstruction

Treatment Approach

- Reduction of incarcerated intestine or visceral segments, resection if necessary
- Closure of the hernial orifice with careful preservation of the often adjacent mesenteric vessels to avoid subsequently impaired perfusion

Further Reading

Amato B, Moja L, Panico S, et al. Shouldice technique versus other open techniques for inguinal hernia repair. Cochrane Database Syst Rev 2009 Oct 7; (4): CD001543. Review

Bittner R, Sauerland S, Schmedt CG. Comparison of endoscopic techniques vs Shouldice and other open nonmesh techniques for inguinal hernia repair: a meta-analysis of randomized controlled trials. Surgical Endoscopy 2005; 19: 605–615

Conze J, Klinge U, Schumpelick V. Narbenhernien. Chirurg 2005; 76: 897–910

Loos MJA, Roumen RMH, Scheltinga MRM. Classifying Postherniorrhaphy Pain Syndromes Following Elective Inguinal Hernia Repair. World J Surg 2007; 31: 1760–1765

Sauerland S, Walgenbach M, Habermalz B, Seiler CM, Miserez M. Laparoscopic versus open surgical techniques for ventral or incisional hernia repair. Cochrane Database Syst Rev 2011 Mar 16; (3): CD007781. Review

Schumpelick V, Klinge U, Rosch R, Junge K. Light weight meshes in incisional hernia repair. J Min Access Surg 2006; 2: 117–123

7

8 Esophagus

M. Voelz

■ Anatomy

- Cervical part, thoracic part, abdominal part

- Elastic tube consisting of smooth and striated muscle between the pharynx and stomach
- Length 23–38 cm between the cricoid cartilage (or 6th cervical vertebra) and 12th thoracic vertebra; ca. 40 cm from the incisor teeth to the gastric inlet
- Cervical part, thoracic part, and abdominal part
- The **arterial supply** in the cervical part is from branches of the inferior thyroid artery, less often from the subclavian artery, common carotid artery,

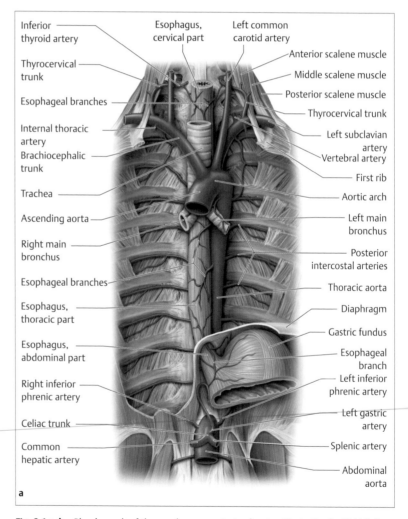

Inferior thyroid artery
Esophagus, cervical part
Left common carotid artery
Thyrocervical trunk
Anterior scalene muscle
Middle scalene muscle
Esophageal branches
Posterior scalene muscle
Thyrocervical trunk
Internal thoracic artery
Left subclavian artery
Brachiocephalic trunk
Vertebral artery
First rib
Trachea
Aortic arch
Ascending aorta
Left main bronchus
Right main bronchus
Posterior intercostal arteries
Esophageal branches
Thoracic aorta
Esophagus, thoracic part
Diaphragm
Esophagus, abdominal part
Gastric fundus
Esophageal branch
Left inferior phrenic artery
Right inferior phrenic artery
Left gastric artery
Celiac trunk
Splenic artery
Common hepatic artery
Abdominal aorta

a

Fig. 8.1 a, b Blood vessels of the esophagus: **a** arteries, **b** veins. Illustration by M. Voll; from Schünke et al. 2006, see p. 413

or thyrocervical trunk (**Fig. 8.1a**). The thoracic part is supplied by direct esophageal branches from the aorta, branches of the bronchial arteries, and rarely by branches of the intercostal arteries on the right. The abdominal part of the esophagus is supplied by branches of the left gastric artery and rarely by direct branches from the celiac trunk.

- **Venous drainage** is from the submucosal plexus into a venous network on the surface of the esophagus (**Fig. 8.1b**). The cervical part drains into the thyroid veins, the thoracic part into the azygos and hemiazygos veins, and the abdominal part into the left gastric vein and the splenic vein.
- **Lymphatic drainage** is to paratracheal lymph nodes and along the internal jugular vein in the cervical part, to paratracheal and parabronchial lymph nodes in the thoracic part, and to paragastric and celiac lymph nodes in the abdominal part.
- The esophagus has no mesentery and no hilum.

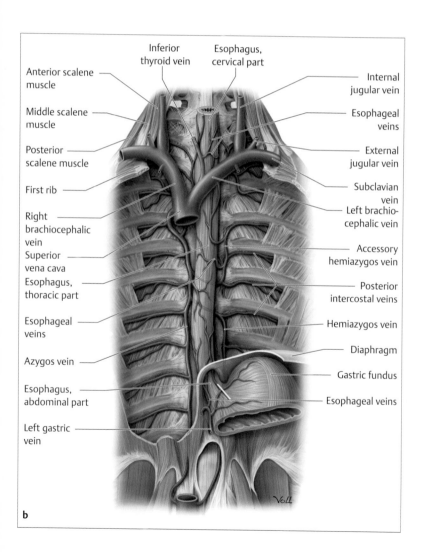

b

8

■ Histology

- Mucosa: squamous epithelium, no serosa, no mesentery

- **Mucosa** consisting of stratified squamous epithelium, which can be distinguished at the cardia from the cylindrical epithelium of the stomach by a wavy demarcation line.
- Beneath it is the **submucosa,** a loose mobile layer containing blood and lymph vessels, nerves, and glands in a connective-tissue matrix.
- **Muscularis:** Inner circular muscle and outer longitudinal muscle layer, upper part consisting of striated muscle, followed distally by skeletal and smooth muscle; after that, the entire muscularis propria consists of smooth muscle.
- The outer connective tissue layer (**adventitia**) penetrates between the muscle layers and carries smaller vessels and nerves. The serosa is absent in the cervical and thoracic parts.

■ Physiology

- Lower esophageal sphincter prevents reflux.

- **Swallowing:** Complex coordinated contractions of the muscles of the mouth and larynx, moving food from the mouth to the esophagus. Under the control of the swallowing center (medulla oblongata); cranial nerves V, IX, X, and XII are involved in this process. Important: correctly timed relaxation of the upper esophageal sphincter.
- Further transport of the food bolus through coordinated propulsive contractions of the esophageal muscle.
- **Lower esophageal sphincter:** The distal 3–4 cm segment of the esophageal smooth muscle is tonically contracted at rest, relaxes when food passes through it, and is subject to various reflex and pharmacological influences (e.g., fat and protein elements of the swallowed food, gastrointestinal hormones, psychotropic drugs). Important for preventing gastroesophageal reflux.

■ Functional Disorders

- Functional disorders of the esophagus are of **neuromuscular** origin.
- They are manifested as alterations from normal peristalsis and function of the lower esophageal sphincter.

Achalasia

- Absence of relaxation of the lower esophageal sphincter

- Rare motor disorder of the esophageal smooth muscle
- Normal relaxation of the lower esophageal sphincter is markedly diminished or completely absent (functional obstruction).
- Instead of normal propulsive motility of the esophagus with wavelike, constantly progressing contractions, manometry shows intermittent simultaneous contractions of small amplitude.
- Primary form of unknown etiology or secondary forms (e.g., in Chagas disease, lymphoma, after radiation, carcinoma)
- Marked reduction in neurons of the myenteric plexus on histology

Symptoms

- Dysphagia
- Retrosternal pain and burning
- Regurgitation of saliva and food remnants
- Esophagitis as a result of retained food with bacterial or fungal colonization of the mucosa; possibly mucosal erosions

• Regurgitation of food, esophagitis, dysphagia

Diagnostic Approach

- **Chest radiograph:** tubular space-occupying lesion in the mediastinum with visible fluid level
- **Barium swallow:** dilatation of proximal esophageal lumen with fluid level, abnormal peristalsis and conical narrowing of the distal esophagus
- **Manometry:** pathological contraction pattern and incomplete or absent relaxation of the lower esophageal sphincter
- **Esophagoscopy:** to rule out carcinoma of the cardia

• Dilatation of the esophagus with production of fluid level in the barium swallow

Treatment Approach

- Calcium antagonists (e.g., sublingual nifedipine before meals)
- Targeted local injection of botulinus toxin
- The treatment of choice is **pneumatic dilatation.**
- Procedure: splinting by a guide wire, introduce balloon dilator and inflate to 200–300 mmHg. Gastrografin swallow to rule out perforation.
- If dilatation is unsuccessful, anterior **Gottstein–Heller myotomy** is performed, but rarely.

• Dilatation and calcium antagonists
• Rarely necessary: surgical myotomy

Anterior Myotomy

Operative Technique

- Laparoscopic approach as for fundoplication or upper median laparotomy
- Retract the esophagus and extend the esophageal hiatus
- Mobilization of the esophagus
- Myotomy, beginning over the stenosis to 2 cm below the cardia
- Loose fundoplication to cover and prevent reflux

8

Other Functional Disorders

Idiopathic Diffuse Esophageal Spasm
- Spastic hyperactivity of the muscle without a histological correlate ("nutcracker esophagus")
- **Treatment** is entirely conservative (butyl scopolamine bromide, e.g., Buscopan, calcium antagonists, nitrates)

■ Esophageal Diverticulum

Definition

- Pulsion diverticulum due to weak points in the wall (Zenker diverticulum)
- Traction diverticulum due to traction from without (inflammatory or embryonic)

- **Pulsion diverticulum** occurs at weak points of the esophageal wall as a result of raised intraluminal pressure aboral to the diverticulum, typically in the vicinity of the upper and lower esophageal sphincters (e.g., in functional disorders).
- **Cervical pulsion diverticulum (Zenker diverticulum)** is the most frequent.
- **Traction diverticulum** is due to traction from without on all layers of the wall, often due to tuberculous lymphadenitis; in addition it can result from embryonic malformation during the separation of esophagus and trachea; typically in peribronchial location.

Symptoms

- Cervical diverticula can compress the esophagus from without and produce a **sensation of a lump** in the throat. Apart from **oral fetor,** retained undigested food in the diverticulum can be **regurgitated**.
- Traction diverticula and epiphrenic diverticula usually become symptomatic only when the inflammatory changes develop in the wall of the diverticulum as a result of retained food, which may result in **perforation**.
- If a **fistula** develops between the diverticulum and the trachea, a chronic **cough** and **aspiration pneumonia** occur.

Diagnostic Approach

- **Barium swallow:** evidence of diverticulum size, retention of contrast
- **Endoscopy:** to assess the indication for endoscopic therapy

Cervical Pulsion Diverticulum (Zenker Diverticulum)

Definition

- Area of reduced muscle (Killian triangle) at the junction of the esophagus and upper pharynx
- Due to increases in pressure in the hypopharynx during swallowing; the mucosa and submucosa of the esophagus bulge out, usually above the cricopharyngeus muscle

Treatment Approach

- Endoscopic or surgical removal with cricomyotomy

- The indication for elimination is established with the diagnosis.
- If possible, removal is performed endoscopically.
- If endoscopic treatment is not possible, treatment is surgical.

Operative Technique

- Head extended and turned to the right
- Incision along the anterior border of the sternocleidomastoid muscle
- The thyroid lobe is pushed away and the esophagus exposed
- The diverticulum is dissected down to its base and clamped

- Extramucosal **cricomyotomy** of the transverse part of the cricopharyngeus distally over a distance of 3–4 cm
- Removal of the diverticulum and closure of its base with interrupted sutures or staples

■ **Complications**

- Recurrent nerve paresis
- Salivary fistula

Epiphrenic Pulsion Diverticulum

Definition

- Located in the distal esophagus, no anatomical weak point
- Probably a functional disorder of the lower esophageal sphincter

Treatment Approach

- **Surgery indicated** only for large diverticula with pain or bleeding

Operative Technique

- Access through a left-sided thoracotomy
- Removal of the diverticulum, splinting the esophagus with a large gastric tube
- Closure of the mucosal defect, cardiomyotomy on anterior wall of esophagus
- Subsequent fundoplication

- Surgical treatment in the event of symptoms, through a left-sided thoracotomy

Traction Diverticulum

Treatment Approach

- **Surgery indicated** only if symptomatic or related to the bronchial system or mediastinum

Operative Technique

- Access through a right-sided thoracotomy
- Exposure of the diverticulum, division of any fibrous strand or fistula to the trachea or bronchial system
- Removal of the diverticulum
- Closure of the defect of the esophageal wall with a gastric tube in place

- Surgical treatment in the event of symptoms, through a right-sided thoracotomy

8

■ Gastroesophageal Reflux Disease (GERD)

Definition

- Collective term (abbreviated GERD) for different conditions that arise from **reflux of gastric** contents into the esophagus
- Most frequent condition: reflux esophagitis, different degrees of severity, end stage **Barrett esophagus**

Manifestations of GERD:
- Purely symptomatic
- Volume reflux
- Bronchitis
- Reflux esophagitis
- Barrett esophagus

- **Chronic bronchitis** due to nocturnal volume reflux without esophagitis
- Purely symptomatic with retrosternal burning, acid regurgitation, and epigastric pain without esophagitis

Classification (Table 8.1)

Table 8.1   Endoscopic classification of esophagitis (after Savary and Miller)

Grade	Description
I	Nonconfluent erosions
II	Confluent epithelial defects
III	Circular loss of epithelium due to erosions and ulcers
IV	Peptic stricture or cicatricial stenosis and columnar epithelial metaplasia (Barrett esophagus)

- Further histological differentiation of metaplastic Barrett esophagus includes absence of dysplasia, presence of dysplasia, and presence of carcinoma (contact a pathology reference center).
- Barrett esophagus is regarded as **precancerous.** How often carcinoma develops is controversial (below 2% up to 10%).

Diagnostic Approach

- Endoscopic assessment and histology are crucial for further therapy.

- **History:** Besides the typical symptoms, consider bronchial symptoms and sleep habits (elevation at night).
- **Endoscopic** assessment of esophagitis/Barrett lesions, if necessary using special light sources and staining methods
- 24-hour esophageal **pH measurement**
- Esophageal **manometry**
- **Biopsy confirmation** (multiple biopsies, pathology reference center), rule out esophageal carcinoma
- Regular **endoscopic follow-up** at least every 1–2 years

Treatment Approach

The treatment approach in reflux disease is **controversial,** both with regard to the indication for individual procedures and with regard to which procedures or conservative therapies should be used. Possible treatments include:
- Long-term drug therapy
- Endoscopic removal of mucosa
- Various methods for ablation of Barrett mucosa (argon beam, photodynamic therapy, endoscopic mucosectomy)
- Reflux surgery (fundoplication)
- Resection of the distal esophagus and cardia

Superficial epithelial defects (**erosions**) can heal fully. Deeper **ulcers** heal with scarring and can lead to a rigid wall. Shrinkage due to scarring can lead to shortening of the longitudinal axis (secondary **brachyesophagus**) and peptic stenosis. Destroyed **squamous epithelium** of the esophagus can be replaced by columnar epithelium of a specialized and intestinal type (Barrett esophagus).

8

■ Indication

Indications for Surgery
- Ulcerative esophagitis, strictures, Barrett esophagus
- Failure or intolerance of drug therapy
- Patient's wish as an alternative to long-term drug therapy
- Volume reflux with chronic bronchitis
- Volume reflux with treatment-resistant regurgitation of food
- An interdisciplinary decision with gastroenterologists should be made.

• Interdisciplinary indication for surgery

■ Conservative Treatment

- Weight reduction
- Sleep with upper body elevated
- Proton pump inhibitors, in ca. 80% freedom from symptoms, healing of the reflux esophagitis almost without exception; often requires lifelong treatment

• Weight reduction, sleeping with upper body elevated, proton pump inhibitors

■ Surgical Treatment

- Laparoscopic Nissen–Rosetti **fundoplication**
- Alternatively, hemifundoplication
- **Hiatoplasty:** posterior narrowing of the esophageal hiatus that has been stretched by the sliding hernia; additionally counteracts reflux by increasing the angle at which the esophagus opens into the stomach
- Additional **fundophrenicopexy** indicated only for upside-down stomach
- With very large sliding hiatal hernias or paraesophageal herniation, use of a **plastic mesh** to close the hernia may be necessary.
- Numerous other procedures are not established for use outside of clinical studies. These include, for instance, heating by radiofrequency therapy, intraluminal mucosal plication, and injection of plastic polymers.

• Standard treatment: laparoscopic fundoplication and hiatoplasty

Laparoscopic Fundoplication

8

Operative Technique

- Position the patient with legs on stirrups and with the buttocks supported.
- Create a pneumoperitoneum and carry out diagnostic laparoscopy (**Fig. 8.2**).
- Then place the patient in semi-seated position with feet lowered and turned slightly to the right side. The surgeon stands between the patient's legs.
- The left lobe of the liver is retracted with a triangle over the trocar from the right costal arch (T5).
- Exposure of the gastroesophageal junction is by incision of the lesser omentum proximal to the accessory left hepatic artery, which is often present.
- Incision of the peritoneal fold over the esophagus
- Dissection of the fundus along the greater curvature of the stomach from adhesions to the spleen (**caution:** short gastric arteries) and in a retroperitoneal direction. Dissection with ultrasonic scissors has proven useful.
- Dissect the esophagus free at the junction with the gastric fundus, protecting the vagal trunks.
- If appropriate, perform dissection of a hiatal hernia in the lower mediastinum.
- Tighten the hiatus, usually by two or three sutures posteriorly using nonabsorbable suture material (hiatus repair; **Fig. 8.3**).
- If appropriate, additional implantation of a plastic mesh after reduction of a large hiatal hernia, paraesophageal hernia or upside-down stomach

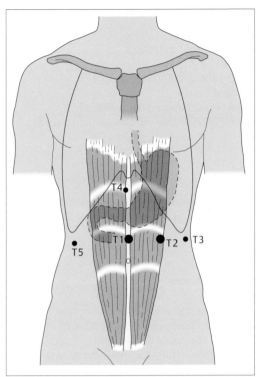

Fig. 8.2 Access routes for laparoscopic fundoplication.
T1: optic trocar
T2: working trocar, surgeon
T3: working trocar, assistant
T4: working trocar, surgeon
T5: working trocar, assistant, for holding the left lobe of the liver (triangle)

- Create a loose fundal cuff around the distal esophagus, drawing the mobilized fundus behind the esophagus.
- Introduction of a large gastric tube to prevent narrowing of the lumen by the fundoplication (this is done only at this time as it would interfere with dissection beforehand)
- Fixation of the cuff by picking up the esophagus with the first suture to prevent the stomach from sliding proximally. Two further sutures are used to form a loose cuff (floppy Nissen; **Fig. 8.4**); all sutures are nonabsorbable.
- Remove the gastric tube and check that the cuff is loose.
- Check for hemostasis, particularly on the spleen and liver.

■ Postoperative Management

- Removal of the gastric tube while still in the operating room
- Light diet the following day, ensuring that it is well masticated
- Check blood count on postoperative days 1 and 3.
- Discharge on postoperative day 3. Reflux symptoms should be eliminated on the day of surgery.

■ Complications

- Dysphagia
- Gas bloat syndrome
- Stenosis
- Recurrence

- Dysphagia and gas bloat syndrome (result of an excessively tight cuff)
- Telescope phenomenon if cuff is not fixed to the esophagus
- Denervation syndrome as a result of injury to vagal branches or vagus trunk
- Reflux recurrence if the cuff loosens
- Cicatricial stenosis at the esophageal hiatus with symptoms of narrowing

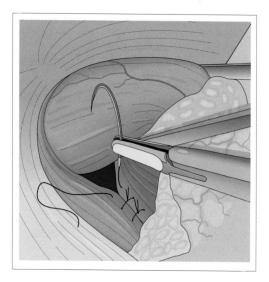

Fig. 8.3 Hiatal repair

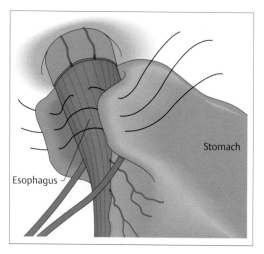

Fig. 8.4 Nissen fundoplication

Esophagus

Stomach

8

■ Esophageal Carcinoma

Epidemiology

- Incidence about 10 per 100 000 population/year
- Predominantly **squamous epithelial carcinomas,** followed by **adenocarcinomas;** incidence of adenocarcinomas of the distal esophagus and gastroesophageal junction has been increasing in recent years.
- Ratio of men to women is 5 : 1.

Etiology

- Rapid metastasis to the local lymph nodes and extensive intramural growth (mucosal margin of the tumor often does not correspond to the tumor margin in the esophageal wall)

- Intramural growth
- Early lymphatogenous metastasis
- Lung and liver metastases
- Peritoneal carcinomatosis

- Distant metastases from proximal tumors especially to the lung and from distal tumors to the liver; skeletal metastases only occur later; with locally advanced distal tumors there is often peritoneal carcinomatosis
- Tumor localization is very important because of the different treatment approaches

Risk Factors
- Smoking
- Alcohol
- Thermal injury (hot foods)
- Cicatricial strictures, for example after acid or alkali corrosive injury, radiation
- Barrett esophagus: precancerous condition for adenocarcinoma of the esophagus

Classification

- Assessment of lymph nodes crucial for staging, prognosis and treatment

- **Squamous epithelial carcinoma:** distinction between cervical, supra- and infrabifurcation
- **Adenocarcinoma** of the distal esophagus is classified with proximal gastric carcinoma as adenocarcinoma of the esophagogastric junction (AEG):
  - ► Type I: distal esophagus (Barrett carcinoma)
  - ► Type II: cardia carcinoma, at the gastroesophageal junction
  - ► Type III: subcardiac gastric carcinoma, infiltrating the cardia from below
- AEG type I tumors are classified as esophageal carcinomas in the TNM classification, and AEG type II and III tumors are classified as gastric carcinomas (**Tables 8.2** and **8.3**).

Table 8.2   TNM classification

Tx	Primary tumor not assessable
T0	No evidence of primary tumor
Tis	Carcinoma in situ
T1	Infiltration of the lamina propria, muscularis mucosae, or submucosa
T2	Infiltration of the muscularis propria
T3	Infiltration of the adventitia
T4	Infiltration of neighboring structures
Nx	Regional lymph nodes not assessable
N0	No regional lymph node metastases
N1	Regional lymph node metastases
M0	No distant metastases
M1	Distant metastases and **nonregional lymph node metastases**
Tumor in the upper thoracic esophagus	
M1a	Metastases in cervical lymph nodes
M1b	Nonregional lymph nodes and/or other distant metastases
Tumor in the middle thoracic esophagus	
M1a	not possible
M1b	Nonregional lymph nodes and/or other distant metastases
Tumor in the lower thoracic esophagus	
M1a	Celiac lymph nodes
M1b	Nonregional lymph nodes and/or other distant metastases

Table 8.3 UICC and AJCC (American Joint Committee on Cancer) staging

Stage 0	Tis, N0, M0
Stage 1	T1, N0, M0
Stage 2a	T2/T3, N0, M0
Stage 2b	T1/T2, N1, M0
Stage 3	T3, N1, M0 and T4, any N, M0
Stage 4	Any T, any N, M1
Stage 4a	Any T, any N, M1a
Stage 4b	Any T, any N, M1b

Depending on the site of the primary tumor, the **regional lymph nodes** are listed below:
- Cervical primary tumor:
  - Scalene lymph nodes
  - Lymph nodes beside the internal jugular vein
  - Upper and lower cervical lymph nodes
  - Peri-esophageal lymph nodes
  - Supraclavicular lymph nodes
- Intrathoracic primary tumor (all thirds)
  - Upper peri-esophageal lymph nodes (above the azygos vein)
  - Subcarinal lymph nodes
  - Lower peri-esophageal lymph nodes (below the azygos vein)
  - Mediastinal lymph nodes
  - Perigastric lymph nodes (with the exception of celiac lymph nodes)

For tumors in the mid-esophagus, the description M1b exclusively is used for metastases in nonregional lymph nodes, as these have an equally poor prognosis as with other distant metastases.

Symptoms

- Dysphagia
- Weight loss
- Retrosternal pain
- Hoarseness

Diagnostic Approach

■ Clinical Examination

- **Lung function tests:** pulmonary reserve for single lung ventilation
- **Cardiac investigations:** echocardiography and stress ECG, high cardiac stress due to two-cavity surgery

■ Laboratory Tests

- **Tumor markers:** CEA, CA 19–9 with adenocarcinoma; SCC with squamous epithelial carcinoma

- Staging and investigation of cardiopulmonary performance are crucial for treatment planning.

8

■ Diagnostic Imaging

- PET-CT is the most important staging investigation and desirable in all patients: essential when tumor stage is unclear.

- **Thoracic CT** and **abdominal CT** with oral and IV contrast. Oral contrast swallow immediately prior to CT obviates the need for barium swallow.
- **PET (positron emission tomography)-CT** allows detection of all distant metastases with one examination, confirms or dispels suspicion of lymph node metastases, and provides evidence of the response to neoadjuvant chemoradiotherapy (second PET-CT after first therapy cycle); the most reliable investigation for distant and lymph node metastasis.
- **Skeletal scintigraphy:** if appropriate when bone metastases are suspected from other imaging procedures or symptoms; not usually necessary if PET-CT is performed.
- **Abdominal ultrasonography:** assessment of the liver (sometimes metastases are visible on ultrasonography that are not visible on CT and vice versa).
- **Endosonography:** depth of penetration into the wall and lymph node status (operator-dependent, often false-positive lymph node assessment. **Caution:** overstaging with the result of not performing indicated surgery)
- Barium swallow is now only used for special queries.

■ Invasive Investigations

- **Endoscopy** with biopsy for histology
- **Bronchoscopy** when involvement of the bronchial system is suspected
- **Mediastinoscopy** when high mediastinal lymph node metastases are suspected
- Diagnostic **laparoscopy** with distal esophageal carcinoma to rule out peritoneal carcinomatosis; if necessary, assessment/biopsy of celiac lymph nodes including laparoscopic ultrasound examination of the liver
- **Colonoscopy** because of the possibility of colon interposition

Treatment Approach

■ Indication

- Mucosal resection rarely indicated
- Esophageal resection for locally controllable cancers
- Indication for neoadjuvant chemoradiotherapy decided individually
- If appropriate: palliative radiation, chemoradiotherapy, stent insertion

- Discussion in **tumor case conference** or consultation with radiotherapist and oncologist, establish the overall treatment plan.
- **Premalignant lesions and early cancers:** Endoscopic mucosal resection is used only for purely intramucosal tumor (T1m, carcinoma in situ), without infiltration of the submucosa, maximum tumor diameter 2 cm, well to moderately differentiated (G1–G2), no ulcer histologically, no lymphatic or venous infiltration, tumor-free resection margins; lymph node metastases in less than 5% of cases; 5-year survival rate over 80%.
- **Disadvantage:** Frequent follow-up and possibly further resection are necessary because of multifocal and metachronous neoplastic changes; long-term complications can be scarring or strictures; **not a general treatment recommendation,** for use only in the context of studies.
- **T1–2, N0, M0:** subtotal esophageal resection with lymphadenectomy; reconstruction by tubular stomach or small bowel/colon interposition
- **Squamous epithelial carcinoma T3, N0, M0:** primary resection as far as possible; if located in the upper esophagus and good general health, neoadjuvant chemoradiotherapy
- **Squamous epithelial carcinoma T1–4, N0–1, M0:** neoadjuvant chemoradiotherapy for proximal carcinomas, indication for neoadjuvant treatment controversial in the case of infrabifurcation carcinomas

- **Adenocarcinoma T2–4, N0, M0; T1–4, N1, M0:** diagnostic laparoscopy to rule out local peritoneal carcinomatosis; surgery if appropriate after neo-adjuvant chemoradiotherapy
- Primary and neoadjuvant **chemoradiotherapy:** with 5-fluorouracil and cis-platin and total dose of 40–50 Gy. Achieves a higher R0 resection rate and longer survival rate. In studies of primary chemoradiotherapy, 5-year surviv-al rates of up to 26% were obtained. Thus, definitive chemoradiotherapy is roughly similar to esophageal resection.
- **Palliative therapy** of metastatic carcinoma: An improvement in swallowing can be achieved by percutaneous radiotherapy on its own. Endoluminal radiation (brachytherapy) is more effective using the afterloading technique. Short-term survival within the first 2 years can be increased by combined **chemoradiotherapy** compared with radiotherapy alone. However, greater toxicity has to be accepted. Endoscopic stent therapy can be used to bridge an area of stenosis.

■ Surgical Treatment

Abdominothoracic Esophageal Resection

- Now widely regarded as the standard procedure with reconstruction by gastric sleeve and intrathoracic anastomosis
- **Advantages:** in particular, specific oncological en bloc resection of esopha-gus, parietal pleura and attached lymph nodes
- Intrathoracic anastomosis offers better quality of life than cervical anasto-mosis (necessary in any case when transmediastinal blunt stripping of the esophagus is performed).
- **Disadvantage:** connection to the pleural cavity in the event of anastomotic leakage with development of pleural empyema
- Two-cavity operation is highly stressful; decide indication carefully with regard to general and cardiopulmonary performance status.
- The anastomosis can also be cervical depending on the level of the tumor and the resulting resection level.

• The most suitable proce-dure as regards radicality and quality of life

8

Operative Technique

Positioning
- Compared with intraoperative repositioning of the patient, we prefer primary positioning in an oblique left-lateral position with a vacuum mattress and supports, so that the patient can be placed in both supine and lateral positions by maximum sideways tilting of the table.
- The entire operation field is draped accordingly, starting with the right half of the thorax and extending over the entire abdomen.
- Depending on the position of the tumor, the operation can start with either **thoracotomy** or **laparotomy.**

Access
- The standard access is a transverse curved upper abdominal laparotomy, if necessary with a short straight extension into the epigastrium, together with a right-sided anterolateral thoracotomy in the 4th to 5th intercostal space (ICS).
- If appropriate, perform a left cervical incision at the anterior border of the sternocleidomastoid muscle.

Abdomen
- Check for operability (e.g., tumor at the esophageal hiatus).
- If not done already during staging laparoscopy, check for peritoneal seeding; intraoperative ultrasonography of the liver.
- Enter the omental bursa, skeletonizing the greater curvature of the stomach and preserving the gastric arcade.
- When intrathoracic anastomosis is planned, the greater curvature is divided transversely at the gastric fundus in the relatively avascular area of the gastric arcade at about the level of the lower pole of the spleen.
- Higher division at the fundus for cervical anastomosis
- Further gradual division using GIA stapler, including the lesser curvature and division of the right gastric artery
- En-bloc resection of proximal stomach and esophagus with central division of the left gastric artery (**Fig. 8.5**). En-bloc resection of the spleen depending on tumor site
- Detachment of the lesser omentum on the hepatic side and division on liver side of an accessory left hepatic artery from the celiac trunk, if present
- Incision of the peritoneal fold at the esophageal hiatus, and circular mobilization of the esophagus from the hiatus; if tumor is located at this site generous removal of the muscle at the hiatus so that any adherent muscle remains with the tumor block
- Completion of lymphadenectomy by removal of the lymph nodes beside the common hepatic artery and in the hepatoduodenal ligament
- Oversewing of the row of staples of the gastric sleeve with a continuous seromuscular suture, and also with interrupted sutures if the length of the gastric sleeve is problematic (less shortening of the gastric sleeve)
- Mobilization of the duodenum (Kocher maneuver) to achieve better extension of the gastric sleeve

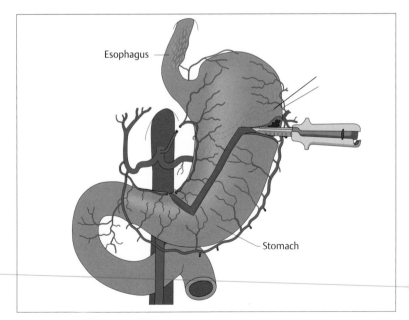

Fig. 8.5   Abdominal site: proximal gastric resection including the lesser curvature.

Thorax
- After repositioning the patient in the left-lateral position by tilting the table, anterolateral thoracotomy is performed in the 4th to 5th ICS (**Fig. 8.6**)
- Single lung ventilation on the left side
- Incision of the parietal pleura anterior and posterior to the esophagus
- Ligation of the azygos vein is optional but nearly always necessary because of the required distance of the resection margin of 7–8 cm from the tumor.
- Circular dissection of the esophagus including the surrounding connective tissue and attached lymph nodes
- Free dissection of the esophagus is most successful after the esophagus has been divided proximally over a purse-string clip.
- Knot the back plate of the circular stapler (cross section 25 mm).
- Frozen section examination to check that resection margins are free from tumor

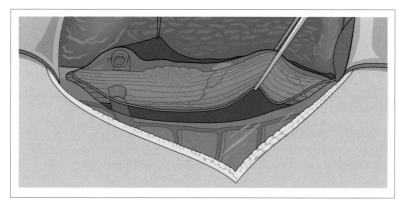

Fig. 8.6 Thoracic site: access through anterolateral thoracotomy in 4th or 5th intercostal space.

8

Reconstruction
- Introduction of the circular stapler abdominally through a longitudinal pylorotomy, which is later closed transversely (Heinicke–Mikulicz pyloroplasty)
- **Advantage:** physiological angle when introducing the circular stapler, no separate gastrotomy necessary in the gastric sleeve, simultaneous pyloroplasty in one step (benefit is controversial)
- Alternatively, after pulling up the gastric sleeve, introduction of the circular stapler in the thorax through a gastrotomy
- Chest drains, closure of the thoracotomy and laparotomy; if the operation field is dry, abdominal drains can be omitted.

Cervical
- When the tumor is in a high location, the esophagus is resected as far as the cervical part (**Fig. 8.7**).
- Oblique incision in front of the sternocleidomastoid muscle with the head extended in right lateral position
- Division of the superficial cervical fascia, deep dissection and division of the middle thyroid vein. The esophagus is located between the thyroid, which is retracted medially, and the neck vessels.

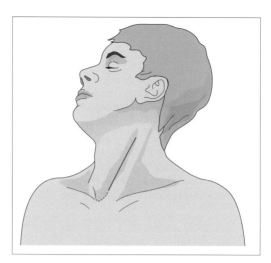

Fig. 8.7 Cervical access

- Circular free dissection and retraction of the esophagus, division over a purse-string suture clip (mechanical anastomosis) or open (manual suture)
- Closure of the cervical fascia and skin suture

Transmediastinal Esophageal Resection

- Blunt stripping of the esophagus in the mediastinum; dubious **from the oncological aspect** so no longer used as a standard procedure

---

Operative Technique

- Surgery is started **abdominally** as in the two-cavity procedure
- Manual, transmediastinal shelling out of the esophagus (splinted with a large gastric tube for better palpation) as far as the tracheal bifurcation. Final stripping is performed bimanually from the abdominal and cervical ends/aspect.
- Then, cervical incision as described above
- The esophagus is divided at the cervical end and pulled through toward the abdomen.
- Anastomosis with gastric sleeve/colon interposition, as above

---

Alternative
- The gastric sleeve/colon is drawn up behind the sternum, rarely used today.
- Digital retrosternal tunneling is performed.
- The prepared interposition graft (gastric sleeve/colon) is drawn upward retrosternally and anastomosed in the neck.

Postoperative Care
- Oral diet gradually from day 5, or tube feeding earlier if a triple lumen tube has been placed at operation
- Chest drains are clamped and removed gradually from day 5.
- Intensive respiratory therapy

- At the least sign of anastomotic leakage (drain fluid, laboratory tests, signs of sepsis) do a CT check with contrast swallow.

- Postoperatively always think of anastomotic leakage.

Palliative Surgery

- For inoperable tumors or when distant metastasis has occurred, palliative surgery may be used to maintain or restore a passage by means of:
  - ➤ endoscopic **stent placement,**
  - ➤ possibly in combination with **radiotherapy,** or
  - ➤ placement of a **PEG tube** for feeding if the patient's esophagus cannot be kept patent.

■ Postoperative Complications

- Secondary hemorrhage
- Tracheal injury
- **Anastomotic leakage**
- Esophagobronchial fistula
- Necrosis of interposition graft
- Cardiopulmonary complications
- Pneumonia

■ Injuries of the Esophagus

Corrosive Injuries

- In childhood due to accidental ingestion of unlabeled or incorrectly labeled aggressive fluids
- In adults often with **suicidal** intent
- **Acids** lead to coagulation necrosis (eschar)
- **Alkalis** lead to colliquative necrosis (liquefaction of the tissue)
- The extent of the tissue damage can range from mucosal edema to ulcers to perforation. Esophageal perforation with acute mediastinitis still has high mortality.

- Ingestion of alkalis or acids

8

Diagnostic Approach

- History and inspection of the mouth and throat
- Chest and abdominal x-ray (free air? mediastinal emphysema?)
- **Thoracic CT** with contrast imaging of the esophagus using water-soluble contrast (e.g., through a proximally placed suction catheter)
- If necessary, radiography with water-soluble contrast
- Endoscopic assessment

- Thoracic CT

Treatment Approach

■ Acute Treatment

- Monitoring in the intensive care unit
- Gastric tube
- High-dose steroid therapy
- Antibiotic cover

- Gastric lavage, attempts at neutralization of the ingested fluid and administration of emetics are **contraindicated.**
- Early bougienage (starting between 6 and 12 days at 2- to 4-day intervals)

■ Surgical Treatment

- Surgery indicated only for perforation or transmural corrosive injury
- Repeated bougienage if necessary for strictures

- The primary **indication for surgery** is confirmed perforation and when there is severe corrosive injury with suspected transmural organ damage.
- With transmural corrosive injury of the esophagus or devitalization of all layers of the wall (extensive circular) resection of the affected segment is indicated.
- The extent of resection and access are determined by the site and extent of the injury.
- Long-term or permanent bougienage is often necessary for corrosive strictures.
- Annual endoscopic follow-up, as corrosive stricture is regarded as **precancerous**

Traumatic Perforation of the Esophagus

- Often **iatrogenic**
- Due to **foreign bodies** (psychiatric patients)
- Stab or gunshot wounds and thoracic trauma
- **Diagnosis** as for corrosive injuries

Treatment Approach

■ Surgical Treatment

- Surgical management by direct suture

- **Direct suture** of the perforation with antibiotic cover
- If necessary, additional covering of the suture site by fundoplication, pleural flap or pedicled diaphragm flap. Direct suture usually suffices.

Spontaneous Esophageal Rupture (Boerhaave Syndrome)

- Rupture of the esophagus due to violent vomiting

- Rupture of the morphologically intact esophagus due to sudden **violent vomiting**. A rapid and large increase in the pressure in the esophagus is responsible pathogenetically for the injury.
- The rupture is nearly always located in the **distal esophagus**.

Symptoms

Clinical features are due to development of **mediastinitis** with mediastinal emphysema:
- Sudden sensation of doom
- Dyspnea
- Retrosternal pain
- Shock symptoms

Diagnostic Approach

- **Thoracic CT** with esophageal imaging by water-soluble contrast, further investigations usually not necessary

Treatment Approach

■ Surgical Treatment

- Confirmation of the diagnosis is an **absolute indication for surgery**.
- The access is guided by the location and direction of the perforation site:
  - ► **Transverse upper abdominal laparotomy** extended into the epigastrium, in the case of perforation, where it passes through or below the diaphragm
  - ► **Left-sided thoracotomy** if thoracic perforation toward the left side
  - ► **Right-sided thoracotomy** if perforation toward the right side
- The operation consists of **direct suture closure** of the site of rupture, if necessary with additional cover provided by fundoplication, pedicled diaphragm or pleural flap. These additional measures are rarely required.
- Irrigation and drainage of the pleural space and mediastinum
- **High-dose antibiotic therapy**

- Immediate surgical repair with direct suture of the esophagus
- Antibiotics

Further Reading

Bennett C, Green S, Barr H, et al. Surgery versus radical endotherapies for early cancer and high grade dysplasia in Barrett's oesophagus. Cochrane Database Syst Rev 2010 May 12; (5): CD007334. Review

Layke JC, Lopez PP. Esophageal Cancer: A Review and Update. Am Fam Physician 2006; 73: 2187–2194

Malthaner RA, Collin S, Fenlon D. Preoperative chemotherapy for resectable thoracic esophageal cancer. Cochrane Database Syst Rev. 2006 Jul 19; 3: CD001556. Review

National Cancer Institute. Esophageal Cancer Treatment. In Internet: http://www.cancer.gov/cancertopics/pdq/treatment/esophageal/healthprofessional/; accessed: 19.05.2011

8

9 Stomach and Duodenum

N.T. Schwarz

■ Anatomy

Arteries

- The excellent perfusion of the stomach allows different forms of resection.

- The stomach is supplied in full and the duodenum in part from the **celiac trunk.** In subtotal distal gastric resection because of carcinoma, the short gastric arteries must be preserved, as otherwise, with obligatory ligature of the left gastric artery at its origin, perfusion of the gastric stump can no longer be ensured.

Veins

- The veins usually run parallel to the arteries. They drain into the portal vein.

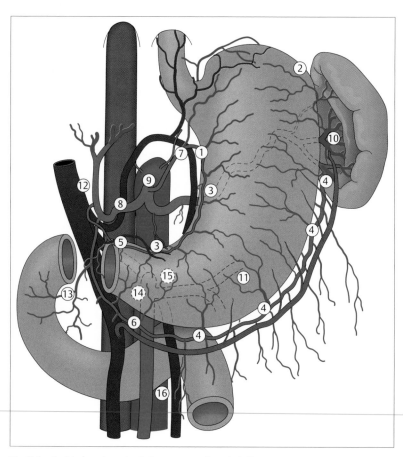

Fig. 9.1 Gastric lymph node stations: compartments I–III.

Lymphatic Drainage, Vagus Nerve (Fig. 9.2)
- From the stomach there are **three lymphatic drainage regions,** which correspond to the three major vessels of the celiac trunk, that is, the left gastric artery, hepatic artery, and splenic artery.
- Lymphatogenous metastasis of gastric carcinoma is initially to the perigastric lymph nodes (LNs) and from there to compartment II along the vessels that originate from the celiac trunk.
- For technical surgical reasons, the LN stations are divided into compartments I, II, and III (**Fig. 9.1**).
  - **Compartment I** (LN groups 1–6), all LNs directly beside the stomach: at the cardia (1, 2), on the lesser and greater curvature (3, 4), and above and below the pylorus (5, 6)
  - **Compartment II** (LN groups 7–11), LNs along the large vessels: left gastric artery (7), common hepatic artery (8), celiac trunk (9), splenic hilum (10), splenic artery (11)
  - **Compartment III** (LN groups 12–16): LNs in the hepatoduodenal ligament (12), behind the head of the pancreas (13), at the root of the mesentery and in the mesentery (14, 15), and along the abdominal aorta (16)

Vagus Nerve
- Above the diaphragm the anterior and posterior branches of the vagus nerve form the **peri-esophageal plexus.**
- Just above the hiatus, the plexus divides into the anterior and posterior **vagal trunks.** Sometimes (16%), the trunks divide into several branches before crossing the diaphragm. In these cases, the vagus nerve is not completely deactivated by truncal vagotomy. Circular dissection of the esophagus is therefore always required.
- The so-called **criminal nerves** branch off from the posterior trunk and pass to the posterior surface of the gastric fundus.

- Injuries of the vagus nerve interfere markedly with quality of life

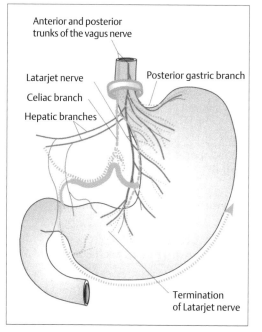

Anterior and posterior trunks of the vagus nerve

Latarjet nerve

Celiac branch

Hepatic branches

Posterior gastric branch

Termination of Latarjet nerve

Fig. 9.2 Course of the vagus nerve.

9

Glands (Fig. 9.3)
- The **anterior branch of the vagus** passes along the anterior surface of the lesser curvature and innervates the anterior wall of the stomach. The hepatic branches, which also innervate the antrum and pylorus, arise from it.
- The **posterior branch of the vagus** runs along the posterior surface of the lesser curvature. It forms the usually prominent celiac branch and innervates the posterior wall of the stomach.

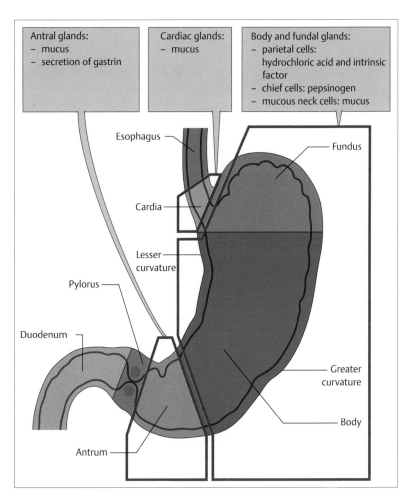

Antral glands:
- mucus
- secretion of gastrin

Cardiac glands:
- mucus

Body and fundal glands:
- parietal cells: hydrochloric acid and intrinsic factor
- chief cells: pepsinogen
- mucous neck cells: mucus

Esophagus

Fundus

Cardia

Lesser curvature

Pylorus

Duodenum

Greater curvature

Body

Antrum

Fig. 9.3   Anatomy of the stomach with distribution of the glands.

■ Ulcer

Definition

- Ulcer: lesion of the mucosa, submucosa, and muscularis mucosae
- Erosion: lesion is limited to the mucosa
- Penetration: the ulcer penetrates a neighboring organ (pancreas, colon)

Epidemiology

- Duodenal ulcer : gastric ulcer = 4 : 1
- The **mortality with perforation** is ca. 10% if there are no other risk factors. In the presence of risk factors (age > 60 years, time between perforation and operation > 8 hours, comorbidities), the mortality is over 30%.
- 65%–80% of **perforated ulcers** are caused by duodenal (or pyloric) ulcers, the remainder by a gastric ulcer. The proportion of perforations caused by gastric carcinoma can be up to 10%.

Duodenal Ulcer
- Peak age: 30–50 years
- 80% of patients are men
- Located almost exclusively in the anterior wall of the duodenal bulb

Gastric Ulcer
- Peak age: 50–70 years
- Men are affected four times more often than women
- Location: 80% are on the lesser curvature, usually at the transitional zone between the antral and the acid-producing mucosa. Only 10% of ulcers develop in the fundus.

Etiology

- The two most important independent factors in the development of an ulcer are *Helicobacter pylori* infection (HP infection) and use of **nonsteroidal anti-inflammatory drugs** (NSAIDs). Without the presence of at least one of these two factors, ulcers only occur exceptionally.
- The cause of ulcers not associated with HP or due to aspirin or NSAIDs is unclear.
- Rare syndromes are known: for example, Zollinger–Ellison syndrome.
- Stress ulcers are due mainly to ischemia.
- The following are **protective:**
  - ➤ Mucosal barrier due to mucus and bicarbonate secretion
  - ➤ Mucosal perfusion, good microcirculation
  - ➤ Prostaglandins
  - ➤ Epithelial regeneration
- The following have an **aggressive** action:
  - ➤ Hydrochloric acid (HCl), pepsin (in duodenal ulcer, the central importance of increased HCl production for the development of an ulcer is undisputed)
  - ➤ *Helicobacter pylori* mucinase → acute gastritis → chronic gastritis B → breakdown of mucosal integrity
  - ➤ Duodenogastric reflux → bile acids and lysolecithin → cell damage
  - ➤ Medications, for example, glucocorticoids or NSAIDs apart from coxibs. They inhibit prostaglandin synthesis. Even diclofenac gel reaches plasma levels that are not significantly lower than those of oral diclofenac.
  - ➤ Alcohol, nicotine
  - ➤ Mucosal ischemia (e.g., due to stress or blood loss)
  - ➤ Stasis as a result of pyloric stenosis → prolonged contact time of food with G cells → increased gastrin production

- Main causes of ulcer development: HP infection and taking NSAIDs

9

Helicobacter Pylori

- The incidence of HP infection is falling.

- Ten years ago, HP was detectable in 70% of all gastric ulcers and 95% of all duodenal ulcers, but the importance of HP in the genesis of ulcers is decreasing today.
- In persons under the age of 30 years, infection with HP is 10%–15%. It is usually acquired in the family and takes place by the age of 50 years in the majority of cases. Presumably, the incidence will not increase in future due to successful eradication.
- HP infection leads initially to acute gastritis and later to chronic gastritis B, and this then leads to a break-up of mucosal integrity.
- However, since only 10% of patients with HP-induced gastritis B develop a peptic ulcer, other factors must still be involved in ulcer development. The exact mechanisms are not known.
  On the one hand, it is still assumed that an imbalance between aggressive and protective mucosal factors is of crucial importance for ulcer pathogenesis ("no ulcer without acid"). A preponderance of the aggressive factors leads via damage to the mucosal barrier to gastritis, damage to the mucosa, and ulcer development.
  On the other hand, complex interactions between bacterial virulence factors and the host's immune response, environmental cofactors, and the increased virulence of some HP strains—and thus the severity of the induced gastritis—are also responsible for ulcer development.
- Dysfunction of the gastric antrum with increased reflux of duodenal juice is also suggested in the development of gastric ulcer.

Aspirin and NSAIDs

- ASA and NSAIDs are mainly responsible for ulcer production.

- Meanwhile, ulcers due to aspirin (acetylsalicylic acid: ASA) and NSAIDs are increasing. The cause is the increasing consumption of NSAIDs. This has led to a massive increase in HP-negative ulcers in recent years, whereas the number of complicated ulcers has remained constant.

Classification

- Postbulbar duodenal ulcer is most common

- **Acute ulcer:**
  - ► Stress ulcer: usually occurs during intensive care treatment, after surgery, polytrauma, burns, renal failure, long-term ventilation → prophylaxis is important
  - ► Simple Dieulafoy ulcer (limited to the mucosa)
  - ► Drug-induced ulcer
- **Chronic ulcer disease:**
  - ► Duodenal ulcer
  - ► Gastric ulcer (**Table 9.1**)

The acid capacity of the stomach diminishes from the pylorus toward the cardia.

Table 9.1   Johnson classification of gastric ulcer

Type I	Ulcer in the body of the stomach, usually on the lesser curvature proximal to the angular incisure without pathological findings in the duodenum and pylorus. The stomach is hypoacidic. Most common form: ca. 60% of cases
Type II	Ulcer in the body of the stomach combined with an ulcer in the duodenum, hyperacidic gastric juice, ca. 20% of cases
Type III	Prepyloric ulcer, hyperacidic

Symptoms

- Gastric ulcer: pain immediately after eating. However, the pain can also occur independent of food intake.
- Duodenal ulcer: pain when fasting, nocturnal pain, late pain; improvement after ingestion of food
- Perforation:
  - ► Ulcer history
  - ► Acute abdomen—signs of peritonitis
- Penetration:
  - ► Usually protracted treatment-resistant pain, rarely acute
  - ► Penetration into the pancreas often causes pancreatitis with raised serum amylase and pain radiating to the back. Jaundice is possible with penetration into the hepatoduodenal ligament
  - ► Occasional fistula development, for example, gastrocolic (accelerated passage of food)

Diagnostic Approach

■ Laboratory Tests

- **Urease rapid test** is equivalent to the histological examination of biopsies. However, it is not reliable with a bleeding ulcer.
- "Test to treat" method in English-speaking countries requires serological HP test initially and endoscopy only if symptoms persist. **"Scope to treat"** is more popular in Central Europe and involves endoscopy initially. The approach reflects the ever-lower prevalence of HP. Performing the serological HP test or noninvasive ^{13}C-urea breath test cannot be recommended for initial diagnosis of HP infection.
- Rule out Zollinger–Ellison syndrome (high basal acid secretion, gastrin is greatly increased basally and after provocation with secretin).
- Stool examination for occult blood
- In the case of penetration: amylase ↑

■ Diagnostic Imaging

- Ultrasonography
- Radiography (contrast GI series)
- Functional diagnostics
- With perforation:
  - ► Plain erect abdominal x-ray, shows free air under the diaphragm in only 70%–80% of cases → **note:** the absence of free air does not rule out perforation
  - ► Abdominal CT with oral water-soluble contrast evidence of the leak
- With penetration: radiography, ultrasonography

- Abdominal x-ray in left lateral position or abdominal CT if gastric perforation is suspected

9

■ Invasive Investigations

- Gastroscopy: biopsy, histology, and bacteriology (testing for HP is an integral part of any endoscopy of the upper GI tract)
- Routine investigations of gastritis: endoscopy and biopsy → two biopsies from the antrum and body, and two further antral biopsies to detect HP by means of the urease rapid test
- Investigations of ulcers: adequate biopsies from the base and margin of the ulcer and from macroscopically normal antrum and fundus

- Endoscopy is the central diagnostic tool to investigate ulcer symptoms.

■ Differential Diagnosis

- Perforation: appendicitis, pancreatitis, perforation of another hollow organ, mesenteric infarction

Treatment Approach

■ Indication

Indication for Surgery

- Perforation: absolute indication for surgery

- Ulcer complications:
  - ► Hemorrhage that cannot be controlled endoscopically (severe, persisting, recurrent)
  - ► Perforation (10% of all gastroduodenal ulcers) is an absolute indication for surgery. An attempt at conservative treatment is possible only in patients with extremely severe comorbidity in whom surgery cannot be justified.
  - ► Gastric outlet stenosis
- Failure of conservative treatment (if the ulcer is not yet healed after more than 8–12 weeks of conservative treatment)
- Chronic recurrent ulcers despite HP eradication
- Suspected carcinoma
- Gastrinoma (Zollinger–Ellison syndrome)

■ Conservative Treatment

- HP eradication should always be complete if there is positive evidence.
- Treatment with PPIs has made conservative ulcer treatment safer.

- Treatment is **primarily conservative.** Carcinoma must first be ruled out endoscopically. Following eradication of *Helicobacter pylori*, gastric ulcers heal in 75%–80% of cases. Recurrence is observed in 2%–5% of cases.
- Helicobacter eradication if HP is found and an ulcer is present by means of **triple therapy (Table 9.2):** treatment regimen is chosen according to any existing allergies
- Elimination of aggressive factors such as nicotine, alcohol, or NSAIDs
- **Drug treatment** with:
  - ► Proton pump inhibitors (PPIs, effective for all ulcers), such as omeprazole (e.g., Losec), pantoprazole (e.g., Protium). Healing rate 70%–90% after 6–8 weeks. Treatment of choice for HP-negative ulcers also
  - ► Antacids
  - ► Aluminum/magnesium hydroxide 10–30 mL after meals
- **Mucosal protection** with:
  - ► Prostaglandin analogues
  - ► Sucralfate
  - ► Roxatidine (e.g., Altat)
  - ► Cimetidine (e.g., Tagamet)

Table 9.2   Treatment of *Helicobacter pylori* infection in ulcer disease[a]

Italian triple therapy	French triple therapy	RAP regimen (reserve regimen)
Clarithromycin 250 mg b.i.d.	Clarithromycin 500 mg b.i.d.	Rifabutin 150 mg b.i.d.
Metronidazole 400 mg b.i.d.	Amoxicillin 1 g b.i.d.	Amoxicillin 1 g b.i.d.
PPI: standard dose b.i.d.[b]	PPI: standard dose b.i.d.[b]	PPI: standard dose b.i.d.[b]

[a] All treatment regimens are for 7 days.
[b] Omeprazole 20 mg, Lansoprazole 30 mg, Pantoprazole 40 mg, Rabeprazole 20 mg, Esomeprazole 20 mg (in this case, half the standard dose is sufficient).
PPI: proton pump inhibitor.

- ► Ranitidine (e.g., Zantac)
- ► Famotidine (e.g., Pepcid)
- **Monitoring** of ulcer healing:
  - ► Gastric ulcer, by endoscopy and biopsy after 4–6 weeks
  - ► Duodenal ulcer, by ^{13}C rapid breath test
- Indication for **gastrin measurement:**
  - ► Rapid ulcer recurrence immediately after treatment
  - ► Multiple ulcers (stomach and duodenum)
  - ► Atypical ulcer manifestation
  - ► Concomitant severe reflux esophagitis
  - ► Diarrhea (which improves on PPI treatment)
- Some perforated ulcers (duodenal ulcer) can be treated conservatively:
  - ► Control shock
  - ► Nasogastric tube, aspiration of stomach
  - ► Antibiotics
- Treatment of **penetration** is primarily conservative: nasogastric tube, PPIs, antibiotics, observation. Surgical treatment if the patient deteriorates: surgical procedure as in uncomplicated ulcer.

■ Surgical Treatment

- Always give calculated antibiotic therapy because of local peritonitis.

Nonresecting Procedures
- Gastric ulcer:
  - ► Closure of perforation: method of choice
  - ► Ulcer excision (for histology) followed by oversewing
  - ► Subsequent drug therapy with PPIs
  - ► Recurrence in HP-positive patients within a year: 5%
- Duodenal ulcer:
  - ► Economical excision, transverse suture; if appropriate, Kocher maneuver to reduce tension
  - ► Pyloric ulcer or pyloric stenosis: Heineke-Mikulicz pyloroplasty (see **Fig. 9.19**)
  - ► Large indurated perforations: Billroth I or rarely Billroth II resection (complicated duodenal ulcer)
  - ► The aim of acid reduction is achieved by PPIs.

- Ulcer excision and over-sewing has become standard since PPIs
- Nonresecting procedures have become accepted for duodenal ulcer.

Resecting Procedures
- Billroth I or Billroth II gastrectomy:
  - ► Billroth I is as effective as Billroth II with fewer side effects and better long-term results.
  - ► Duodenogastric reflux nearly always occurs after both procedures. This results in pathological changes of the mucosa, including carcinoma. On the other hand, fewer recurrent ulcers are observed because of the buffering of gastric acid.
  - ► Mortality: 1%–2%
  - ► Functional disorders after Billroth II: 20%
  - ► Recurrence: 2%
  - ► Incidence of carcinoma in gastric stump, four times higher with Billroth II than with Billroth I
- **Vagotomy** has been abandoned in view of the effectiveness of the PPIs and the frequency of recurrence.

- Treatment with PPIs has replaced intraoperative vagotomy.

9

- Combined procedures
- Anti-reflux reconstruction procedures: rare, as Roux-en-Y or small bowel interposition

Operative Tactics

The surgical procedure is selected according to the location of the ulcer.
- Excision of the ulcer (**Fig. 9.4**) is fundamental, as unrecognized carcinoma is present in 2%–5% of cases. If tumor is found at surgery, an oncologically adequate operation is performed.
- Larger perforations require gastric resection (**Fig. 9.5**; atypical resection, Billroth I, or rarely Billroth II), and rarely a gastrectomy in the case of location in the fundus or cardia.
- Ulcer perforation can also be treated laparoscopically in principle. Patients with peritonitis, shock, or unsuitable ulcer location need a conventional laparotomy.
- Mortality is 4%–9% after both conventional and laparoscopic surgery.
- Recurrent ulcer after Bilroth II or Bilroth I resection is always suspicious for tumor.

Suture Techniques in the Stomach and Duodenum

Manual Suture
- Material: absorbable sutures, braided or monofilament, 3–0 to 4–0
- One or two rows of sutures, continuous or interrupted
- A single row of interrupted or continuous sero-submucosal sutures has become popular. The submucosa must be included to ensure hemostasis, and the mucosa can be spared. "Take lots of serosa and little mucosa." Healing takes ca. 6 days.
- Tension-free suture and adequate perfusion of the wound margins must be ensured.
- Manual suture can be performed anywhere.

Stapling
- For extensive resections (gastric resection, to form a stomach replacement) or to construct difficult and potentially complicated anastomoses (e.g., esophagojejunostomy)
- **Straight stapling devices:** TA, GIA (gastrointestinal anastanosis) → everted row of sutures
  - ► Construction of gastric sleeve as esophageal replacement with the GIA
  - ► Construction of replacement stomach with the GIA
  - ► Simple duodenal stump closure (especially in cancer surgery). In ulcer surgery and for complicated duodenal closure, there are often massive mural changes so manual suture is essential.
  - ► Hemostatic sutures may be required.
  - ► The need for serosal stapling is controversial.
- **Circular stapling devices:** EEA (end-to-end-anastanosis) → inverted row of sutures
  - ► Esophagojejunostomy: considerable reduction in rate of leakage to under 10%
  - ► Roux-en-Y reconstruction: the stapling device confers hardly any advantages

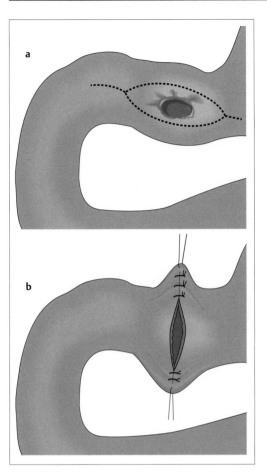

Fig. 9.4 a, b
a Perforated pyloric ulcer, excision for primary repair.
b Transverse closure with interrupted sutures after ulcer excision. Duodenum mobilized.

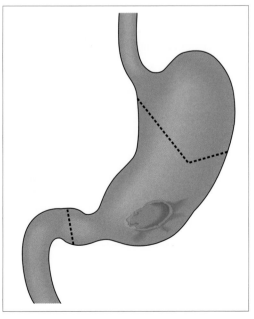

Fig. 9.5 Large perforated gastric ulcer in the body of the stomach toward the greater curvature: incisions for resection of ⅔ of the stomach.

9

Distal Gastric Resection

Indications
- Gastric ulcer
- Complicated duodenal ulcer

Operative Technique

Access Routes
- Transverse right-sided upper abdominal laparotomy
- Upper paramedian incision
- Left paramedian incision, also on the right for Billroth I

Skeletonization of the Greater Curvature (Fig. 9.6)
- The skeletonization begins below the gastroepiploic adventitia; stay within the arcade, close to the stomach. Skeletonization proceeds proximally as far as the gastroepiploic adventitia (confluence of the right and left gastroepiploic arteries).
- Distal skeletonization continues ca. 2–3 cm beyond the pylorus as far as the peritoneal reflection on the head of the pancreas.

Kocher Mobilization of the Duodenum (Fig. 9.7)
- Not essential: a means of relieving tension in Billroth I or for difficult duodenal stump closure

Skeletonization of the Lesser Curvature
- Begin by ligating the right gastric artery, protecting the gastroduodenal ligament and the pancreas.
- Skeletonization of the lesser curvature to ca. 5 cm below the cardia.
- **Resect the stomach** ca. 2 cm distal to the pylorus using a stapler or with open procedure (duodenotamy).
- Place retaining sutures on the duodenum.
- Wrap the gastric stump in an abdominal towel.
- Fold the stomach up out of the operation field.
- Close the duodenum when Billroth II reconstruction is planned.
- **Establish the resection line in the stomach** and place retaining sutures in the lesser curvature.
- Transverse division of the stomach on the greater curvature side at the level of the anastomosis to give a length that corresponds roughly to the lumen of the duodenum. If Billroth II reconstruction is planned, the stomach is narrowed to about one-third of its width. The width of the anastomosis should be ca. 6 cm.
- The **resection line** runs obliquely from this corner toward the lesser curvature to ca. 5 cm below the cardia (**Fig. 9.8**).
- **Excision of the remainder of the stomach** and closure of the lesser curvature with the TA90. Serosal closure over the staples with seromuscular interrupted (or continuous) suture. Alternatively, closure of the blind sac portion on the lesser curvature side with two rows of manual sutures (inner row: continuous all-layer absorbable 3–0 suture; outer row: seroserous interrupted sutures (**Fig. 9.9**).

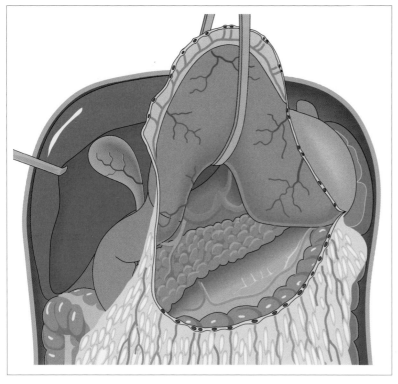

Fig. 9.6   Skeletonization of the greater curvature as far as the gastroepiploic adventitia.

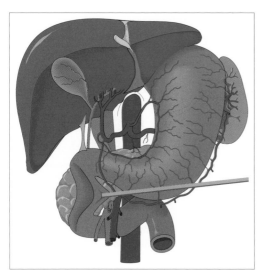

Fig. 9.7   Kocher mobilization of the duodenum.

9

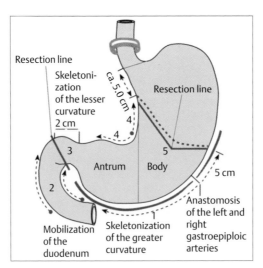

Fig. 9.8 Resection line in the stomach in distal gastric resection.

Resection line

Skeletonization of the lesser curvature 2 cm

ca. 5.0 cm

Resection line

4

4

3

5

Antrum   Body

2

5 cm

Anastomosis of the left and right gastroepiploic arteries

Mobilization of the duodenum

Skeletonization of the greater curvature

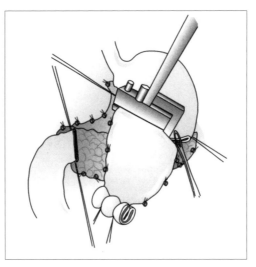

Fig. 9.9 Excision of the stomach (Billroth).

Billroth I Reconstruction

Operative Technique

- Billroth I reconstruction is preferable functionally to Billroth II.

- Distal gastric resection
- Closure of the lesser curvature
- Creation of gastroduodenostomy using a double row of manual sutures. A single row of interrupted sutures through all layers is also possible (**Fig. 9.10**).
- Place the seromuscular sutures in the posterior wall: the duodenum is fixed end-to-end with absorbable sutures (posterior suture). The distance between the sutures and between the sutures and the resection margin is ca. 0.5 cm (**Fig. 9.11**).
- Absorbable 3–0 suture (interrupted or continuous) of the posterior wall, 0.5 cm between the interrupted sutures
- Absorbable 3–0 suture (interrupted or continuous) of the anterior wall of the anastomosis, 0.5 cm between the interrupted sutures (**Fig. 9.12**)

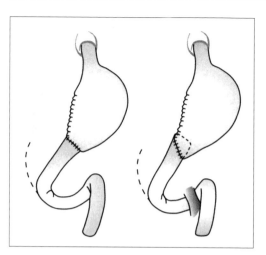

Fig. 9.10 Reconstruction after Billroth I resection. End-to-end or end-to-side gastro-duodenostomy.

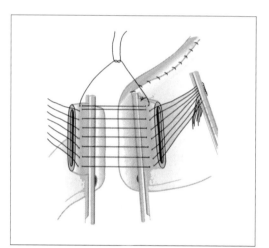

Fig. 9.11 Placement of the posterior wall sutures.

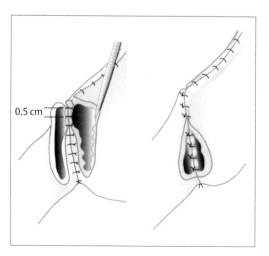

0.5 cm

Fig. 9.12 Posterior wall sutures. Suture of the anterior wall.

9

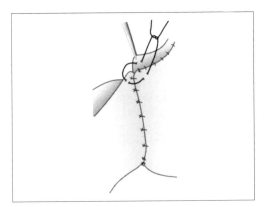

Fig. 9.13   Securing the "angle of sorrow."

- Second inverting row of sutures, absorbable polyfilament or monofilament, starting on the lesser curvature side, three-point suture of the "angle of sorrow" (**Fig. 9.13**)
- Nasogastric tube in the stomach/duodenum, triple-lumen tube if appropriate for early enteral feeding
- Subhepatic easy-flow drain, close to the anastomosis

Billroth II Reconstruction

Methods
- **Antecolic-Anisoperistaltic**
  - ► Braun anastomosis between afferent and efferent jejunal loops is necessary (also relieves the duodenal stump).
  - ► Less reflux → more ulcer recurrence → fewer carcinomas
- **Retrocolic-Anisoperistaltic** (Polya–Reichel see Hoffmeister–Finsterer):
  - ► Short afferent loop, possibly no Braun anastomosis necessary
  - ► Without Braun anastomosis: total bile reflux and alkaline duodenal juice → carcinomas more frequent

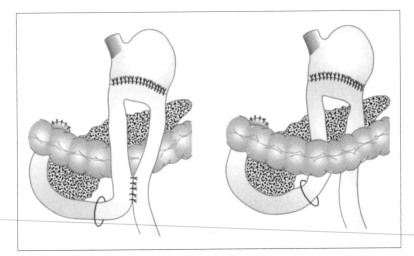

Fig. 9.14   Antecolic or retrocolic Billroth II reconstruction.

Operative Technique

- Distal gastric resection
- Closure of the duodenal stump:
  - ► Staple with TA, which can include serosal closure, or
  - ► place double row of manual sutures: all-layer suture, secured by interrupted seromuscular sutures, or
  - ► perform a continuous lock-stitch suture, which can be covered with the pancreas capsule (rare).
- Closure of the lesser curvature
- Selection of the proximal jejunal loop:
  - ► Find the duodenojejunal flexure and pull the jejunum forward just behind the duodenum (see **Fig. 9.15** for dimensions).

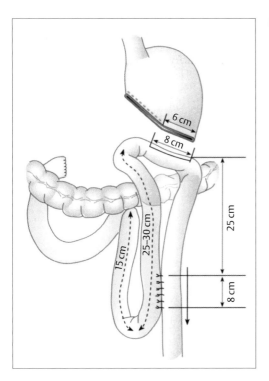

Fig. 9.15   Billroth I resection

- ► Pull the loop up in front of or behind the colon.
- ► Fix afferent loop to the lesser curvature.
- Antimesenteric incision of the jejunal segment selected for anastomosis
- **Gastrojejunostomy** (partial, antecolic, anisoperistaltic):
  - ► Place closely spaced interrupted sutures through all layers, first in the posterior wall, then in the anterior wall (taking a lot of serosa and little mucosa), or
  - ► use staples.
- Secure the poles by three-point sutures.
- **Braun anastomosis** ca. 25 cm below the gastroenterostomy; width ca. 6 cm; single row of sutures through all layers or staples

9

Posterior Wall Ulcers with Penetration into the Pancreas

- Duodenal stump leakage difficult to treat surgically

- Closure of the duodenal stump is difficult in the presence of posterior wall ulcers penetrating the pancreas. In this situation a free duodenal margin for closing the stump is missing.

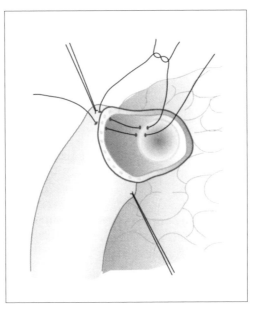

Fig. 9.16 Suture of the lower border of the ulcer and anterior wall of the duodenum.

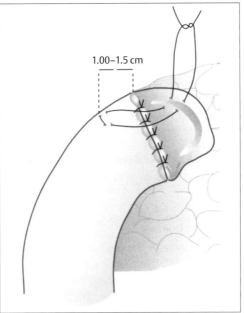

1.00–1.5 cm

Fig. 9.17 Second row of sutures: upper border of the ulcer-anterior wall of the duodenum with U-sutures.

Operative Technique

- Skeletonization of the distal stomach as usual
- Mobilization of the upper duodenum

- Open excision of the ulcer-bearing segment below the ulcer or even transversely through the ulcer. Close the gastric stump with a clamp and reflect it upward.
  Variant: incise the anterior wall of the duodenum at the level of the lower border of the ulcer and cut around the penetrating ulcer.
- Closely spaced interrupted sutures between the lower border of the ulcer and anterior wall of the duodenum (absorbable or nonabsorbable) (**Fig. 9.16**)
- Second row of sutures: upper border of the ulcer and anterior wall of the duodenum with U-sutures (**Fig. 9.17**). Cover with free omentum tip.

Roux-en-Y Reconstruction (Fig. 9.18)

Principle
- Distal gastric resection
- Closure of the duodenal stump
- End-to-side Roux anastomosis ca. 40 cm aboral from the gastrojejunostomy in a single row of all-layer sutures; alternatively use staples

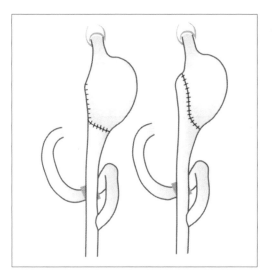

Fig. 9.18 Roux reconstruction

Drainage Operations and Procedures

- Widening the gastric outlet by pyloroplasty leads to
  - ► Accelerated gastric emptying, which promotes dumping and diarrhea
  - ► Increased duodenogastric reflux
  - ► A reduction in the mixing and grinding of solid food; maldigestion and dyspeptic symptoms can be the result
- Careful observation of **strict indications** is therefore necessary.

Dilation Procedures
- Open dilation
- Closed dilation
- Endoscopic dilation

9

Extramucosal Pyloromyectomy (Closed)
- **Indications:** supplement to total or selective gastric vagotomy, so rarely performed (pediatric surgery)

Operative Technique

- Longitudinal oval incision of the serosa on the anterior side of the pylorus
- Dissect off the serosa together with the muscle from the mucosa without opening the mucosa.
- Close the muscle defect transversely by interrupted seromuscular sutures using absorbable material.

Heinecke–Mikulicz (Open) Pyloroplasty

- **Pyloroplasty is often necessary with postpyloric ulcers.**

- **Indications:**
  - ► Pyloric stenosis
  - ► Gastroduodenal hemorrhage when longitudinal opening of the pyloroduodenal junction is necessary to locate the source of bleeding
  - ► Postpyloric ulcers

Operative Technique

- Longitudinal opening of the anterior antro-duodenal wall for a distance of 6–8 cm. All layers of the wall are divided.
- Transverse suture through all layers with fine absorbable sutures from the retracted ends to the middle (**Fig. 9.19**)

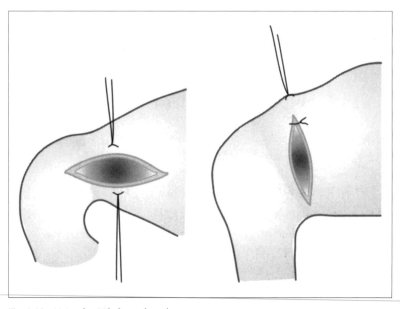

Fig. 9.19 Heinecke–Mikulicz pyloroplasty

Finney and Jaboulay Gastroduodenostomy
- Short-circuit between the proximal duodenum and the distal stomach. This provides a wide passage from the antrum into the duodenum. An ulcer in the anterior wall can be resected at the same time.
- The disadvantages are an increased rate of dumping, increased bile reflux, and increased diarrhea.
- The **Finney** method includes the pylorus in the anastomosis (**Fig. 9.20**).

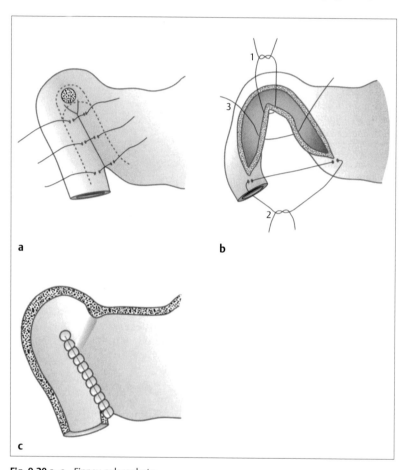

Fig. 9.20 a–c   Finney pyloroplasty

- In the **Jaboulay** technique, the pylorus is preserved (**Fig. 9.21**).
- **Indications:**
  - Severe scarring in the pylorus region
  - Long segments of stenosis

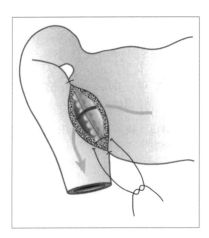

Fig. 9.21 Jaboulay technique

Operative Technique

- Mobilization of the duodenum
- Approximation of the duodenum to the stomach, approximating sutures
- U-shaped incision of the stomach and duodenum; an anterior wall ulcer, if present, is excised.
- Suture of posterior and anterior wall with a single row of absorbable sutures through all layers

---

Vagotomy Procedures

- Vagotomy has become obsolete in the era of PPIs.

These procedures are hardly ever used today and will therefore not be described in detail. The principle of vagotomy is denervation of the parietal cells. A reduction in acid of ca. 60%–70% is achieved with the various forms of vagotomy. Selective proximal vagotomy (SPV) was performed most frequently, leaving the anterior and posterior Latarjet nerve.

■ Postoperative Care after Gastric Resection

- Early enteral feeding possible through triple-lumen tube.

- **Day of surgery:** infusion therapy (electrolyte solution), analgesia
- **From day 1:** enteral feeding through a triple-lumen tube, mobilization, physiotherapy and breathing exercises
- **Day 4:** if no triple-lumen tube, clamp nasogastric tube; remove when less than 400 mL of secretion drains; tea ad libitum.
- **Day 5:** gradually increase diet, 6–8 small meals over 24 hours.
- **By day 8:** remove target drain.
- **Day 10–12:** remove sutures.

■ Complications

Perioperative Complications after Gastric Resections

Secondary Hemorrhage
- Intraluminal:
  - ► Revision if there is persisting bleeding that affects Hb level and causes circulatory reactions; first attempt endoscopic hemostasis.

- ► Relaparotomy: open the stomach 4 cm proximal to the anastomosis and purse-string suture the bleeding source.
- Extraluminal: relaparotomy and treat the bleeding source in the typical way.

Suture Leakage
- Suture leakage at the anastomosis occurs in 3%–4% of cases after Billroth I operations.
- **Postoperative gastric atony** can last 3–7 days. Signs of peritonitis with prolonged gastric atony indicate suture leakage.
- If there are local signs of peritonitis and normal peristalsis and the drain and nasogastric tube are draining fully, it is possible to wait. Give parenteral nutrition. Spontaneous closure of the fistula occurs frequently, possibly after gradual withdrawal of the drain.
- With progression of the disease—**paralytic ileus** → relaparotomy:
  - ► If the sutures are intact: close the leak with a single row of sutures through all layers; cover the suture with omentum; place intraluminal and peritoneal drains.
  - ► If the wound margins cannot be sutured: attempt local excision and suture; place a drain.
  - ► If local repair is not possible: resection of the anastomosis, closure of the duodenal stump, fashion a Billroth II or Roux-en-Y gastrojejunostomy.
  - ► If immediate repair is not possible with severe peritonitis: seal stomach and duodenum with balloon catheters, Witzel fistula, definitive management later.
  - ► Peritonitis: copious irrigation and drainage

- Suture leakage in the stomach can often be treated conservatively.

Postoperative Stenosis of the Anastomosis
This is often the result of edema of the anastomosis. Spontaneous resolution after 8–14 days.

Late Complications after Gastric Resection
- Reflux gastritis
- Atrophic gastritis

Afferent Loop Syndrome
Occurs rarely, after Billroth II resections.
- **Pathogenesis** (two types):
  - ► Outflow of the afferent loop is too narrow, so pancreas secretion and bile stagnate.
  - ► The gastric contents empty into the afferent instead of the efferent loop.
- **Symptoms:** bloating, nausea, and bilious vomiting, which produces instant relief
- **Investigations:** gastroscopy, GI contrast series
- **Treatment:**
  - ► Creation of a Braun anastomosis or Roux-en-Y anastomosis
  - ► Conversion of Billroth II to Billroth I

Efferent Loop Syndrome
Obstruction of the efferent loop of the jejunum after gastric resection or gastroenterostomy (GE). This complication may occur hours to years after the operation.

9

- **Pathogenesis:**
  - ► Acute: internal hernia, technical surgical problems in the area of the anastomosis
  - ► Chronic: ulcers, scarring in the region of the anastomosis, adhesions, internal hernias or jejunogastric intussusception
- **Symptoms:**
  - ► Acute:
    - – Cramps, usually localized around the umbilicus
    - – Vomiting of large volumes of fluid containing bile
  - ► Chronic: intermittent vomiting similar to afferent loop syndrome. It is only the presence of large lumps of food that allows differentiation.
- **Investigations:** radiographic examination provides the diagnosis. However, the chronic form is difficult to diagnose.
- **Treatment:**
  - ► If the efferent loop is closed in the region of the anastomosis, it is possible to wait.
  - ► **Indications for surgery** are an acute syndrome, signs of an acute abdomen, jejunogastric intussusception, and incarceration of internal hernias.
  - ► **Reintervention** should never take place before day 7 and ideally should only be performed after several weeks.
  - ► **Operative options** for stenosis in the region of the GE:
    - – Second antecolic GE above the first GE
    - – Resection with creation of a new GE
    - – If there is a concomitant afferent loop syndrome: enteroenterostomy

Early Dumping

This can occur after 3–4 weeks, mainly following Billroth II or Roux-en-Y resection. The gastrointestinal and cardiovascular symptoms start 10–30 minutes after ingesting food.

- **Pathogenesis:**
  - ► Sudden gastric emptying due to an excessively small gastric remnant and an excessively wide anastomosis. This leads to rapid severe overstretching of the efferent loop resulting in the release of vasoactive substances from the wall of the small intestine (serotonin, kallikrein, bradykinin, insulin, gastric inhibitory polypeptide).
  - ► Due to the hyperosmolarity of the chyme, especially after meals with a high carbohydrate content, there is an influx of secretion into the jejunum with a drop in plasma volume and temporary hypovolemia.
- **Symptoms:** 10–30 minutes after eating: bloating, nausea, upper abdominal pain, retching, possibly diarrhea, palpitations, sweating, dizziness, weakness, fainting, shock
- **Investigations:**
  - ► History
  - ► Standard high-glucose meal to provoke symptoms
  - ► Endoscopy and radiology to rule out other causes
- **Treatment:**
  - ► Conservative:
    - – High protein and fat diet, avoidance of foods high in carbohydrates
    - – Frequent small meals
    - – No liquids with meals
    - – Spasmolytic agents if necessary

- Conversion of Billroth II to Billroth I is the treatment for early dumping.

9

- ► Surgical:
  - – Conversion of Billroth II to Billroth I
- ► Rarely:
  - – Jejunum interposition between the stomach and duodenum after Billroth I resection to enlarge the gastric reservoir
  - – Fashioning of a substitute stomach

Late Dumping

The rare, late dumping syndrome can begin ca. 6 months postoperatively. The hypoglycemic attacks usually occur 2–3 hours after eating.

- **Pathogenesis:** rapid passage of food, rapid carbohydrate absorption. This results in reactive hypoglycemia due to increased insulin secretion after meals high in carbohydrates.
- **Symptoms:** sweating, weakness, hunger, collapse, loss of consciousness due to hypoglycemia
- **Investigation:** The oral glucose tolerance test provokes the typical symptoms.
- **Treatment:**
  - ► Conservative:
    - – Dietetic measures, low-carbohydrate diet
    - – Glucose in an attack
  - ► Surgical (exceptional cases):
    - – Conversion of Billroth II to Billroth I
    - – Delay of gastric emptying, for instance, by anisoperistaltic jejunal interposition

• Treatment of late dumping by dietary regulation

Gastric Stump Carcinoma

Carcinoma may develop in the stomach remnant after gastrectomy. Two-thirds of carcinomas arise in the region of the anastomosis.

- **Pathogenesis:**
  - ► The cancer may be caused by the chronic atrophic gastritis that develops in the resected stomach after a few days, probably also as a result of bile reflux.
  - ► The type of the original ulcer also influences the incidence. Carcinoma occurs in the gastric stump more often after resection of a gastric ulcer.
  - ► The overall incidence is 6%–16%. The latency between resection and the development of carcinoma is ca. 15 years. Endoscopy should therefore be performed regularly from the 10th postoperative year.
- **Investigations:** endoscopy, radiology
- **Treatment:**
  - ► Gastrectomy, if operable
  - ► Otherwise palliative surgery

• Gastric stump carcinoma in up to 16% of cases

9

Overall, the prognosis is poor. It depends on the time of diagnosis.

Recurrent Ulcer

- **Pathogenesis:**
  - ► Deficient acid depression due to:
    - – Inconsistent postoperative treatment with PPI or eradication
    - – Inadequate resection with residual stomach too big
    - – Antrum remnant left at the duodenal stump in a Billroth II resection
    - – Hypersecretion (increased gastrin production) due to persistent alkaline milieu on account of the lack of an "acid brake"
    - – Zollinger–Ellison syndrome (unrecognized gastrinoma), rare, 1.8%

• Postoperative treatment with PPI prevents ulcer recurrence.

- **Incidence:**
  - ▸ 1%–5% after Billroth I and Billroth II resections
  - ▸ Five to 10 times more frequent in men
  - ▸ More frequent after a duodenal ulcer than after a gastric ulcer
- **Investigations:**
  - ▸ Endoscopy, GI contrast series, blood in the stool
  - ▸ Rule out Zollinger–Ellison syndrome by measuring serum gastrin.
- **Complications:**
  - ▸ Perforation
  - ▸ Penetration into the colon with development of a gastrojejunocolic fistula
  - ▸ Bleeding
- **Treatment:** Attempt **conservative treatment initially** (as with preoperative ulcer). If conservative therapy unsuccessful:
  - ▸ After **Billroth II resection:**
    - – Further resection with conversion to Billroth I if there is a large gastric remnant; PPI treatment
    - – Further resection and new Billroth II construction or Roux-en-Y reconstruction; PPI treatment
  - ▸ After **Billroth I resection:**
    - – Further resection and PPI treatment
    - – Further resection with Billroth II reconstruction or Roux-en-Y reconstruction and PPI treatment
  - ▸ **Isolated gastrinoma:** Can be treated by partial resection of the pancreas. Otherwise, treat conservatively with PPIs or octreotide in the case of metastases. Gastrectomy following unsuccessful treatment is hardly ever necessary today.

■ Bleeding from the Stomach and Duodenum

Epidemiology

Sources of Bleeding

- Bleeding ulcers often only become clinically apparent at an advanced stage.

- Peptic ulcers in 30% of cases, followed by esophageal varices, gastritis, and Mallory–Weiss tears
- Esophageal varices 12%, of which > 60% with liver cirrhosis
- 30%–50% of all patients have no ulcer symptoms prior to the ulcer bleed.
- Bleeding occurs in 20% of patients with ulcers.

Prognostic Factors

- 80% of all bleeds cease spontaneously without treatment.
- 5%–10% of bleeds cannot be controlled without endoscopic or surgical intervention.
- Tendency to recurrent bleeding (see also **Table 9.3**):
  - ▸ Forrest I and II: ca. 30%
  - ▸ Forrest II: little susceptibility to recurrence
  - ▸ In 15%–20% of cases, recurrent bleeding usually occurs in the first 2–3 days (early recurrence).

Etiology

Risk Factors for Recurrent Upper GI Tract Hemorrhage

- Forrest Ia or Ib hemorrhage
- Vessel diameter > 2 mm
- Ulcer diameter > 2 cm
- Hemorrhage and circulatory instability
- Ulcer of the posterior duodenal wall
- Elderly patient
- Comorbidities such as cirrhosis, coagulation disorders (drug-induced)

- Mortality is highest with Forrest Ia hemorrhages.

Mortality

- Upper GI hemorrhage overall: 5.3%–14%
- The mortality depends on the intensity of the bleeding (severe bleeding is over 1000 mL/24 hour); the mortality is about twice as high when the initial Hb is below 5–7 gm/dl compared with a higher initial Hb. It increases with the number of transfused units. In patients who require more than 6 units/24 hours to stabilize their circulation, mortality is twice as high as in those given fewer than 6 units.
- Forrest Ia: up to 40%
- Forrest Ib: ca. 10%; much better prognosis since bleeding is more easily controlled endoscopically
- Forrest IIa: ca. 10%
- As a result of negative selection of surgical patients (usually with a prior attempt at endoscopic hemostasis), surgical hemostasis is associated with greater mortality.

Classification (Table 9.3)

Table 9.3   Bleeding activity according to Forrest

Forrest I		Forrest II		Forrest III
Actively bleeding lesion		Inactive bleeding		Lesion without signs of bleeding, history of bleeding
Ia	arterial spurting	IIa	visible vessel stump	
Ib	venous oozing	IIb	ulcer covered with clot	
		IIc	ulcer covered with hematin	

9

Symptoms

- Anemia due to bleeding or hemorrhagic shock with massive bleeding
- Hematemesis with gastric ulcer (not essential)
- Red blood: more severe upper GI bleeding, esophageal?
- "Coffee grounds" blood: delayed upper GI bleeding
- Melena

Diagnostic Approach (Fig. 9.22)

- Chronic bleeding:
  - ► History of ulcer
  - ► Hemoccult test
  - ► Laboratory tests

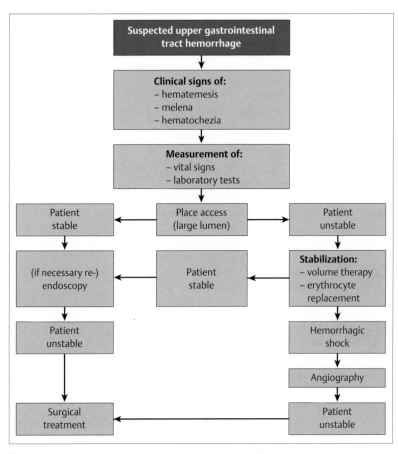

Fig. 9.22   Procedure for suspected bleeding in the upper GI tract.

- Acute bleeding:
  - ► Nasogastric tube, aspiration—evidence of blood
  - ► Shock index, central venous pressure, laboratory tests
  - ► Emergency endoscopy to confirm diagnosis and for risk assessment of the bleeding, and to determine the treatment: endoscopic or surgical

Treatment Approach

■ Indication

Endoscopic Treatment
- **Forrest I:** endoscopic hemostasis
- **Forrest II:** prophylactic endoscopic treatment to avoid recurrent bleeding ("programmed repeated endoscopic treatment")
- **Recurrent bleeding** can also be managed endoscopically.

Surgical Treatment
- Transfusion requirement of > 6 units/24 hours with unstable circulatory status, which does not improve even with short-term intensive shock therapy → absolute indication for surgery

- Surgery indicated with blood transfusion > 6 units/24 hours or unsuccessful endoscopic treatment

9

- Further need for transfusion after endoscopic hemostasis
- Massive bleeding from the duodenal bulb (endoscopic hemostasis usually not possible)
- Deep ulcers in the posterior wall of the duodenal bulb
- Bleeding ulcers associated with perforation
- Increased risk of recurrent bleeding—agreed with the endoscopist (see recurrence risks)

Selective Angiographic Embolization
- Source of bleeding not identifiable on endoscopy
- Patients with increased comorbidity and therefore increased surgical risk

■ Surgical Treatment

Endoscopic Treatment
- Treatment of upper GI bleeding is **primarily endoscopic** nowadays.
- Success rate is 80%–90%, up to 57% with recurrent bleeding.
- Recurrent bleeding occurs in ca. 15%–20%. Recurrent bleeding after initial endoscopic hemostasis represents a life-threatening emergency.

• Treatment of bleeding ulcer is primarily endoscopic.

Contraindications
- Deep penetrating ulcers of the posterior wall of the duodenal bulb
- Ulcers with bleeding from major arteries

Methods
- Laser coagulation, electrocoagulation
- Injection therapy with epinephrine solution and polidocanol, fibrin glue, alcohol or hypertonic saline with epinephrine

Early Surgery To Prevent Recurrent Bleeding
- The necessity of an early operation, that is, surgery within 48 hours after hemostasis, is controversial and depends on the patient's risk factors (see above) and the endoscopic possibilities.

• Ulcer surgery is primarily organ-preserving without extensive resection.

Bleeding from a Gastric Ulcer
- In the stomach usually excision of the ulcer with oversewing, followed by treatment with PPIs. Rarely, partial gastrectomy (rate < 10%)
- A **Dieulafoy ulcer** on the posterior wall of the fundus is usually managed endoscopically.
- Non-ulcer bleeding, for example, in the Mallory–Weiss syndrome, is generally managed endoscopically.

Unknown Bleeding Source (Fig. 9.23)
- Selective angiography; if exploration is unsuccessful, attempt to locate the ulcer by palpation; rule out another bleeding source.
- If localization is unsuccessful: gastrotomy at the junction of the body and antrum parallel to the lesser curvature, transversely in the fundus, and possibly postpyloric in the duodenum also.
- Further procedure depends on ulcer location: see below.

Bleeding from a Duodenal Ulcer
- Bleeding ulcers that require surgery are in the posterior wall of the duodenal bulb in 35%–65% of cases (deep, penetrating **posterior wall ulcer**).

9

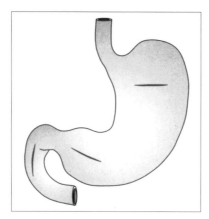

Fig. 9.23   Possible access routes for unknown bleeding source.

Operative Technique

- Opening of the duodenum ca. 3–4 cm beyond the pylorus, longitudinal or transverse
- **Intraluminal** purse-string suture of the ulcer (**Fig. 9.24**)
- **Extraluminal** ligature of the gastroduodenal artery at its origin from the common hepatic artery at the upper border of the duodenum. If necessary, extraluminal ligation of the superior, anterior, and posterior pancreaticoduodenal arteries and of the right gastroepiploic artery at the lower border of the duodenum. This is often unsuccessful because of adhesions, in this case intraluminal purse-string suture only (**Fig. 9.25**).
- Closure of the duodenotomy by a single row of interrupted sutures through all layers (3–0 absorbable). Pyloroplasty: depends on site and extent.

Selective Angiographic Embolization

Complications

- Angiographic embolization as a possible alternative treatment
- Rate of recurrent bleeding significantly increased at 27%
- Ischemia or necrosis of neighboring organs, rare

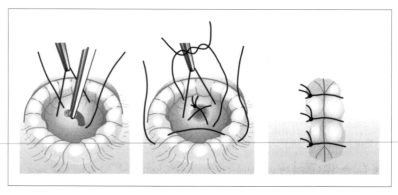

Fig. 9.24   Intraluminal purse-string suture of the ulcer.

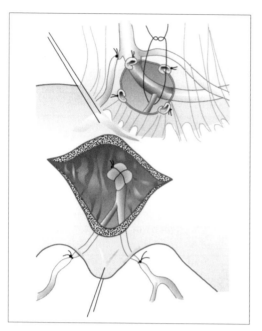

Fig. 9.25 Extraluminal ligation of the pancreaticoduodenal artery, right gastroepiploic artery, and gastroduodenal artery.

■ Gastric Carcinoma

Epidemiology

- Second most frequent cancer-related cause of death worldwide
- Incidence and mortality are falling in Europe and the USA, but adenocarcinoma of the esophagogastric junction (AEG) is increasing.
- Men : women = 2 : 1, blood group A predominance
- Peak incidence between the ages of 50 and 70 years

- The incidence of gastric carcinoma is falling.

Etiology

Main Locations
- Lesser curvature, antrum, more rarely on the greater curvature

Risk Groups and Precancerous Conditions
- Chronic gastritis with proliferative intestinal metaplasia
- Pathogenetic association of HP-induced chronic gastritis B with gastric carcinoma has been confirmed in large epidemiological studies. Changes in dietary habits and widespread HP eradication are the reasons for the falling incidence. Prophylactic eradication therapy is not currently recommended.
- Pernicious anemia with chronic atrophic gastritis
- Gastric polyps, familial cancer predisposition
- Ménétrier disease (8%)
- Operated stomach (Billroth I or II, GE) after ca. 15 years
- Gastric ulcer

9

Classification (Tables 9.4, 9.5, 9.6)

Lauren Classification (Histological Differentiation)

* Intestinal type
* Diffuse type

* Intestinal type is the most frequent histologically.

Table 9.4   Histological classification (WHO)

Description	Frequency
Adenocarcinoma	95%
Papillary, tubular, mucinous, signet ring carcinoma, adenosquamous carcinoma	4%
Squamous epithelial carcinoma	< 1%
Undifferentiated carcinoma	< 1%
Unclassified carcinoma	< 1%

Table 9.5   TNM classification

T—Primary tumor	
Tx	Primary tumor not assessable
T0	No evidence of primary tumor
Tis	Carcinoma in situ: intraepithelial tumor without infiltration of the lamina propria
T1	Tumor infiltrates lamina propria, muscularis mucosae, or submucosa
T2	Tumor infiltrates muscularis propria
T2a	Tumor infiltrates muscularis propria
T3	Tumor infiltrates subserosa
T4a	Tumor breaches the serosa (visceral peritoneum) but does not infiltrate neighboring structures
T4b	Tumor infiltrates neighboring structures
N—Regional lymph nodes	
Nx	Regional lymph nodes not assessable
N0	No regional lymph node metastases
N1	Metastases in 1–2 regional lymph nodes
N2	Metastases in 3–6 regional lymph nodes
N3	Metastases in > 7 regional lymph nodes
M—distant metastases	
M0	No distant metastases
M1	Distant metastases
Histopathological grading	
Gx	Degree of differentiation not assessable
G1	Well (highly) differentiated
G2	Moderately differentiated
G3	Poorly differentiated
R classification	
Rx	Residual tumor not assessable
R0	No residual tumor
R1	Microscopic residual tumor
R2	Macroscopic residual tumor

9

Table 9.6   Staging according to the International Union Against Cancer (UICC)

Stage 0	Tis	N0	M0
Stage IA	T1	N0	M0
Stage IB	T1	N1	M0
	T2	N0	M0
Stage II	T1	N2	M0
	T2	N1	M0
	T3	N0	M0
Stage IIIA	T2	N2	M0
	T3	N1	M0
	T4	N0	M0
Stage IIIB	T3	N2	M0
Stage IV	T1	N3	M0
	T2	N3	M0
	T3	N3	M0

Early Gastric Carcinoma

- **Early carcinoma** is limited to the mucosa and submucosa of the stomach, independent of the presence or absence of regional lymph node metastases. It is diagnosed in 15%–20% of gastric carcinoma in Europe and has a good chance of cure after surgical removal (**Fig. 9.26**).

- Early gastric carcinoma in only 15%–20% of diagnoses of gastric carcinoma in Europe

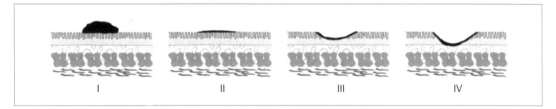

I   II   III   IV

Fig. 9.26   Classification of early carcinoma.

Advanced Gastric Carcinoma

- Borrmann's classification is used (**Fig. 9.27**).

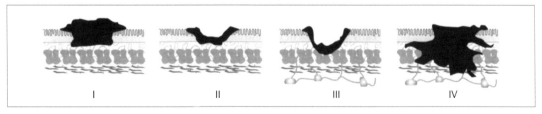

I   II   III   IV

Fig. 9.27   Borrmann classification

Symptoms

- History
- Anorexia, sensation of bloating
- Aversion to meat

9

R0 resection is thus not justified currently outside studies, especially as it is often less well or poorly tolerated in gastrectomy patients with weight loss.

- In a prospective randomized study (Intergroup-116), a survival advantage was found for patients with locally advanced gastric carcinoma who received adjuvant chemoradiotherapy compared with surgical treatment alone. However, the study has method-related difficulties, for example, because many of these patients did not have adequate (D2) LN resection.

Neoadjuvant Chemotherapy

- Might be superior to adjuvant therapy for the following reasons:
  - ► The general and nutritional status of the patients is better preoperatively.
  - ► Downsizing of the tumor might result in a higher rate of R0 resections.
  - ► The tumor cells can be tackled earlier by starting systemic treatment preoperatively.
- Neoadjuvant chemotherapy is not yet standard for locally advanced and potentially R0 resectable tumors. In this case, too, there are method-related difficulties in the available prospective randomized phase II and III studies (e.g., UK MAGIC trial).
- Whether to employ the therapy—for example, to try to downsize a tumor that is not initially definitely R0-resectable or to treat a nonresectable gastric carcinoma in order ultimately to achieve R0 resection—must be decided on an individual basis.

It is not yet possible to assess which concept will become established as standard for locally advanced gastric carcinoma. Whether adjuvant chemoradiotherapy or neoadjuvant radiotherapy is useful should be investigated by including the patients in randomized phase III studies.

■ Surgical Treatment

Principles of Curative Surgery of Gastric Carcinoma

- D2 lymphadenectomy is standard in gastric carcinoma.
- Splenectomy is rarely indicated.

- In principle, R0 resection is the key to curative treatment.
- The tubular extent of resection is guided by the Lauren histological subtype, the location of the tumor, and the tumor stage. In principle the greater and lesser omentum and the regional lymph drainage regions are removed.
- Respect **safety margins:**
  - ► Intestinal type: 4–5 cm proximal safety margin
  - ► Diffuse type: 8–10 cm proximal safety margin, so usually total gastrectomy
  - ► Distal safety margin includes a duodenal cuff of ca. 3 cm in situ.
- **Standard lymphadenectomy** includes compartments I and II (see **Fig. 9.1**). Extended lymphadenectomy (compartment III) is not required by the UICC (International Union Against Cancer) for pN classification. It is not routine treatment. An improvement in survival due to lymphadenectomy can be expected only for patients with N1 or early N2 metastasis, equivalent to tumor stages II and IIIa.
- Remove the anterior layer of the mesocolon and the anterior capsule of the pancreas.
- Extended D2 lymphadenectomy. No advantage for D3 lymphadenectomy. The LNs of compartment III are regarded as distant metastases. The benefit of lymphadenectomy has not been confirmed beyond doubt; at best, minor LN metastases benefit from consistent lymphadenectomy.

- Splenectomy if strictly indicated: direct tumor penetration into the hilum of the spleen or splenic vessels, tumor involving the entire stomach; tumor in the greater curvature close to the spleen with obligatory lymph drainage through the splenic hilum is a relative indication.

Laparoscopic and Endoscopic Procedures

Endoscopic Mucosal Resection (EMR)
- The mucosa with the tumor is first aspirated and then resected endoscopically.

Laparoscopic Intragastric Mucosal Resection
- The tumor is marked gastroscopically.
- Insertion of three trocars into the lumen of the stomach, introduction of the laparoscope into the stomach, tumor inspection, and determination of resection boundaries
- Elevation of the mucosa by injection of saline
- En-bloc resection of the tumor with thermocautery or ultrasonic dissector
- Removal of the specimen through the gastroscope

This method is employed when EMR is technically too difficult. Through the simultaneous use of the laparoscope and gastroscope, the resection boundaries and thus adequate safety margins can be determined exactly.

Laparoscopic Endoscopic Local Wedge Excision
- Laparoscopic tangential resection of the gastric wall (wedge resection) using the "lesion-lifting" method. The tumor is marked gastroscopically. A T-lifter is advanced through the abdominal wall into the lumen of the stomach. The tumor must not be penetrated. With the T-lifter, the tumor is elevated and then resected tangentially with the stapling device under endoscopic control.
- The specimen is removed in a retrieval bag.

This method can be used when EMR is too difficult technically. Laparoscopic intragastric mucosal resection is preferable. The advantages are avoidance of R1 resection and a postoperative ulcer due to wedge resection.

9

Gastrectomy for Gastric Carcinoma

Operative Technique

- Typical **extent of resection:** from the level of the cardia to ca. 3 cm distal to the pylorus. Removal of the greater omentum en bloc with the stomach. Standard D2 lymphadenectomy of compartments I and II.
- **Access routes:**
  - ➤ Transverse upper abdominal laparotomy
  - ➤ Upper median laparotomy, if necessary with incision around the left of the umbilicus
- **Exploration:**
  - ➤ Tumor size and position
  - ➤ Resectability
  - ➤ Exclusion of metastases, intraoperative ultrasonography (open/laparoscopic)

- Sharp division of the greater omentum with the gastrocolic ligament from the transverse colon taking the anterior layer of the mesocolon. Dissection as far as the lower border of the pancreas. Division of the duodenocolic and splenocolic ligaments
- Division of the right gastroepiploic artery at its origin from the gastroduodenal artery at the lower border of the duodenum (pylorus)
- Kocherization of the duodenum. Dissection of the parapyloric LN (LN 5 + 6)
- Ligation of the right gastric artery at its root
- Removal of the lesser omentum as close as possible to the liver and as far as the cardia
- Excision of the duodenum two fingerbreadths (3 cm) distal to the pylorus. TA stapler or open excision with retaining sutures. Closure of the duodenal stump (see below) depending on the planned reconstruction method
- Removal of the LNs along the common hepatic artery and celiac trunk (LN 8 + 9)
- Division of the left gastric artery near its origin, double ligature (LN 7)
- Blunt circular mobilization of the esophagus including paracardiac LNs (LN 1 + 3)
- Dissection toward the left along the splenic artery (LN 11), splenectomy if indicated
- Truncal division of the vagus; the esophagus can then be better mobilized into the abdomen
- Division of the esophagus, usually after placing a clamp for a purse-string suture

Consequences of Total Gastrectomy

- Regular vitamin B12 replacement is important after gastrectomy.

- Severe treatment-resistant reflux esophagitis
- Dumping syndrome
- Loss of reservoir function and absence of sensation of hunger and appetite
- Iron deficiency anemia and megaloblastic anemia. Therefore vitamin B12 replacement 1000 µg every 3 months
- If splenectomy is performed, pneumococcal vaccination is given 2–3 weeks postoperatively.

Distal Gastric Resection

Operative Technique

- Typical extent of resection: resection of distal four-fifths (**Fig. 9.28**). On the lesser curvature to 1–2 cm distal to the cardia; on the greater curvature depending on tumor site. Safety margin: distally at least 2 cm beyond the pylorus. Removal of the greater omentum en bloc with the stomach. D2 lymphadenectomy of compartments I and II.
- Procedure as in total gastrectomy
- No splenectomy because of the perfusion of the gastric stump (see **Fig. 9.1**)
- Reconstruction as in Billroth II resection:
  - ► Antecolic-anisoperistaltic (or isoperistaltic) gastrojejunostomy, Braun anastomosis between afferent and efferent loops
  - ► Roux gastrojejunostomy

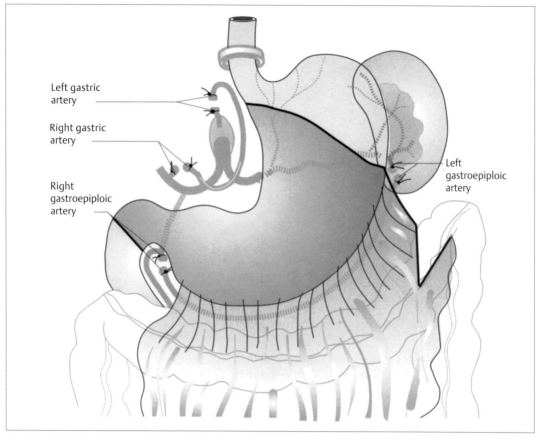

Fig. 9.28 Distal gastrectomy, typical extent of resection.

Left gastric
artery

Right gastric
artery

Right
gastroepiploic
artery

Left
gastroepiploic
artery

Multivisceral Resection

Distal Pancreatectomy
- **Indications:**
    - Carcinomas penetrating the posterior wall of the stomach that have infiltrated the tail or body of the pancreas
    - Isolated LN metastases in stations 14 and 16. These can be removed completely by distal pancreatectomy.

Operative Technique

- Removal of the spleen (**Fig. 9.29**):
    - Dissect the spleen from the left from fetal adhesions. It is elevated from its bed and held medially under tension.
    - Expose and ligate the splenic artery and vein.
- Blunt dissection of the pancreas from its bed; lateral capsule is divided with scissors (**Fig. 9.30**)
- Fishmouth excision of the pancreas (together with the spleen) to the left of the superior mesenteric vein (**Fig. 9.31**)

9

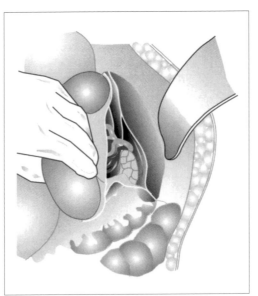

Fig. 9.29   Dissection of the spleen.

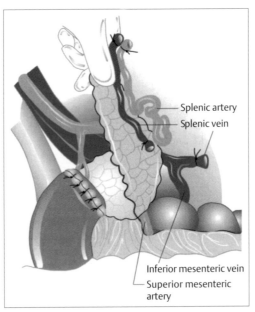

Fig. 9.30   Dissection of the pancreas.

Splenic artery
Splenic vein
Inferior mesenteric vein
Superior mesenteric artery

9

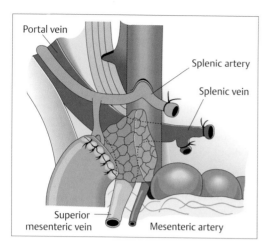

Fig. 9.31 The pancreas is excised.

- The pancreatic resection surface is managed with purse-string sutures and the pancreatic duct is closed with a Z-suture.
- Adenectomy of LN stations 14 and 16 (para-aortic, left renal hilum)
- Easy-Flow drain at the pancreatic stump to treat potential fistulas

Segmental Resection of the Transverse Colon
- **Indication:** tumor infiltration of the mesocolon or transverse colon

Operative Technique

- Mobilization of the hepatic and splenic flexure
- Resection of the segment containing tumor, ligature of the middle colic artery at its root
- Wedge-shaped resection of the corresponding part of the mesocolon
- Single row end-to-end anastomosis

Reconstruction Methods after Gastrectomy (Overview)

A distinction is made between
- preservation of duodenal passage or exclusion of duodenal passage, and
- pouch creation or omission of pouch creation.

In over 75% of clinics, reconstruction is performed by a simple Roux-en-Y end-to-side esophagojejunostomy. Creation of a pouch has shown marginal advantages for quality of life in a few studies.

Small bowel interposition (Longmire method) is performed in only one in every seven or eight patients. The esophageal reflux of bile is a disadvantage. If the use of jejunum is not possible, large bowel is used in rare cases. No functional advantages have been found for any of these methods compared with the technically simpler and lower-risk Roux-en-Y reconstruction.

Functions of the Substitute Stomach
- Reservoir function (most important)
- Avoidance of esophageal reflux

9

- Roux-en-Y reconstruction is the most frequent method of restoring continuity/passage.

- Portioned passage of food into the small bowel without accelerated enteral passage

Restoration of Continuity

- No advantages were found in studies for restoration of the passage to the duodenum.

- **Without duodenal passage** (**Fig. 9.32**):
  - ► The first substitute stomach procedure, without duodenal passage, was performed by Schlatter. This was an end-to-side esophagojejunostomy, but this is now obsolete because of the excessive reflux.
  - ► Roux popularized the Y anastomosis of the afferent loop, which is now implanted at least 40 cm distal to the esophagojejunostomy to prevent reflux.
  - ► Hunt supplemented this technique by forming a pouch. Protection of the gastrojejunal anastomosis by different kinds of jejunoplication followed later.
- **With duodenal passage** (**Fig. 9.33**):
  - ► Creation of a substitute stomach with duodenal passage using jejunal interposition was first described by Seo and developed by Longmire, Gütgemann (lengthening of the loop to enlarge the reservoir), and Schreiber (jejunoplication to cover the esophagojejunal anastomosis).
  - ► Apart from the supposed physiological conditions, preservation of duodenal passage has not been shown to confer any significant pathophysiological benefits, such as improved glucose metabolism, increased absorption of iron and calcium, or better pancreatic function. The interposed loop of jejunum should be long (ca. 40 cm), on the one hand to increase the reservoir and on the other hand to avoid the frequent reflux.
  - ► The Merendino operation for AEG tumors is an exception. In essence, this consists of anisoperistaltic interposition of a segment of jejunum with a vascular pedicle and has been experiencing a renaissance in recent years.

Tactical Considerations

- The choice of procedure is guided by the patient's condition, the radicality of the operation, the surgeon's operative experience, and the prognosis.
- Nowadays, the Roux-en-Y reconstruction is preferred for carcinomas that are resectable for cure.
- Roux-en-Y reconstruction rather than an interposition operation is also feasible in palliative surgery or in risk patients.

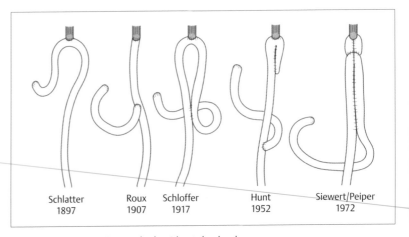

| Schlatter 1897 | Roux 1907 | Schloffer 1917 | Hunt 1952 | Siewert/Peiper 1972 |

Fig. 9.32 Reconstruction methods without duodenal passage.

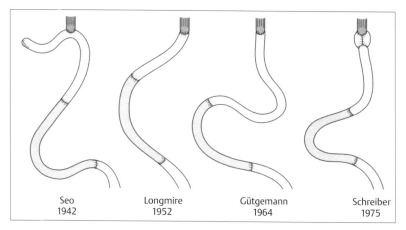

| Seo | Longmire | Gütgemann | Schreiber |
| 1942 | 1952 | 1964 | 1975 |

Fig. 9.33   Reconstruction methods with duodenal passage.

Jejunum Interposition (Isoperistaltic) after Seo, Longmire, Gütgemann, Schreiber

Operative Technique

Obtaining the Interposition Graft
- Selection of the 2nd jejunal loop ca. 15–20 cm distal to the ligament of Treitz. Graft length: ca. 35–45 cm. The resection boundaries are determined by the vascular supply. This is checked with diaphanoscopy. The interposition graft must be supplied by a substantial mesenteric artery through arcades (**Fig. 9.34**).
- Division of the mesentery and mobilization of the interposition graft preserving the marginal arcade
- Excision of the jejunal loop between rows of staples

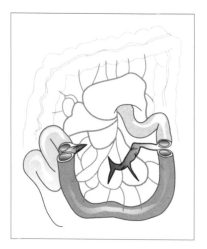

Fig. 9.34   Selection of the 2nd jejunal loop.

9

Placement of the Interposition Graft
- Incise the mesocolon in a region free of blood vessels and draw the jejunal loop up behind the colon (**Fig. 9.35**).

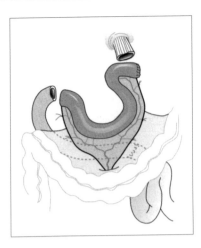

Fig. 9.35 Placement of the interposition graft.

- End-to-end jejunojejunostomy of the site of removal
- Closure of the opening in the mesentery (3–0 absorbable)

Esophagojejunostomy
- **End-to-side esophagojejunostomy using staples (Fig. 9.36):**
  - ► Resection of the oral row of staples of the interposition graft; check the perfusion in the region of the anastomosis, further resection if necessary
  - ► Stretch the oral end of the interposition graft with dressing forceps; introduce the CEEA stapler, magazine size 25–28 mm; short incision of the interposition graft on the antimesenteric side 7 cm distal to the oral end or 15 cm if jejunoplication is planned; purse-string suture; pass the spike through this incision
  - ► Purse-string suture in the distal esophagus; concentric stretching with dressing forceps; insertion of back plate for the CEEA device in the distal esophagus; tie the purse-string suture
  - ► Approximation of the stapler, connection with the back plate, close the instrument and fire to complete the anastomosis
  - ► Check for leaks by insufflation of air or intraluminal blue dye
  - ► Insertion of a triple-lumen tube during end-to-end jejunoduodenostomy in single-row suture through all layers

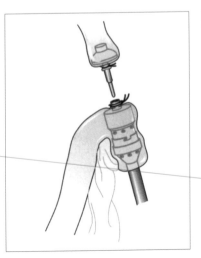

Fig. 9.36 End-to-side esophagojejunostomy (staple technique).

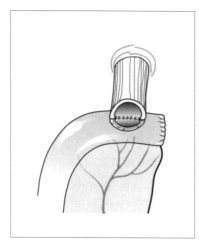

Fig. 9.37 End-to-side esophagojejunostomy (manual suture technique).

- **End-to-side esophagojejunostomy with manual sutures** (Fig. 9.37):
  - ► Attach the jejunum to the posterior wall of the esophagus with 3–0 monofilament absorbable sutures (the suture includes serosa and muscularis of the jejunum and adventitia and muscularis of the esophagus).
  - ► Incision of the jejunum 3–5 cm wide, 4–6 cm from the blind end, or 15 cm from the blind end if jejunoplication is planned
  - ► Suture of the posterior wall in all layers, close together, 3-mm distance between sutures, 5-mm distance from wound margin. The sutures are first placed, then tied. The knots are intraluminal.
  - ► Similar single row of sutures through all layers in the anterior wall. The knots are extraluminal.
  - ► Check the anastomosis for leaks. It must be tension-free and well perfused.
  - ► Rarely: with jejunoplication, insertion of a triple-lumen tube during end-to-end jejunoduodenostomy in a single row of sutures through all layers

Roux Esophagojejunostomy (Fig. 9.38)

Operative Technique

- Closure of the duodenal stump with staples or two-layer interrupted sutures
- Select the 2nd jejunal loop.
- Divide the jejunum between staples at least 20 cm distal to the ligament of Treitz. Dissect the adjacent mesentery, preserving the marginal arcade.
- The distal, blindly closed jejunal loop is drawn up behind the colon.
- End-to-side or end-to-end anastomosis with the esophagus, possibly jejunoplication
- At least 40 cm and up to 60 cm below the esophagojejunostomy, the loop of small bowel coming from the duodenum is anastomosed end-to-side in the form of a Roux-en-Y anastomosis (using a stapler or manual suture through all layers with absorbable 3–0 monofilament).
- Fixation of the small bowel during closure of the opening in the mesocolon

- Roux-en-Y reconstruction is possible with pouch formation or jejunoplication.

9

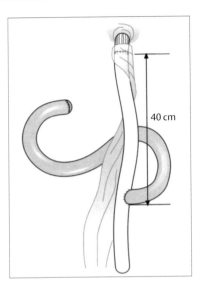

Fig. 9.38 Roux-en-Y esophagojejunostomy

40 cm

Stomach Substitution with Creation of a Pouch

Hunt–Lawrence–Rodino Operation
- Modification of the Roux-en-Y substitute stomach
- End-to-side esophagojejunostomy, the protruding segment is ca. 15 cm long
- Side-to-side enteroenterostomy between the protruding segment and the jejunum, ca. 15 cm long (no jejunoplication)

Herfarth Operation
- Hunt–Lawrence–Rodino pouch supplemented by jejunoplication
- A freely mobile 50-cm loop of upper jejunum is pulled up behind the colon.
- A 15-cm parallel enteroenterostomy is fashioned leaving a centrally mobile loop of intestine.
- Transverse incision of the efferent loop of jejunum at the level of the upper suture pole
- Esophageal anastomosis
- Formation of jejunoplication with the mobile segment of intestine above the anastomosis
- Plication fixed by interrupted sutures

Siewert–Peiper Operation
- Selection of a readily mobile upper loop of jejunum; the loop is pulled up to the upper abdomen behind the colon.
- Creation of a broad, side-to-side enteroenterostomy leaving a mobile loop cranially 6–8 cm in length; the upper pole of the anterior enteroenterostomy is left open and the esophagus is sutured here.
- Formation of the jejunoplication with the loop of bowel remaining free above the anastomosis; the plication is fixed by interrupted sutures.

Kremer Operation
- Selection of a readily mobile upper loop of jejunum 50 cm long; the loop is pulled up to the upper abdomen behind the colon.

- Creation of a broad, side-to-side enteroenterostomy as described above, leaving a mobile 6–8 cm loop cranially
- Division of the loop toward the afferent end with the GIA device
- Perform the anastomosis between the efferent segment and the esophagus with the EEA device as described above.
- Cover the anastomosis with the afferent segment to form a jejunoplication and fix the cuff with interrupted sutures.

■ Palliative Measures

- If residual microscopic tumor remains after presumed R0 resection (R1 resection without distant metastases), further resection should be performed (R0 resection).
- After R2 resection or in the case of gastric carcinoma with distant metastases, purely palliative chemotherapy is indicated.
- Current combinations for palliative chemotherapy:
  - ► **ECF** (epirubicin/cisplatin/5-FU)
  - ► **FLP** (5-FU/folinic acid/[= Leucoverin]/cisplatin)
  - ► **MCF** (mitomycin/cisplatin/5-FU)
  - ► Patients in poor general condition: 5-FU and folinic acid

Palliative Surgery
The goal is restoration of the passage of food in the case of a **stenosing** or **bleeding** and **nonresectable** carcinoma. Several methods are available:
- **Gastroenterostomy** (for stenosis in the distal half of the stomach; **Fig. 9.39**)
- **Esophagogastrostomy,** Heyrowsky method (with stenosis in the upper half of the stomach; **Fig. 9.40**)
- **Tube,** surgical or endoscopic, metal stent, possibly coated:
  - ► Häring (**Fig. 9.41**)
  - ► Celestin
- Witzel fistula (**Fig. 9.42**)
- PEG (percutaneous endoscopic gastrostomy): a transcutaneous external gastric fistula is created under endoscopic control.

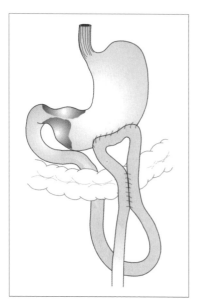

Fig. 9.39 Gastroenterostomy, antecolic with Braun anastomosis.

9

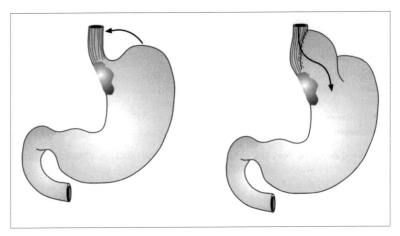

Fig. 9.40   Heyrowsky esophagogastrostomy

Fig. 9.41   Häring tube

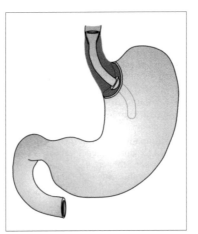

Fig. 9.42   Witzel fistula

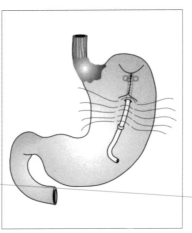

9

Postoperative Care

- Tumor follow-up is guided by the symptoms.
- Since further surgical resection is quite feasible for early recurrences at the anastomosis, regular tumor follow-up is nevertheless recommended.

Prognosis

UICC 5-year survival rates:
- Stage I 70%
- Stage II 30%
- Stage III 10%
- Stage IV 1%

The prognosis in Japan is better, probably because of different biological behavior patterns and a higher proportion of early gastric carcinomas.

■ MALT Lymphoma

Definition

- MALT = mucosa associated lymphatic tissue
- Non-Hodgkin lymphomas are classified into nodal and primary extranodal lymphomas. The MALT lymphomas are among the **primary extranodal non-Hodgkin lymphomas.** Most primary lymphomas of the stomach are MALT lymphomas. There is a close causal association with HP infection.

- MALT lymphomas are associated with HP.

Location

- The extranodal lymphomas are manifested predominantly in the GI tract, with the stomach most frequently affected in 60%–70% of cases.
- The stomach has no primary lymphatic tissue (unlike the physiological MALT of the large and small intestine). Gastric MALT is acquired secondarily. It nearly always arises on the basis of an immune reaction in chronic HP-induced gastritis. This leads to the formation of B lymphatic follicles in the mucosa.
- MALT lymphomas exhibit organ-bound growth for a long time. If metastasis occurs, other MALT organs are affected first, for example, the rest of the GI tract or the tonsils. LN involvement or generalized spread only occurs later in the disease.

9

Histology

- On histopathology, a distinction is made between low-malignancy and highly malignant B-cell lymphomas of the MALT. Moreover, the very rare aggressive T-cell non-Hodgkin lymphomas of the stomach must also be distinguished from B-cell MALT lymphomas (by immunohistochemistry).

Classification

Classification of the Primary Gastrointestinal non-Hodgkin Lymphomas after Isaacson

- **B-cell lymphomas:**
  - ► Lymphomas of the MALT type
  - ► Low-malignancy lymphomas (mainly in the stomach)
  - ► Highly malignant lymphomas with or without a low-malignancy component (mainly in the stomach)
  - ► Immunoproliferative small intestinal disease (IPSID), low, mixed, and highly malignant
  - ► Mantle cell lymphoma (lymphomatous polyposis)
  - ► Burkitt and Burkitt-like lymphoma
  - ► Other B-cell lymphomas that correspond to equivalent nodal lymphomas
- **T-cell lymphomas:**
  - ► Enteropathy-associated T-cell lymphomas (EATLs)
  - ► Other nonenteropathy-associated types

Diagnostic Approach

- History, clinical examination
- Laboratory tests:
  - ► Complete blood count, lactate dehydrogenase (LDH), transaminases, electrophoresis, cholestasis-indicating enzymes, urea, creatinine, electrolytes, urinalysis, paraproteins
  - ► HIV status
  - ► Vitamin B12, folic acid, serum iron, ferritin
- Histopathological classification with distinction of B-cell MALT from highly malignant non-Hodgkin lymphomas and from carcinoma. *Helicobacter pylori* status
- Chest x-ray, ultrasonography of the abdomen, CT of the abdomen and thorax
- Endosonography to determine the depth of infiltration
- Endoscopy with multiple biopsies from suspicious and nonsuspicious areas
- Bone marrow biopsy

Treatment Approach

■ Indication

• MALT lymphomas are treated mainly conservatively.

- A general treatment strategy cannot yet be stated because of the lack of appropriate data. The treatment strategies are still controversial. The main question is: surgical or conservative treatment?
- Because of a lack of experience, the treatment should as far as possible be given only in the framework of controlled studies.

Low-Malignancy Lymphomas (Table 9.7)
- In EII lymphomas according to more recent studies, HP eradication alone appears to be adequate (complete remission in 60%) but follow-up is required (10% remission). Otherwise, R0 resection is recommended in EI1 and EII2 lymphomas with postoperative radiotherapy. Radiation alone is given in the case of inoperability.
- EIII and EIV lymphomas: chemotherapy and radiotherapy are recommended, possibly palliative surgery.

Table 9.7   Staging of lymphoma (modified from Musshoff)

Stage	Description
EI1	Uni- or multilocular involvement of the stomach, the lymphoma is limited to the mucosa and submucosa (so-called early lymphoma)
EI2	As EI1, but the lymphoma passes the submucosa (infiltration of the muscularis propria or serosa) or spread by continuity into an organ
EII1	Uni- or multilocular involvement of the stomach of any infiltration depth including organ involvement by continuity and/or synchronous involvement of the intestine of the same extent and additional involvement of the regional lymph nodes (compartments 1 and 2)
EII2	As EII1, but involvement of the lymph nodes in compartment 3
EIII	Lymphoma involvement of the stomach and lymphoma involvement of both sides of the diaphragm including further localized organ involvement in the gastrointestinal tract including the Waldeyer ring
EIV	Gastric lymphoma, all corresponding lymph nodes involved and diffuse disseminated involvement of one or more extragastric organs

Highly Malignant Lymphomas
- EI1 and EII2 lymphomas: chemotherapy, possibly resection
- EIII and EIV lymphomas: chemotherapy and radiotherapy

■ Conservative Treatment

Chemotherapy
- The CHOP or CVI regimen is employed (cyclophosphamide, vincristine, prednisolone).
- Good results were achieved in highly malignant nodal lymphomas. There is as yet insufficient information about the results in MALT lymphoma.

Radiotherapy
- Postoperative radiotherapy is established with low-malignancy gastric lymphoma grades EI and EII.

■ Surgical Treatment

Surgery has therapeutic and diagnostic purposes. Depending on the tumor location, subtotal gastrectomy or total gastrectomy including lymph node dissection of compartments I and II.

Further Reading

Guglielmi A, Ruzzenente A, Sandri M, et al. Risk assessment and prediction of rebleeding in bleeding gastroduodenal ulcer. Endoscopy 2002; 34: 778–786

Ripoll C, Banares R, Beceiro I, et al. Comparison of transcatheter arterial embolization and surgery for treatment of bleeding peptic ulcer after endoscopic treatment failure. J Vasc Interv Radiol 2004; 15: 447–450

Tytgat GNJ, Tytgat SHAJ. Grading and Staging in Gastroenterology. Stuttgart: Thieme; 2008

Van Leerdam ME, Vreeburg EM, Rauws EA, et al. Acute upper GI bleeding: did anything change? Time trend analysis of incidence and outcome of acute upper GI bleeding between 1993/1994 and 2000. Am J Gastroenterol 2003; 98: 1494–1499

Wu AW, Xu GW, Wang HY, Ji JF, Tang JL. Neoadjuvant chemotherapy versus none for resectable gastric cancer. Cochrane Database Syst Rev 2007 Apr 18; (2): CD005047. Review

Wagner AD, Unverzagt S, Grothe W, et al. Chemotherapy for advanced gastric cancer. Cochrane Database Syst Rev 2010 Mar 17; (3): CD004064

9

10 Small Intestine

I.L. Schmalbach

■ Anatomy

- Jejunum and ileum, length ca. 4–6 m
- Blood supply by branches of the superior mesenteric artery in several arcade levels

- The small intestine consists anatomically of the duodenum, jejunum, and ileum but surgically it comprises the jejunum and ileum, extending from the duodenojejunal flexure (ligament of Treitz) to the ileocecal valve (Bauhin valve).
- Intraperitoneal position: highly mobile due to flexible mesentery
- Extensive blood supply through branches of the superior mesenteric artery: jejunal and ileal arteries with up to five arcade levels
- Duodenum: branches of the celiac trunk
- Venous drainage through branches of the superior mesenteric vein into the portal vein
- Lymphatic drainage alongside the arteries
- Extrinsic nerve fibers from the celiac and superior mesenteric plexus accompany the arteries.
- Layers of the bowel wall (from within outward): mucosa (Kerckring folds, which diminish from the jejunum to the ileum), submucosa (vascular layer of the mucosa, Peyer patches in the ileum are mucosa-associated lymphatic tissue), circular muscle layer and longitudinal muscle layer with the myenteric plexus between them, serosa

■ Crohn Disease

Definition

- Granulomatous inflammation of the entire bowel wall, which can occur in the entire gastrointestinal tract from the lips to the anus.

- Chronic inflammatory bowel disease (CIBD) of unclear etiology
- Granulomatous inflammatory reaction involving the entire bowel wall including the mesenteric fat (typical macroscopic sign: "creeping fat" extending into the bowel wall) and regional lymph nodes
- Relapsing disease course with highly acute symptomatic phases and remission periods of varying length
- All parts of the gastrointestinal tract (lips to anus) can be involved; typically discontinuous segmental involvement ("skip lesions").
- Frequency of involvement: terminal ileum up to 80% (terminal ileitis, rectum involved at the same time in 20%), colon only 30% (Crohn colitis), ileocecal 30% (regional enterocolitis), proximal small intestine 5%–10%, stomach/duodenum 2%–3%, esophagus 0–1% (see **Fig. 10.1**)

Epidemiology

- Incidence 7–9/100 000 per year
- Prevalence 200/100 000

- Prevalence (increasing in the past 20 years) 200 per 100 000 population; incidence 7–9 per 100 000 population per year
- Men and women affected equally often

- Onset usually between the ages of 16 and 35 years or after the age of 60 years
- Familial and ethnic prevalence: white-skinned persons develop the disease about twice as often as dark-skinned.

Etiology

Suggested possible causal/predisposing factors include:
- Autoimmune processes
- Nicotine (abstention has a favorable effect on the disease course, but this is not the case in ulcerative colitis)
- Gene defects (NOD 2/CARD 15, chromosome 16)
- *Mycobacterium pseudotuberculosis*
- Altered bowel flora
- Diet (excessive fat and meat)
- Excessive hygiene
- Psychosomatic
- Overall, there is an imbalance between pro- and anti-inflammatory factors.

- CIBD of unclear etiology

Classification

Crohn Disease Activity Index (CDAI) after Best (Table 10.1)
- Instrument for classifying Crohn disease into degrees of severity, expression of disease activity
- Assessment of disease course and efficacy of medication
- CDAI up to 150 points: remission
- CDAI 150–220 points: mild to moderate inflammatory activity
- CDAI 220–450 points: moderate to severe inflammatory activity
- CDAI over 450 points: very severe inflammatory activity
- A positive response to therapy is assumed when the CDAI decreases by more than 100 points.

- CDAI to determine Crohn activity and for monitoring course

Table 10.1 Determination of the CDAI using eight criteria and their weighting

Clinical variable/laboratory parameter	Weighting factor
Average number of liquid or soft stools daily over 7 days	× 2
Average abdominal pain (grade 0–3) over 7 days	× 5
Average subjective general condition (grade 0–4) over 7 days	× 7
Presence of complications or extraintestinal manifestations[a]	× 20
Use of opiates as antidiarrheal agent	× 30
Presence of abdominal guarding (0 for none, 2 for doubtful, 5 for definite)	× 10
Alteration in hematocrit (47% in men, 42% in women)	× 6
Percentage difference from standard weight	× 1

[a] One point is given for each of the following complications: arthralgia or arthritis; iritis or uveitis; erythema nodosum, pyoderma gangrenosum, aphthous ulcers; anal fissures, fistulas, abscesses; other fistulas; fever in the previous week (>37.8°C).

10

Symptoms

- Right lower abdominal pain, diarrhea without blood, abscesses, fistulas

- Abdominal pain, often in the right lower abdomen (mimics appendicitis)
- Nausea, vomiting, weight loss, anorexia
- Palpable guarding/loop in right lower abdomen
- Moderate pyrexia
- Diarrhea, usually *not* mixed with blood, in contrast to ulcerative colitis
- With chronic course recurrent (sub-)ileus states, septic temperatures, abscess formation, fistula formation
- Bile acid loss syndrome: cholelithiasis, chologenic fatty stools, nephrolithiasis
- Extraintestinal manifestations in 10–20% of Crohn patients: arthritis of the large joints 4%–16%, sacroiliitis 4%–20%, gallstones up to 30%, kidney stones 10%, fibrosing alveolitis, erythema nodosum 15%–25%, pyoderma gangrenosum, aphthous stomatitis 10%–20%, conjunctivitis, uveitis, and iritis

Diagnostic Approach

■ Laboratory Tests

- Assessment of disease activity and treatment course, for differential diagnosis
- Raised CRP level and ESR, leukocytosis, anemia, vitamin B12 deficiency, iron deficiency, ANA, ANCA, antibodies to *Saccharomyces cerevisiae* (differential diagnosis from ulcerative colitis)
- Stool cultures with serology: detection of pathogenic microorganisms, exclusion of sprue (gliadin antibodies)

■ Diagnostic Imaging

Radiography (Gastrointestinal Series, Colon Contrast Enema, CT)
- Segmental pattern of involvement, in contrast to ulcerative colitis
- Macroscopic cobblestone pattern, threadlike discontinuous stenoses, wall rigidity ("garden hose" appearance due to fibrosis), linear ulcers
- Assessment of extent and degree of stenosis morphologically and functionally
- Conglomerate masses, abscesses, wall thickening, differential diagnosis

Ultrasonography
- Imaging of abscesses, wall thickening, stenosis, free fluid
- Evidence of differential diagnoses

■ Invasive Investigations

Endoscopy (Incl. Terminal Ileum)
- Alternating healthy and inflamed mucosa, discontinuous extension
- Characteristic lesions: erosions, aphthous ulcers, "cobblestone pattern," fistulas, longitudinal ulcers, inflammatory stenosis
- Biopsy, histology: lymphocytes, eosinophilic granulocytes, histiocytes, epithelioid cell granulomas, microgranulomas, multinucleated giant cells

- Most important investigation: endoscopy with biopsy and histological confirmation
- Discontinuous involvement, in contrast to ulcerative colitis

10

■ **Differential Diagnosis**

* Most important differential diagnosis is ulcerative colitis (**Fig. 10.1** and **Table 10.2**; see also Chapter 12)
* Appendicitis, diverticulitis
* Ischemic, infectious, drug-induced, radiation-induced, postoperative colitis
* Irritable bowel syndrome

Treatment Approach (Fig. 10.2)

■ **Indication**

* Cure of Crohn disease is not possible, conservative therapy should be continued as long as possible and useful.
* Complications often represent an indication for surgery.

* Surgery often indicated for complications

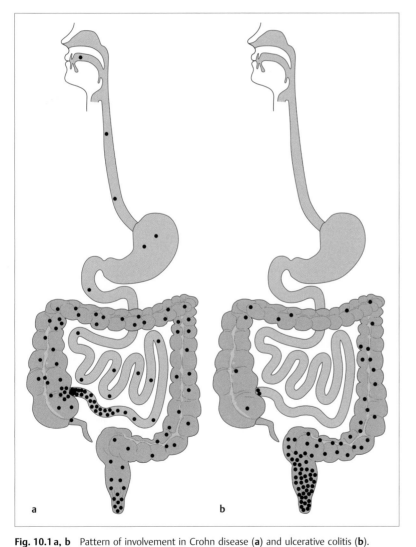

Fig. 10.1 a, b   Pattern of involvement in Crohn disease (**a**) and ulcerative colitis (**b**).

10

Table 10.2 **Differential diagnosis of the inflammatory bowel diseases, Crohn disease / ulcerative colitis**

Criterion	Crohn disease	Ulcerative colitis
Location (**Fig. 10.1**)	Entire GI tract possible, predominantly ileum and ascending colon	Rectum and colon (ascending) only
Inflammation level	Entire bowel wall	Mucosa only
Rectal involvement	20%	Obligatory
Ileal involvement	Up to 80%	Rarely as "backwash ileitis"
Extent	Discontinuous/segmental	Continuous, ascending
Symptoms, clinical signs	Non-bloody diarrhea, palpable loop in right lower abdomen	Bloody/mucous diarrhea
Extraintestinal manifestations	Frequent	Rare
Radiographic signs	Cobblestone pattern Wall rigidity ("garden hose") Stenoses Longitudinal ulcers	Collar stud ulcers Pseudopolyps Atonic dilatation Toxic megacolon
Endoscopic signs	Aphthous lesions Sharp ulcerations Cobblestone pattern Stenoses Fistulas	Diffuse mucosal erythema Unsharp ulcers Pseudopolyps Vulnerability Contact bleeding
Histology	Epithelioid cell granulomas Giant cells	Crypt abscesses Reduction in goblet cells
Typical complications	Fistulas Stenosis Abscesses Conglomerate masses	Toxic megacolon Bleeding/anemia
Cure	Not possible	Possible by proctocolectomy with ileoanal anastomosis

10

- Disease-modifying therapy: local therapy with mesalazine or, ideally, budesonide
- Systemic corticosteroids (prednisolone) and/or immunosuppressants (azathioprine, 6-mercaptopurine) in severe cases
- A further alternative: anti-TNFα antibody

■ **Conservative Treatment**

The type of treatment depends on:
- The current disease situation (cf. CDAI): acute relapse, remission, chronic activity
- The course: chronic recurrent or active, complicated, steroid-refractory
- The pattern of involvement: terminal ileitis, Crohn colitis, extraintestinal

The success of treatment is assessed from the clinical course and not from the intestinal morphology, and also from a drop in the CDAI by at least 100 points.

Acute Relapse with Mild to Moderate Activity
(All stated doses apply for adults.)
- Mesalazine (5-aminosalicylic acid: 5-ASA, for example Pentasa, Salofalk, Claversal): 3–4 g/d
- When involvement is predominantly ileocecal: budesonide (e.g., Entocort capsules or suppositories, Budenofalk capsules or rectal foam): 9 mg/d

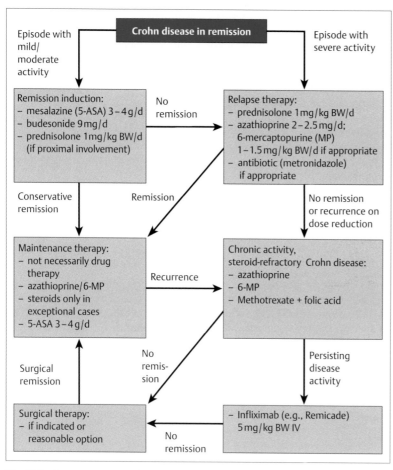

Fig. 10.2   Treatment regimen for Crohn disease.

- Alternatively or with proximal involvement: prednisolone 1 mg/kg body weight (BW) per day

Acute Relapse with Severe Activity
- Prednisolone 1mg/kg BW per day
- With frequent relapses (over two per year): azathioprine (e.g., Imuran): 2–2.5 mg/kg BW per day or 6-mercaptopurine (e.g., Puri Nethol): 1–1.5 mg/kg BW per day in addition
- Parenteral nutrition or residue-free liquid diet if appropriate
- In the case of fistulas, abscesses, colon or rectal involvement: metronidazole (e.g., Flagyl), 500 mg b.d. IV

Chronic Active Form, Steroid-Refractory Crohn Disease
- Defined as persistent or recurrent symptoms for 6 months with previous adequate therapy
- Long-term use of azathioprine or 6-mercaptopurine
- The drug of second choice is methotrexate: 25 mg/week IM, and 15 mg after remission; folic acid 2.5–5 mg/week in addition.

10

- Infliximab 5 mg/kg IV per day (e.g., Remicade, anti-TNFα monoclonal antibody): reserve medication for persistent high disease activity despite adequate medication with steroids and azathioprine (steroid-refractory Crohn disease)
- Replacement of calories, proteins, electrolytes, vitamins, and iron in malabsorption syndrome
- Surgical treatment when indicated

Long-Term Treatment / Maintenance of Remission
- No general treatment recommendation for all patients
- Indication, choice of medication, and duration of therapy are determined individually
- Important: abstention from nicotine
- Steroids unsuitable
- Patients with complex disease course: azathioprine/6-mercaptopurine
- Alternatively: methotrexate or anti-TNF-α antibody

■ Surgical Treatment

- A surgical cure is not possible.
- Surgery is indicated only for complications.

Crohn disease cannot be cured by surgery. However, an operative procedure will be necessary sooner or later in 90% of patients because of a complication (p. 183). Because of the high recurrence rate, most of the affected patients have to undergo surgery repeatedly in the course of their disease.

Principles of Surgical Treatment
- Conservative therapy as long as possible
- Strict indication for surgery, only in the case of complications
- With small bowel resections, always strive for as little as possible, as much as necessary.
- Strive for the least possible trauma.
- Perform skeletonization close to the bowel wall.
- Anastomoses are always end-to-end, as end-to-side anastomoses lead to blind loop syndromes with recurrence of Crohn disease in them.
- Preferably use single row, all-layer (possibly extramucosal) continuous suture techniques with absorbable monofilament material to avoid fistulas.
- Do not use staplers (they cause fistulas).
- As far as possible, do not use intra-abdominal drains (they cause fistulas).
- If appropriate, defunction the affected segments of bowel/operation areas by creating a stoma.

Stenosis in the Duodenum
- Perform bypass operation with gastrojejunostomy or duodenojejunostomy.
- Depending on position, stricture repair may also be adequate (longitudinal opening of the bowel, transverse single row continuous suture; frequent measure for small bowel stenosis).

Stenosis in the Small Bowel or Colon/Rectum
- Sparing segmental resection or ileocecal resection with anastomosis
- Hartmann discontinuous resection for isolated rectal involvement
- Creation of a protective stoma, if appropriate
- Stricture repair, if appropriate

Fistulas

Always strive for a sparing resection of the diseased bowel segment with the origin of the fistula plus:

- Curetting of the fistula with a sharp curette or excision outward (enterocutaneous)
- Excision and oversewing of the fistula opening in healthy bowel (entero-enteric)
- Oversewing of the fistula opening in the bladder (enterovesical) or vagina (enterovaginal)
- Insertion of a mesh plug retroperitoneally after draining the abscess (retroperitoneal fistula)
- Incision of the abscess and if appropriate laying open the fistula in the case of perianal fistulas; create a diverting stoma if there is a risk of sphincter damage, and also if there is an extensive fistula system.

- Strive for minimal tissue trauma and extent of surgery; resect sparingly.

Complications

Stenosis

- Due to scarring of the inflamed segments of bowel
- Most frequent indication for surgery in Crohn disease when there are increasing symptoms of intestinal obstruction

- Stenosis, fistula, abscess, and perforation are frequently indications for surgery.

Fistulas

- **Perianal fistulas:**
  - ► Most frequent complication of Crohn disease, often the first manifestation
  - ► High rate of spontaneous healing or good healing after minor surgery, but high recurrence rate
  - ► Simple fistulas extend from the submucosal dentate line to the skin and can simply be opened.
  - ► Complex fistulas (high fistulas) originate from the intestine or rectum and require more complex treatment and surgical concepts (see Chapter 14).
- **Enterocutaneous fistulas:**
  - ► Relatively rare, usually a result of suture failure or anastomotic recurrence
  - ► Usually located before a stenosis
  - ► Surgery is usually indicated for definitive healing.
- **Entero-enteric fistulas:**
  - ► Often asymptomatic for a long time
  - ► Can lead to a malabsorption or maldigestion syndrome
- **Enterovesical fistulas:**
  - ► Cause cystitis or pyelonephritis
  - ► Absolute indication for surgery
- **Enterogenital fistulas**
  - ► Usually manifested as enterovaginal fistulas
  - ► Absolute indication for surgery
- **Retroperitoneal fistulas**
  - ► Blindly ending fistulas with retroperitoneal abscess formation
  - ► Surgery indicated if symptomatic

Abscess Formation

- Intra-abdominal, retroperitoneal, perianal, entero-enteric loop abscesses, subcutaneous, epifascial

10

Perforations
- As free perforation with rapid progression of inflammation ("hot Crohn's") and (still) lack of cover by adjacent tissue
- Emergency surgery is indicated for toxic dilatation of the bowel similar to toxic megacolon.

■ Meckel Diverticulum

- Possible complications: bleeding, perforation, inflammation, ileus, intussusception, volvulus
- In childhood always removed when discovered during appendectomy

- Fetal yolk stalk remnant due to failure of the omphalomesenteric duct to obliterate
- Located in the ileum, 60–90 cm above the ileocecal valve, antimesenteric
- Incidence: 2%–3% of the population
- Usually an incidental finding at appendectomy: clinical signs can be identical, and if the appendix is normal, a Meckel diverticulum must be sought.
- Characteristic: presence of ectopic gastric mucosa or pancreatic tissue in the diverticulum
- Complications: bleeding, perforation, inflammation, ileus, intussusception, volvulus
- Complication rate decreases with increasing age.
- Treatment: removal of the diverticulum by wedge resection or resection of a segment of the small intestine
- An incidentally discovered Meckel diverticulum is always removed in childhood, but in adulthood it can be left in situ in the definite absence of complications.

■ Jejunal Diverticulum

- Usually asymptomatic in the upper jejunum; serious complications can be caused especially by bleeding and perforation.

- Small bowel diverticula are rare (0.5%–1% of the population).
- They occur in the duodenum and upper jejunum, in about two-thirds of cases as diverticulosis on the mesenteric side of the jejunum.
- Congenital, true diverticula, and acquired pseudodiverticula may occur.
- Usually an asymptomatic finding
- Symptoms with complications: diverticulitis, bleeding, perforation, peritonitis, ileus, fistula formation
- In pure diverticulitis, conservative therapy with intravenous antibiotics
- Surgical treatment by resection of the segment of small intestine with the diverticula, end-to-end anastomosis; if appropriate placement of a jejunal tube through the anastomosis for early enteral nutrition

Further Reading

De Cruz P, Prideaux L, Wagner J, et al. Characterization of the gastrointestinal microbiota in health and inflammatory bowel disease. Inflamm Bowel Dis 2011 May 20. doi: 10.1002/ibd.21751. [Epub ahead of print]

Messmann H. Atlas of Colonoscopy: Examination Techniques and Diagnosis. Stuttgart; Thieme: 2005

Schumpelick V. Atlas of General Surgery. Stuttgart: Thieme; 2009

Strong SA, Koltun WA, Hyman NH, Buie WD; Standards Practice Task Force of The American Society of Colon and Rectal Surgeons. Practice parameters for the surgical management of Crohn's disease. Dis Colon Rectum 2007 Nov; 50(11): 1735–1746

10

11 Vermiform Appendix

I.L. Schmalbach

■ Anatomy

- The appendix is an intestinal appendage, 2–20 cm long and 0.5–1 cm thick, that is situated at the fundus of the cecum, thus forming part of the large intestine.
- Numerous lymph follicles in its wall provide evidence of its immune defence function, especially in early childhood development ("intestinal tonsil").
- Its origin/base is at the junction of the three taeniae coli: omental taenia, free taenia, and mesocolic taenia.
- Intraperitoneal location, mesoappendix (mesentery) with the appendicular artery from the ileocolic artery
- Lymphatic drainage and venous drainage correspond to the region of the ascending colon.
- Variations in position: retrocecal, medial, or lateral to the cecum, in the pelvis (pouch of Douglas), right upper abdomen (e.g., in pregnancy), left lower abdomen (very rarely with situs inversus)

- Part of the large intestine
- Originates at the junction of the taeniae, intraperitoneal

■ Acute Appendicitis

The clinical picture of acute appendicitis can mask nearly any intra-abdominal disease, from harmless gastroenteritis to cancer of the appendix. Acute appendicitis is therefore called the surgical chameleon. The history and clinical symptoms remain the most important criteria for deciding on conservative or surgical treatment.

- Most common differential diagnosis with right-sided lower abdominal pain
- Surgical chameleon

Epidemiology

- In Western countries, 1 person in 10 gets acute appendicitis in the course of his or her life, usually between the ages of 10 and 30 years, and men are affected twice as often as women.

Etiology

Penetration of pathogenic microorganisms into the appendix wall, favored by:
- Stagnation of secretions due to fecaliths/viscous feces or undigested food (most frequent cause)
- Scarring, adhesions
- Parasites: *Enterobius* is found in 3%–5% of children, rarely *Schistosoma* and *Entamoeba*.
- Lymphatic hyperplasia (in childhood)
- Very long appendix with a narrow lumen
- Increase in virulence of otherwise physiological bowel flora due to stasis; mucosal ulceration develops because of the increase in tissue pressure and hypoxia, especially at the tip of the appendix, where perfusion is poorest.

- Increase in virulence due to stasis

11

Classification

Clinical

- Unperforated, perforated, perityphlitic abscess

- Acute
- Subacute
- Chronic recurrent with episodic course

Histopathological
- Catarrhal: hyperemia, swelling, inflammatory exudate
- Ulcerophlegmonous: mucosal erosions, in addition, inflammatory reaction in all layers of the wall
- Gangrenous: irretrievable tissue destruction
- Perforated (closed or free): obvious defect in the wall
- Perityphlitic abscess: collection of pus outside the appendix lumen
- Neurogenic appendicopathy: neural proliferation in the appendix wall

Rare Conditions (see pp. 193–194)
- Endometriosis of the appendix
- Crohn disease
- Diverticulitis of the appendix
- Appendix carcinoid
- Mucinous cystadenoma
- Pseudomyxoma peritonei
- Carcinoma of the appendix

Symptoms

- Onset of pain in epigastrium, later concentrated in right lower abdomen
- Variations in old age, children, and pregnant women

- Classically starts with dull epigastric/right upper abdominal pain ("upset stomach"; visceral pain)
- After 12–24 hours the pain moves to the right lower abdomen as a sharp, stabbing pain (somatic pain).
- Frequent initial concomitant symptoms: nausea, vomiting, anorexia, constipation for feces, and flatus
- Rare concomitant symptom: diarrhea (rather suggests gastroenteritis)
- Pain on shaking when traveling by car or on a stretcher
- Lumbar pain when the appendix is in retrocecal position, alleviated by drawing up the right leg (relieves psoas irritation)
- Mittelschmerz when located in the pouch of Douglas
- Frequently in children: general listlessness, appears quiet and phlegmatic, dark circles around the eyes
- Frequently at an advanced age: mild symptoms sometimes even with advanced disease (50% of cases of appendicitis in the over-60s are already perforated when the diagnosis is made)
- With perforation there may be a pain-free interval of up to a few hours.

Diagnostic Approach

■ Clinical Examination

- Decisive criteria still: clinical signs and examiner's clinical experience

Classical signs of appendicitis and pain points (**Fig. 11.1**):
- **Sherren triangle:** tenderness in the right lower abdomen between the umbilicus, symphysis and right flank
- **McBurney point:** tender point at the middle of an imaginary line (Monro line) between the umbilicus and the anterior superior iliac spine

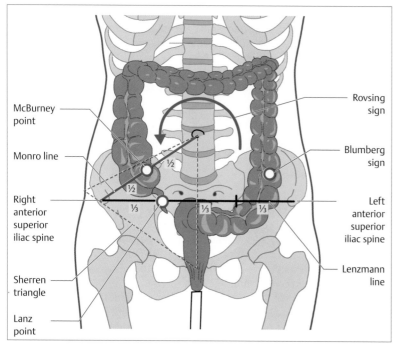

McBurney
point

Monro line

Right
anterior
superior
iliac spine

Sherren
triangle

Lanz
point

Rovsing
sign

Blumberg
sign

Left
anterior
superior
iliac spine

Lenzmann
line

Fig. 11.1   Clinical signs of appendicitis.

- **Lanz point:** tender point at the junction of the middle and right lateral thirds of a line joining the two anterior superior iliac spines (Lenzmann line)
- **Blumberg sign:** pain at McBurney point on abrupt release of contralateral steady pressure over the left lower abdomen
- **Rovsing sign:** pain at McBurney point, when pushing colonic content against cecum
- **Psoas sign:** pain in the right lower abdomen when the extended right leg is elevated against resistance
- **Tenderness in the pouch of Douglas:** present on digital rectal examination on anterior palpation (in young women, obtain gynecologic consultation to rule out pregnancy, ovarian cysts, adnexitis, extrauterine pregnancy, tubo-varian abscess)
- **Vibration pain:** pain in the right lower abdomen when the examination trolley is shaken or when the patient drops onto the heels after standing on tiptoe
- In pregnancy: diagnosis more difficult due to displacement of the appendix into the right upper abdomen; symptoms and laboratory changes often explicable by pregnancy alone
- Graduations of pain intensity on examination: pain on deep palpation, on superficial palpation, local or generalized percussion tenderness, guarding, local or generalized peritonism

11

■ Laboratory Tests

- Leukocytes, CRP, and temperature are the most important markers.

- Leukocytosis > 10/nL with left shift, > 20/nL tends to indicate a different inflammatory event (enteritis, pneumonia, pancreatitis)
- Raised CRP level
- Lipase elevation in pancreatitis as differential diagnosis
- Urine: urinary tract infection as differential diagnosis or signs of appendicitis close to the bladder
- Temperature: axillary temperature > 38°C with a recto-axillary temperature difference > 1°C
- In children: eosinophilia > 5% would suggest enteritis due to worms.

■ Diagnostic Imaging

Ultrasonography (Fig. 11.2)

- There is a close positive correlation between the examiner's experience and relevance of findings.
- **Caution:** failure to image the appendix does not rule out appendicitis.
- CT and MRI can be used in cases of doubt.

- Sensitivity: 75%–93%, specificity 90%–99%, very highly operator-dependent
- Tubular (longitudinal) or targetlike (transverse), fluid-filled, hyporeflecting structure in the right lower abdomen without peristalsis, hardly or not compressible
- Maximum tenderness over aforementioned pathological structure
- Appendix diameter > 6–8 mm
- Free fluid in the right lower abdomen and/or pouch of Douglas
- Decreased peristalsis in the right lower abdomen with peritoneal irritation
- Exclusion of disease of other organs (liver, gallbladder, kidneys, bladder, colon, uterus, ovary)

Radiography

- Appendicography with colon contrast imaging is now obsolete.
- Plain abdominal x-ray in left lateral position: when other findings are unclear, to exclude free intra-abdominal air, detect ileus and possible signs of peritoneal irritation in the right lower abdomen
- CT of abdomen: only in genuine cases of doubt to rule out malignancy, diverticulitis, and abscess. Should be used more liberally when there is high operative risk and findings are unclear, for example, advanced age. Obsolete in children and young women.

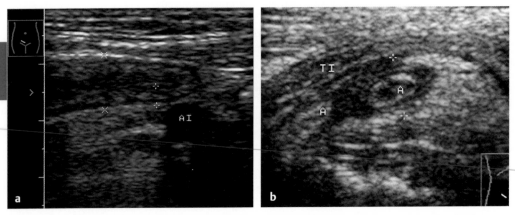

Fig. 11.2a, b   Acute appendicitis on ultrasound: **a** transverse, **b** longitudinal. (From Schmidt 2003, see p. 413.)

■ Differential Diagnosis

Urological
- Acute cystitis/pyelonephritis
- Uretero-/nephrolithiasis
- Torsion of the testis
- Epididymitis
- Prostatitis

- In case of doubt, perform further investigations, consult with other specialists.

Gynecological
- Pregnancy / extrauterine pregnancy
- Dysmenorrhea
- Endometriosis
- Ovarian cysts
- Follicular bleeding
- Ovarian torsion
- Adnexitis
- Tubovarian abscess
- Ovarian malignancy

Surgical/Gastroenterological
- Fecal impaction
- Gastroenteritis
- Crohn colitis / ulcerative colitis
- Diverticulitis
- Meckel diverticulum
- Perforated gastric ulcer
- Cholecystitis
- Pancreatitis
- Ileus due to adhesions
- Mesenteric ischemia
- Right-sided colon carcinoma

Other
- Internal or external hernia
- Rectus sheath hematoma
- Psoas abscess or hemorrhage
- Diabetic pseudoappendicitis
- Torsion of parts of the greater omentum or appendices epiploicae

Treatment Approach

■ Indications

Indication for Conservative Treatment when Symptoms Are Subacute
- Untypical history and moderate clinical signs
- Few or no laboratory changes
- Absence of ultrasonographic signs

11

Indication for Surgery
If acute appendicitis is present or likely from the history and clinical signs and if this is supported by laboratory tests and ultrasonography, surgical appendectomy is the treatment of choice. Aim: removal of the infection focus and prevention of abscess formation/perforation/peritonitis. The operation should

- Operation is the treatment of choice to control infection and prevent complications such as abscess and peritonitis.

therefore be performed promptly when indicated and is preferable to conservative treatment in the case of doubt. The operation method (open or laparoscopic) depends on the department. In numerous hospitals, laparoscopic surgery is now the method of choice. When surgery is indicated, immediate administration of antibiotics is also indicated (while the patient is still in the outpatient unit or emergency room); depending on the operative findings, they are continued or consist of single-shot antibiotic therapy.

■ Conservative Treatment

• Close monitoring

- In-patient monitoring
- Patient kept fasting
- Infusion
- Restrained use of analgesia
- Ice bladder if appropriate
- Laxatives if appropriate
- Clinical, laboratory, and ultrasound review
- A decision on how to proceed must be made within 6–8 hours.

■ Surgical Treatment

Laparoscopic Appendectomy

Advantages
- Entire abdominal cavity can be inspected.
- Treatment of concomitant findings is possible through the same access: adhesions, ovarian cysts, endometriosis, tubovarian abscess.
- Shorter unfitness for work due to illness
- Better cosmetic result
- Easier technically in obese patients

Disadvantages
- Average operating time somewhat longer
- Higher material requirements, higher costs
- Greater risk of thermal tissue injury due to bipolar current
- Greater surgical experience necessary
- Difficulty in deciding when a switch to open surgery is indicated, for instance, with bleeding, poor visibility, cecal pole involvement, other unexpected findings, organ damage that cannot be repaired laparoscopically

(Relative) Contraindications

• Note contraindications and indications for switching.

- Patients who are too small
- Adhesions anticipated after previous surgery
- Presence of abdominal hernias that must also be managed
- Excessive cardiac risk for pneumoperitoneum

11

Operative Technique

- For positioning of surgeon, assistant, scrub nurse, screen and ports, see **Fig. 11.3**.
- Port for the camera trocar (usually 10 mm, 5 mm possible also) is transverse below or longitudinal above the umbilicus.
- Create pneumoperitoneum (12–14 mmHg) through Veress needle or minilaparotomy.

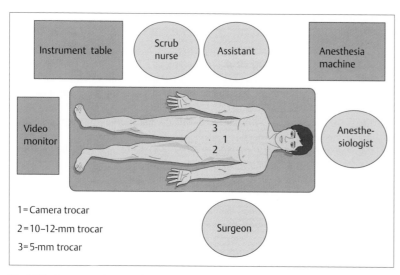

1 = Camera trocar
2 = 10–12-mm trocar
3 = 5-mm trocar

Fig. 11.3   Laparoscopic appendectomy—operating room arrangement.

- First, camera survey to assess position, rule out intra-abdominal injuries due to access
- Placement of further trocars: 10–12 mm in the left mid-abdomen, 5 mm in right mid-abdomen
- Exposure of the appendix, if necessary lowering the patient's head, aspiration of purulent fluid if present
- Dissection and exposure of the mesentery, clip ligature of the appendicular artery and skeletonizing of the appendix to its base (point where the three taeniae meet)
- Division of the appendix at its base using Röder loop or Endo-GIA
- Extraction of the appendix in a specimen bag through the 10–12 mm trocar in the left mid-abdomen. Each specimen is examined histopathologically so as not to overlook malignancy.
- Copious intra-abdominal irrigation in accordance with findings, especially of the pouch of Douglas (3–10 L)
- Search for Meckel diverticulum
- Place a drain and/or decide on postoperative antibiotic therapy for advanced disease (turbid fluid, perforation, abscess, peritonitis).
- If appropriate, schedule a planned second-look laparoscopy for further irrigation and inspection of the stump
- Release pneumoperitoneum and remove trocars.
- Skin closure with interrupted sutures or continuous intracutaneous suture
- Elegant and safe procedure when the surgeon has adequate expertise, with broader options if unexpected conditions are encountered
- Ideal training procedure in laparoscopic technique when uncomplicated

11

Conventional Appendectomy

Operative Technique

- Classical method using few materials
- Can be performed safely in hospitals in nonindustrialized countries

- McBurney muscle-splitting incision or pararectal incision / lower midline laparotomy (latter is better in an extremely obese patient and when the differential diagnosis is unclear as it can be extended more readily. Disadvantage: greater risk of incisional hernia)
- The cecal pole is rotated and delivered with identification of the appendix base where the taeniae coli meet.
- Depending on findings, antegrade or retrograde skeletonizing of the appendix, ligature of the appendicular artery, exposure of the appendix base
- Crush the appendix base from proximal to distal, positioning the clamp and ligature close to the base.
- Divide the appendix between clamp and ligature with a scalpel on a moist sponge, pass specimen with attached clamp for histopathological examination.
- Bury the stump by a purse-string suture, secured further with a Z-suture.
- If appendix is normal, look for a Meckel diverticulum, explore the terminal ileum, look for mesenteric lymphadenitis, if possible inspect the female internal genitalia.
- Irrigation locally and in the pouch of Douglas (not much more is possible with open surgery)
- Decide on placement of a drain, antibiotic therapy, and whether a second-look operation should be performed (as in laparoscopic appendectomy).
- Wound closure in layers, skin closure with interrupted sutures or staples

■ Postoperative Care

- In case of doubt, decide promptly whether a second-look operation is indicated.

- Continue antibiotics according to intraoperative findings, intravenous fluid replacement.
- Gradual increase of diet from the first postoperative day, sips to drink as soon as anesthetic has worn off
- Monitor clinical condition, infection parameters, temperature, drain secretion.
- Second-look operation if clinical signs persist or infection parameters remain persistently high
- Prompt mobilization
- Monitor any concomitant diseases present.

■ Complications

Perioperative Complications

Intraoperative

- **Caution:** aortic injury when creating access for the camera in the laparoscopic technique

- Intestinal injury, development of (fecal) peritonitis if this goes unnoticed
- Bladder injury (development of urinoma, urine loss through drain)
- Vascular injury or accidental ligature (iliac artery, mesenteric vessels) with consequent reduced perfusion or intraoperative bleeding
- Ureter injury (hydronephrosis or urine loss through drain or development of urinoma)

Postoperative
- Superficial wound healing disorders, wound seroma, abscess
- Subfascial abdominal wall abscess
- Intraperitoneal abscess: cecal region, inter-enteric, pouch of Douglas, subhepatic, subphrenic
- Secondary hemorrhage (appendicular artery, mesenteric vessels)
- Stump leak due to peri-appendicitis inflammatory reaction, thermal intestinal wall injury, purse-string / Z-suture too tight or too deep
- Necrosis of cecal pole due to ligature of branches of the ileocolic/right colic artery
- Early ileus (up to 4 weeks postoperatively in 0.7% of cases)

Late Complications

- Late ileus (3% of cases)
- Fistula development (in Crohn disease, due to nonabsorbable suture material)
- Incisional hernias
- Late abscesses
- Persisting wound pain, wound neuroma

> • Most frequent complications are wound infections, hematomas, abscesses, and peritonitis.

■ Rare Diseases of the Appendix

Endometriosis of the Appendix

- Appendectomy must be performed. Further foci in the parietal or visceral peritoneum are possible and these must be coagulated if possible.

Crohn Disease

- Isolated involvement of the appendix is very rare: manifestation as appendicitis, intestinal hemorrhage, chronic recurrent right-sided lower abdominal pain, incidental finding in appendectomy specimen
- With intraoperative diagnosis resection is usually not performed (to avoid inducing a fistula) and drug therapy is instituted (see Chapter 7).
- With isolated appendix involvement there are often no other sites of manifestation of Crohn disease for very long periods of time.

> • The treatment of first choice is conservative.

Diverticulitis of the Appendix

- Very rare, but found more often in elderly patients as a cause of acute appendicitis

11

Appendix Carcinoid

- The most common of all appendix tumors, accounting for 85% of cases (see Chapter 22).
- Incidental finding in 0.7% of all appendectomy specimens, usually located at the appendix tip.
- 80% of appendix carcinoids are incidental findings in appendectomy performed because of appendicitis.
- 50% of all carcinoids of the entire gastrointestinal tract arise in the appendix.

Treatment Approach

- Tumors up to 1 cm in size: appendectomy is safely sufficient.
- Tumors over 2 cm in size: right hemicolectomy with lymphadenectomy
- Evidence of or suspected lymph node metastases: right hemicolectomy with lymphadenectomy
- Tumors between 1 and 2 cm in size: decide on an individual basis, perform hemicolectomy if mesoappendix is infiltrated

■ Postoperative Care

- With tumors over 1 cm in size, think of secondary operation, check other sites of manifestation.

- Chromogranin A and the respective hormone levels in blood and urine are used as follow-up parameters.
- Up to 80% of neuroendocrine tumors express somatostatin receptors so that other or new tumor manifestations can be diagnosed, for example, with the somatostatin analogue octreotide using receptor scintigraphy.

Prognosis

- The 5-year survival rate of 90% is much better than with neuroendocrine tumors of the small intestine (69%).
- Lymph node metastases can be expected in 30%–50% of cases where the tumor is greater than 2 cm in size.

Mucinous Cystadenoma / Pseudomyxoma Peritonei

- The treatment of choice is repeated surgery but the prognosis is poor.

- Second most common tumor of the appendix
- When found incidentally in an appendectomy specimen, two-stage right hemicolectomy appears to improve the 10-year survival rate.
- In up to 50% of cases, there are already intra-abdominal manifestations when the diagnosis is made.
- In a third of cases a pseudomyxoma peritonei is present:
  - ► Collection of masses of mucus in the peritoneal cavity; the sites of origin can be the appendix, ovary, uterus and colon.
  - ► The treatment is radical surgery, and repeated procedures are necessary.
  - ► The usefulness of radiotherapy and/or chemotherapy is so far doubtful.
  - ► The 5-year survival rate is very poor at 6%.

Appendix Carcinoma (Fig. 11.4)

- Treatment as in colon carcinoma

- Incidental finding in 0.01%–0.08% of appendectomy specimens
- On histology, adenocarcinomas of the colon type are found
- Necessary therapy: right hemicolectomy with lymphadenectomy (like colon cancer)
- The rules for colon cancer apply for adjuvant and palliative therapy and follow-up (see Chapter 12).

11

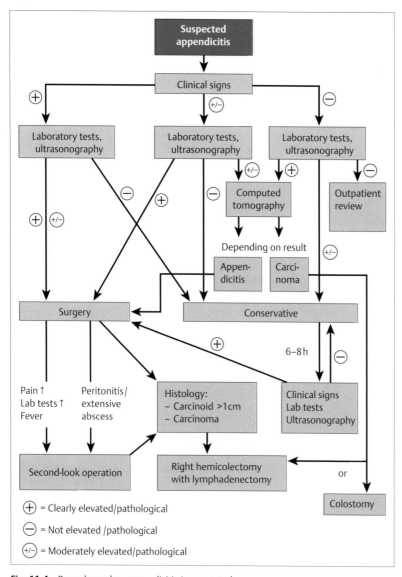

Fig. 11.4   Procedure when appendicitis is suspected.

Further Reading

Chiang DT, Tan EI, Birks D. "To have ... or not to have". Should computed tomography and ultrasonography be implemented as a routine work-up for patients with suspected acute appendicitis in a regional hospital? Ann R Coll Surg Engl 2008; 90(1): 17–21

Sauerland S, Jaschinski T, Neugebauer EA. Laparoscopic versus open surgery for suspected appendicitis. Cochrane Database Syst Rev 2010 Oct 6; (10): CD001546. Review

Sauerland S, Lefering R, Neugebauer EAM. Laparoscopic versus open surgery for suspected appendicitis. Cochrane Database Syst Rev 2004: CD001546. DOI: 10.1002/14651858.CD001546.pub2

11

12 Colon

J.M. Mayer

■ Anatomy

The colon can be divided into five sections:
- The **cecum** is a blind pouch below the junction with the small intestine. It can be adherent with the parietal peritoneum (fixed cecum, rare) or be mobile on a mesocolon. The boundary with the ascending colon is arbitrary; it is usually considered to start at the end of the ileum.
- The **ascending colon** is retroperitoneal. The right colic flexure forms the junction with the transverse colon.
- The **transverse colon** is intraperitoneal. It varies in form and position. The transverse mesocolon is fixed to the posterior abdominal wall at about the level of the right renal hilum, duodenum (descending part), and the head of the pancreas. The left colic flexure forms the junction with the descending colon.
- The **descending colon** is retroperitoneal. It becomes the sigmoid colon at about the level of the iliac crest.
- The **sigmoid colon** is intraperitoneal. The boundary between the colon and rectum is at about the level of the 3rd sacral vertebra in the region of the peritoneal reflection. This corresponds to a proctoscopic level of ca. 16 cm.

Arteries

- Very variable in origin and course
- Frequent interruption of continuity of the marginal artery (e.g., left colic flexure)

There are numerous variants (**Fig. 12.1**):
- Cecum and ascending colon: ileocolic artery (1) from the superior mesenteric artery, right colic artery (2) from the superior mesenteric artery
- Transverse colon: middle colic artery (3) from the superior mesenteric artery
- Descending colon: left colic artery (4) from the inferior mesenteric artery (5)
- Sigmoid colon: sigmoid arteries (6) from the inferior mesenteric artery

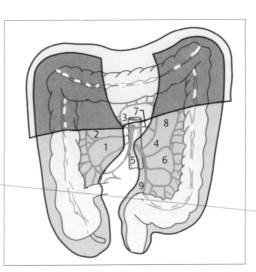

Fig. 12.1 Arterial supply and lymphatic drainage regions.

- **Special features:**
  - ► The anastomosis of Riolan (7) is an inconstant collateral that connects the superior mesenteric artery with the inferior mesenteric artery.
  - ► The vascular arcade running parallel to the intestine is called the Drummond arcade (8); also called the marginal artery. There is often a break in continuity in the region of the left colic flexure.
  - ► Through these vascular connections, the arterial supply from the superior mesenteric artery can extend as far as the sigmoid region. If the inferior mesenteric artery is ligated centrally during sigmoid resection, the descending colon is perfused through these connections. If there is no anastomosis of Riolan and if the continuity of the marginal artery is interrupted at the left colic flexure, the descending colon will no longer be adequately perfused after central ligature of the inferior mesenteric artery.
  - ► The Sudeck point (9): There is no anastomosing marginal artery between the most distal sigmoid artery and the superior rectal artery. If the intestine is not resected sufficiently distally during sigmoid resection with central ligature of the inferior mesenteric artery, the remaining rectal stump may be underperfused, which involves a risk of anastomotic failure. However, adequate perfusion through distal collaterals is usually preserved.

Veins
- The veins essentially follow the arteries and drain into the portal vein.

Lymphatic Drainage
- Lymphatic drainage is alongside the corresponding arteries.
- A distinction is made between epicolic, paracolic (in the region of the marginal arcade), intermediate (along the main vessels), and central lymph nodes (in the region of the aorta).
- Because of the lymphatic vessels along the marginal artery, lymph node metastasis upward and downward, parallel to the intestine is possible (10 cm safety margin in oncological resection).

- Lymph drainage along the arteries
- **Caution:** metastases up to 10 cm laterally along the marginal artery

■ Anastomosis Techniques

Overview

- End-to-end, end-to-side, or side-to-side anastomosis
- Manual suture:
  - ► One to three rows
  - ► Extramucosal or all-layer
  - ► Interrupted sutures or continuous technique
- Stapling techniques
- Compression techniques

12

General Principles

- Adequate mobilization of the intestine is important for a tension-free anastomosis.
- When an ileocolostomy is performed as an end-to-end anastomosis, the resection line in the small intestine is oblique and it is straight in the large intestine to compensate for the difference in lumen.

- Qualities of an anastomosis: patent, not leaking, tension-free, well-perfused

- Skeletonization should be performed sparingly to obtain well-vascularized bowel ends (skeletonize about 1.5 cm of the small intestine, not at all or at most 0.5–1 cm of the large intestine).
- Check the perfusion of the bowel ends before constructing the anastomosis.
- **End-to-end anastomosis** is best. It is preferable, whenever possible.
- Single layer of sutures: less risk of ischemia and later stenosis compared with multiple layers
- Continuous suture: less time-consuming and more economical
- All-layer interrupted sutures are advisable for technically demanding anastomoses (place the sutures first) or when inflammation is present.
- Suture material: absorbable, monofilament, synthetic sutures
- Avoid intramural hematomas.
- A triple layer of sutures is hardly ever used now.

Single-Row Intestinal Suture

Interrupted Suture

- Monofilament seromuscular or all-layer suture
- Useful when there is swelling due to inflammation or for demanding anastomoses

- Suture material: monofilament, 3–0 or 4–0
- Stay sutures are placed at the poles.
- Interrupted sutures through all layers close together. The mucosa is included only at the edge. Some authors prefer extramucosal/seromuscular suture.
- The posterior wall can be sutured from the lumen and the knots are then on the mucosa. It is also possible to suture the posterior wall from the outside (external interrupted sutures), but in this case, a rotation maneuver is required after suturing half the circumference.

Continuous Suture

- Monofilament seromuscular or all-layer suture
- Advantage: even suture tension

- Suture material: double-armed suture, monofilament, 3–0 or 4–0
- Start the suture at the mesenteric attachment (seromuscular). Tie the suture, using one-half of the suture as a stay thread.
- Place a stay suture at the opposite antimesenteric end.
- Continuous extramucosal/seromuscular or all-layer suture with oblique stitches as far as the antimesenteric pole. The continuous suture is locked here by an interrupted suture. Loose and even approximation of the bowel ends is important and the suture must not be tightened too much. The needle entry sites must be ca. 4–5 mm apart and ca. 5 mm from the resection margin.
- Rotation maneuver and continuous suture with the second half of the thread from the mesenteric to the antimesenteric side
- Tie the suture ends with six throws (to secure the knot with a monofilament suture), if necessary securing the knot with a metal clip over the sixth throw.

Stapling Technique

Colon anastomoses (ileocolostomy or colo-colostomy) can be fashioned as side-to-side anastomoses with linear stapling devices.

- If necessary, close both ends of the intestine to be anastomosed with a linear stapler.
- Place the antimesenteric surfaces of the bowel ends next to one another.
- The antimesenteric ends of the rows of staples are cut off so widely that one limb of a GIA device can be inserted in each. Fire the mechanism.
- The two intestinal lumens are closed with the GIA device.
- If necessary, secure the ends of the stapled anastomosis with additional interrupted sutures.

12

Colorectal anastomoses are performed as simple stapled anastomoses or using a double stapler method (see Chapter 13).

■ Minimally Invasive Colon Surgery

Indications

Benign Colorectal Diseases

- Diverticulosis, diverticulitis (especially in a free interval)
- Colovesical fistulas
- Chronic inflammatory bowel disease (ulcerative colitis)
- Post-inflammatory stenosis
- Adhesions
- Polyps that cannot be removed by colonoscopy

• All nonmalignant diseases

Malignant Colorectal Diseases

- Laparoscopic resection of colon carcinoma is equivalent to open resection from the oncological aspect.
- This also appears to apply to rectal carcinoma, but evidence from studies is still lacking.
- The precondition for laparoscopic cancer surgery is that oncological principles are followed:
  - ► Resection margins are observed.
  - ► Radicality in lymphadenectomy with central vascular ligature; total removal of the mesorectum with all rectal carcinomas in the middle and lower thirds
  - ► Avoid injection metastases at the trocar entry site (port site metastases) by using specimen bags.
  - ► Avoid seeding of tumor cells by adequate operation technique, observation of a "no-touch" technique.

• Colon carcinoma, probably also rectal carcinoma
• Observe oncological principles as in open surgery.

Resection Procedures

- For laparoscopic dissection, along with electrical instruments and clips, **ultrasonic dissectors,** which can safely divide vessels with a diameter of up to several millimeters, are suitable (Ligasure Atlas up to 7 mm).
- A distinction can be made among several laparoscopic colon resection procedures:
  - ► Laparoscopically assisted resection
  - ► Nearly complete laparoscopic resection
  - ► Complete laparoscopic resection
  - ► Combined laparoscopic resection

Laparoscopically Assisted Resection

Of all minimally invasive surgical techniques on the colon, this is used most often today. Resection and anastomosis are performed outside the body.

- The colon is mobilized and dissected laparoscopically.
- A small abdominal incision is then made, through which the segment of intestine to be resected is pulled outside the abdominal wall.
- The extracorporeal resection and anastomosis are performed as usual.
- This technique allows the use of a comparatively small abdominal incision.

12

Nearly Complete Laparoscopic Resection

Resection and anastomosis are performed laparoscopically inside the body.
- Laparoscopic dissection and division of the intestine.
- The dissected intestine is dislocated in front of the abdominal wall through a small incision (usually an enlarged trocar port), resected, and finally the anvil for the stapled anastomosis is inserted in the proximal bowel end.
- Since the stapler is introduced through the anus, the procedure is so far possible only in the left hemicolon.

Complete Laparoscopic Resection

Resection and anastomosis are performed laparoscopically inside the body.
- The resected specimen is extracted through the intestinal lumen or through a 33-mm trocar (with intra-abdominal morcellation of the specimen, if necessary).
- Since the stapler is introduced through the anus, the procedure is so far possible only in the left hemicolon.

Combined Laparoscopic Resection

- Combination of conventional and laparoscopic techniques, for instance, in abdominoperineal rectal resection

■ Diverticulosis and Diverticulitis

Definition

- Diverticulosis: asymptomatic diverticula
- Diverticular disease: diverticulitis or diverticular bleeding

- **Diverticulum:** outpouching of the bowel wall
  - ▶ True diverticulum: outpouching of the entire bowel wall
  - ▶ Pseudodiverticulum: outpouching of the mucosa and submucosa through gaps in the muscle
- **Diverticulitis:** symptomatic inflammation of diverticula
- **Diverticular disease:** all diseases cause by diverticula

Epidemiology

- Diverticulosis is the most common benign condition in the GI tract.
- 10%–25% of patients develop diverticular disease

- Diverticulosis is the most common benign condition of the gastrointestinal tract.
- The prevalence rises with increasing age. While it is rare in the under-40s, it occurs in ca. 30% of 60-year-olds and ca. 65% of 85-year-olds.
- Men and women are affected equally.
- Only ca. 10%–25% of persons with diverticula develop diverticular disease, and complicated diverticular disease occurs in 5%.
- The incidence of diverticulitis is 80–126/100 000 population per year.

Etiology

- Multifactorial: diminished resistance of the bowel wall, increased intraluminal pressure due to age and genetic predisposition, diet

- The pathogenesis of diverticulosis is multifactorial. The diverticula develop due to reduced resistance of the intestinal wall and increased intraluminal pressure. In over 90% of cases, they form in the sigmoid colon. An increase in pressure occurs due to a low-fiber diet with a high proportion of meat and fat, along with a lack of exercise. Genetic factors and age also lead to flaccidity of the intestinal wall.

12

- A further explanation for the development of diverticula in the sigmoid colon is the circumstance that sphincter characteristics are ascribed to the rectosigmoid junction and the upstream sigmoid colon is thus a high-pressure area, which favors the development of diverticula.
- Muscle gaps at vessel entry sites through the muscle are sites of predilection for the development of diverticula so that outpouching of the mucosa and submucosa occurs at these sites. These therefore are **pseudodiverticula** (pulsion diverticula).
- True diverticula are rare, usually congenital and often affect the right hemicolon.
- Diverticulitis arises due to constipation with consequent bacterial growth in the diverticulum, producing inflammation of a variable degree.
- Diverticular bleeding occurs in ca. 5% of patients with diverticula and is manifested independent of diverticulitis. Risk factors are advanced age, nonsteroidal anti-inflammatory drugs and right-sided diverticula.

- Usually pseudodiverticula in the sigmoid colon
- Diverticulitis due to constipation and consequent inflammation

Symptoms

- Diverticulosis is asymptomatic and is of no disease significance.
- Diverticulitis is characterized by left-sided lower abdominal pain, which is often of abrupt onset and rapidly progressive. Fever, nausea and vomiting, dysuria, change in bowel habit, and blood in the stool can also occur.
- Complications:
  - ► Abscess
  - ► Perforation and peritonitis
  - ► Stenosis
  - ► Fistula
- Diverticular bleeding clinically consists of painless rectal bleeding, which can be persistent or intermittent. The bleeding ceases spontaneously in 80% of cases.

- Diverticulosis: asymptomatic
- Diverticulitis: left-sided lower abdominal pain, fever, blood in the stool
- With perforation: acute abdomen
- Diverticular bleeding: painless rectal bleeding

Classification (Table 12.1)

Table 12.1   Classification of diverticulosis and diverticulitis

Condition	Hansen and Stock	Hinchey
Diverticulosis	0	
Acute uncomplicated diverticulitis	I	
Peridiverticulitis, phlegmon	IIa	
Pericolic, mesocolic abscess	IIb	I
Distant abscess (e.g., pelvic floor)	IIc	II
Free perforation, purulent peritonitis	IIc	III
Free perforation, fecal peritonitis	IIc	IV
Chronic recurrent peritonitis	III	

Diagnostic Approach

■ Clinical Examination

- Tenderness in the left lower abdomen
- Palpable loop
- Meteorism

- Tenderness in the left lower abdomen, palpable loop up to acute abdomen

12

- With advanced inflammation: local percussion tenderness and guarding
- After perforation with diffuse peritonitis: acute abdomen

■ Laboratory Tests

- Raised inflammatory parameters

- Leukocytosis with neutrophilia
- Elevated C-reactive protein (CRP) level
- Raised erythrocyte sedimentation rate (ESR)
- With sepsis: raised procalcitonin

■ Diagnostic Imaging

Ultrasonography

- Bowel wall thickening, abscesses, free fluid

- Diverticulitis is apparent as hypoechoic thickening of the bowel wall. The **dome sign** is highly specific, a hypoechoic lesion located eccentrically beside the bowel wall, which corresponds to an inflamed diverticulum. In addition, pericolic fat insudations, abscesses, and free fluid can also be diagnosed.

Computed Tomography

- "Gold standard" for exact imaging of the degree of the inflammation

- CT with IV contrast injection and rectal contrast enema: This is the standard diagnostic imaging method, particularly when complicated diverticulitis is suspected. The presence of diverticula, thickened bowel wall including the surrounding inflammatory insudations, abscesses, and free fluid or air can be demonstrated. A classification into stages can also be made.

Colonoscopy

- Rule out other diseases in the free interval

- Colonoscopy plays no part in the acutely inflamed situation (**caution:** risk of perforation). However, after inflammation has subsided, interval colonoscopy should be performed to rule out other colon diseases (especially colon carcinoma).
- **Diverticular bleeding** is demonstrated by colonoscopy in 70%–90% of cases. It should be noted that detection is usually unsuccessful in the bleeding-free interval. Angiographic or CT diagnosis is possible when there is high bleeding activity.

■ Differential Diagnosis

- Irritable bowel syndrome
- Chronic inflammatory bowel disease
- Infectious colitis
- Ischemic colitis
- Polyps/carcinoma
- Diseases of the urogenital tract

Treatment Approach

■ Indications (Fig. 12.2)

- **Emergency surgery:**
  - ► Perforation with peritonitis (Hansen and Stock stage IIc)
  - ► Abscess with signs of sepsis
  - ► Obstruction due to stenosis
  - ► Uncontrollable bleeding (p. 205)

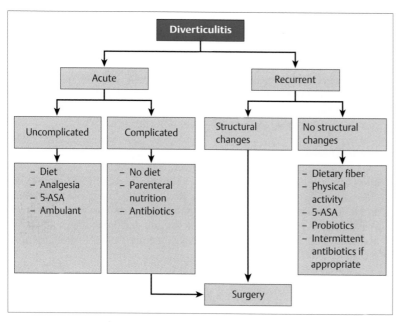

Fig. 12.2 Treatment approach in diverticulitis.

- **Early elective surgery:**
  - ► Phlegmonous diverticulitis (Hansen and Stock stage IIa)
  - ► Closed perforated diverticulitis (Hansen and Stock stage IIb)
- **Elective interval surgery:**
  - ► Chronic recurrent diverticulitis with structural changes (Hansen and Stock stage III)
  - ► Fistula
  - ► Stenosis without obstruction

■ Conservative Treatment

- Initial conservative treatment of uncomplicated diverticulitis is successful in 70%–100% of patients. **Fasting from food** for 2–3 days usually suffices in uncomplicated diverticulitis (fluids and liquid diet absorbable in the small intestine can be given). Antibiotic therapy is not absolutely essential at this stage. The patient should also be given adequate analgesia and spasmolytic treatment. 5-Aminosalicylate (5-ASA) can be given as supportive therapy.
- Elective interval surgery is not indicated in the uncomplicated stage, even in young patients (exception: immunosuppression), since complications due to diverticulitis are not to be expected subsequently.
- In the complicated stage, parenteral nutrition should be given until the patient is asymptomatic. **Broad-spectrum antibiotic therapy** should also be given, parenterally at first: acylamino penicillins + β-lactamase inhibitors; second, third or fourth generation cephalosporins + metronidazole; second or third generation fluoroquinolones + metronidazole, and carbapenems can be used.
- The indication for early elective surgery or interval surgery should be considered.

- Uncomplicated diverticulitis: short-term fasting from food, no antibiotics, no interval surgery
- Complicated diverticulitis: fasting, antibiotics, interval surgery

12

■ Surgical Treatment

- Principle: removal of the inflamed segment of intestine, including the upper rectum in the case of sigmoid diverticulitis

- The basis of the surgical treatment of complicated diverticulitis is removal of the inflamed segment of intestine.
- The distal resection margin should be in the upper rectum (below the peritoneal reflection), which can significantly reduce the risk of recurrence (complete removal of the high-pressure area). Persistence of isolated diverticula proximal to the proximal anastomosis in the descending colon has, in contrast, no influence on the probability of recurrence.

Conventional Versus Laparoscopic Procedure

- Laparoscopic procedure has less access trauma.
- Not suitable with severe inflammation, abscess, peritonitis, or fistula

- Laparoscopic sigmoid resection has lower overall morbidity compared with open surgery. This is attributed to the lower access trauma but more favorable patient selection may also play a part. In Hansen and Stock stages IIa and III, the laparoscopic procedure is standard in many places.
- When there is marked inflammation in Hansen and Stock stages IIb and IIc and with fistulas and inflammatory conglomerate masses, a primary open procedure is often a rational choice.

Timing of Operation

Emergency Surgery

- One-stage: resection with primary anastomosis
- Two-stage: Hartmann discontinuity resection or resection with primary anastomosis and proximal protective stoma
- Three-stage: obsolete

- **Timing:**
  - ► One-stage: Resection of the diverticulum-bearing segment of intestine with primary anastomosis.
  - ► Two-stage: Resection of the diverticulum-bearing segment of intestine, bringing out a terminal descending colostomy (Hartmann operation) or resection of the diverticulum-bearing segment of intestine with primary anastomosis and fashioning of a proximal protective stoma (e.g., transverse colostomy).
    Restoration of intestinal continuity or closure of the protective stoma takes place after the inflammation has healed (e.g., after 3 months).
  - ► Three-stage: Obsolete.
- With large abscesses, an emergency operation can be avoided by interventional drain insertion combined with antibiotic therapy. The resecting procedure can be performed as early elective surgery after the acute inflammation has subsided.

Early Elective Surgery (7–10 Days after Onset of Symptoms)

- One-stage sigmoid resection with primary anastomosis between the descending colon and rectum is the procedure of choice. This requires a well-perfused tension-free anastomosis in an uninflamed segment of bowel.
- If in doubt: fashion a protective stoma.

Elective Interval Surgery (after 4 or More Weeks)

- According to recent knowledge, the probability of future complications depends on the finding of structural changes (e.g., abscess formation, scar stenosis) and not on the number of previous attacks of diverticulitis. In particular, recurrent uncomplicated diverticulitis is not associated with an increasing likelihood of complications. The indication for surgery in Hansen and Stock stage III should therefore depend on CT evidence of structural changes in conjunction with individual factors (age, comorbidity).
- Sigmoid resection is performed as a one-stage procedure with primary anastomosis between the descending colon and rectum.

Diverticular Bleeding

- Since clinically significant blood losses can occur, close monitoring of the circulation and blood count is indicated initially, in an intensive care unit if necessary. Adequate blood units should be available.
- Since 80% of bleeding episodes cease spontaneously, nothing needs to be done in these cases apart from monitoring. If bleeding persists, endoscopic hemostasis (epinephrine injection, clip application, coagulation) is the procedure of choice. If this is not successful, angiographic selective embolization can be attempted if there is high bleeding activity. Segmental colon resection is indicated as a last resort when there is circulatory depression despite supportive medications and transfusion of four or more units of erythrocyte concentrate per 24 hours.
- Elective segmental resection of the colon is justified after the second recurrent episode of bleeding.

- Close circulatory monitoring, 80% of bleeds cease spontaneously
- If bleeding persists: endoscopic hemostasis or angiographic embolization
- Last resort: resection

Prevention

- Patients with diverticula should ensure that their diet is high in fiber and low in fat and that they have adequate physical activity. Nicotine, nonsteroidal anti-inflammatory drugs and paracetamol should be avoided in addition.

- High-fiber, low-fat diet, exercise

Prognosis

- The postoperative mortality is 0.9% with elective and early elective surgery, 3.2% with closed perforation, and over 20% with diffuse peritonitis. The corresponding overall morbidity is 17%, 30%, and 44%.
- In the longer term, postoperative recurrence of diverticulitis can be expected in 1%–11% of cases and further surgery in 0–3%.

■ Ulcerative Colitis

Definition

- Chronic inflammatory disease of the colon with continuous spread and with the development of mucosal ulcerations of unclear etiology
- It is possibly an autoimmune disease due to a genetic predisposition, which is activated by a specific trigger (infection, stress).

- Chronic inflammatory colon disease of the mucosa with continuous spread from distally, of unclear etiology

Epidemiology

- Incidence ca. 6/100 000 population per year
- Peak incidence between the ages of 20 and 35 years
- Women affected slightly more often than men
- There is both a familial and ethnic increased incidence (white population, especially those of Jewish descent).

12

Pathogenesis

• Acute: inflamed edematous mucosa, contact bleeding, crypt abscesses
• Chronic: loss of mucosa, carcinomatous degeneration

• The inflammation always starts in the rectum and spreads continuously in a proximal direction. It affects only the mucosa of the colon and rectum. In rare cases, the terminal ileum can also be involved ("backwash ileitis").
• In the acute stage, inflamed, erythematous, edematous mucosa is seen, with a tendency to contact bleeding. Granulocytic crypt abscesses are seen on microscopy.
• In the chronic advanced stage there is destruction of the mucosa with loss of the physiological fold relief. Residual islands of mucosa look like pseudopolyps. Lymphocyte and histiocyte infiltration is seen microscopically. Epithelial dysplasia, which is a precursor of carcinomatous degeneration, can also occur.

Symptoms

• Bloody slimy diarrhea

• Bloody slimy diarrhea (lead symptom)
• Abdominal pain, tenesmus
• Fever

Complications

• **Caution:** carcinomatous degeneration

• Massive bleeding
• Toxic megacolon
• Carcinoma risk
• Weight loss, growth disorder
• Extraintestinal:
  ► Skin: aphthous ulcers, erythema nodosum, pyoderma gangrenosum
  ► Eyes: iritis, uveitis, episcleritis
  ► Joints: arthritis, ankylosing spondylitis (usually HLA-B27 positive)
  ► Liver: primary sclerosing cholangitis

Course

• **Chronic relapsing** (85%): recurrent exacerbations alternating with periods of complete remission; usually only the distal colon and rectum affected
• **Chronic continuous** without complete remission (10%): symptoms of varying intensity without asymptomatic periods
• **Acute fulminant** course (5%): sudden disease onset with tenesmus, diarrhea, septic temperatures, and shock. Complication: toxic megacolon, mortality 30%

Diagnostic Approach

■ Clinical Examination

• Inspection of the anus
• Digital rectal examination: evidence of blood
• Look for extraintestinal manifestations, especially in the skin.

12

■ Laboratory Tests

• Raised inflammatory parameters
• Finding of pANCA

• Leukocytosis
• CRP elevation
• Raised ESR
• Thrombocytosis with severe inflammation

- Rise in α_2-globulin with severe inflammation
- Anemia with bleeding
- Detection of perinuclear antineutrophil cytoplasmic antibodies (pANCA) in 60%–70% of cases
- Increase in alkaline phosphatase (AP) and γ-glutamyl transferase (γGT) with primary sclerosing cholangitis

■ Diagnostic Imaging

- **Double contrast enema:** loss of mucosal relief and haustrations or even "bicycle tube" appearance finding of pseudopolyps
- **Ultrasonography:** thickened bowel wall

■ Invasive Diagnostic Investigations

- **Endoscopy:** rectosigmoidoscopy/colonoscopy with biopsies at different levels (**caution:** risk of perforation with acute inflammation)

  • Colonoscopy with step biopsies

■ Differential Diagnosis

- Crohn disease
- Diverticulitis
- Infectious colitis
- Ischemic colitis
- Microscopic colitis
- Drug-induced toxic colitis
- Colon carcinoma
- Irritable bowel syndrome

Treatment Approach

■ Indications

- **Emergency surgery:**
  - ► Perforation with peritonitis
  - ► Massive bleeding
- **Urgent surgery:**
  - ► Fulminant episode refractory to drug treatment
  - ► Toxic megacolon
  - ► Bleeding refractory to endoscopic treatment
- **Elective surgery:**
  - ► Colorectal carcinoma
  - ► High-grade intraepithelial neoplasia
  - ► Stenosis suspicious for carcinoma
  - ► Recurrent disease interfering with quality of life (relative)
  - ► Low-grade intraepithelial neoplasia (relative)

■ Conservative Treatment

Acute Episode
- **Distal colitis:**
  - ► Mild to moderate activity: topical **aminosalicylates** (suppositories, enema) for distal disease, oral therapy with 5-ASA 3–4 g/d for proximal disease; if topical use of steroids fails, oral administration also if applicable
  - ► High activity: combined therapy with topical aminosalicylates and oral steroids (prednisolone 40–60 mg/d); IV steroid therapy for very severe episode

  • Aminosalicylates, possibly combined with prednisolone orally or IV

12

- **Marked colitis:**
  - ► Mild to moderate activity: oral therapy with aminosalicylates (3–4.8 g/d); if unsuccessful, oral steroid therapy (prednisolone 40–60 mg/d)
  - ► High activity: systemic steroid therapy (prednisolone 40–60 mg/d orally or IV) combined with oral aminosalicylate therapy

Fulminant Episode

- Prednisolone IV and fasting, followed by azathioprine
- Last resort: proctocolectomy

- A fulminant episode requires interdisciplinary treatment. Close cooperation between gastroenterologists and surgeons is needed.
- If surgical therapy is not indicated, systemic **steroid** therapy is begun immediately (prednisolone 1.0–1.5 mg/kg BW per day). If steroids are not tolerated or treatment is unsuccessful, ciclosporin A (2–4 mg/kg BW per day IV) is employed. Parenteral nutrition should be given if gastrointestinal passage is disturbed. Antibiotic treatment is indicated only if infection is suspected.
- After the acute phase has been controlled, it should be followed by maintenance therapy with oral azathioprine (2–2.5 mg/kg BW per day) for 3–6 months.
- Surgery is indicated if conservative therapy fails.

Chronic Active Course

- Azathioprine or 6-mercaptopurine; alternatively, proctocolectomy

- **Immunosuppression** for 3–5 years with azathioprine (2–2.5 mg/kg BW per day) or 6-mercaptopurine (1–1.5 mg/kg BW per day). Topical steroids can be employed in addition for distal colitis. Long-term systemic steroid treatment is not justified because of the side effects.
- Alternatively, proctocolectomy can be considered.

Maintenance of Remission

- Aminosalicylates, possibly azathioprine or 6-mercaptopurine

- The treatment of choice is oral **aminosalicylates** (e.g., 5-ASA 1.5 g/d), with topical aminosalicylate application (suppositories, foam, enema) in addition if proctitis or left-sided colitis is present. Maintenance therapy should be continued for at least 2 years.
- If this fails, treatment with azathioprine or 6-mercaptopurine can be attempted. Steroids are not suitable for long-term therapy.

Cancer Prophylaxis

- Annual colonoscopy with step biopsies
- Proctocolectomy indicated if there is high-grade intraepithelial neoplasia

- The risk of developing colorectal carcinoma is significantly increased in patients with ulcerative colitis. Annual colonoscopy is necessary, with biopsies at different levels, especially when the disease has been present for a long time. In addition, the risk of carcinoma can be reduced by long-term aminosalicylate treatment.
- The possibility of proctocolectomy should be raised with the patient. If high-grade intraepithelial neoplasia is found at colonoscopy, proctocolectomy is indicated.

■ Surgical Treatment

Proctocolectomy

- Standard procedure: continence-preserving proctocolectomy with ileoanal (pouch) anastomosis

- The standard procedure is continence-preserving proctocolectomy with an ileoanal (pouch) anastomosis and fashioning of a temporary protective ileostomy. Alternatively, a terminal ileostomy can be created.
- In certain cases, a colectomy can be performed with ileorectal anastomosis, but annual proctoscopy is then necessary. If carcinoma is found, oncological criteria are followed, including any prior treatment or after-treatment.

Creation of a Brooke Terminal Ileostomy (Fig. 12.3)

- Since ileal stool causes considerable skin irritation, the ileostomy must be prominent so that the stool can empty directly into the stoma bag.
- If creation of an ileostomy is definitely necessary, even preoperatively, the site where it passes through the abdominal wall is prepared first.

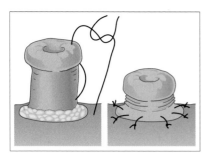

Fig. 12.3   Terminal ileostomy

Operative Technique

- Preoperative marking of the location on the lower abdomen with the patient standing, sitting, and lying
- Excise a circle of skin ca. 2 cm in diameter.
- Longitudinal splitting of the rectus sheath. Blunt separation of the fibers of the rectus abdominis muscle. The posterior layer of the rectus sheath and the peritoneum are opened together by a cross incision. The stoma opening should admit two fingers.
- About 4 cm of ileum are pulled through the abdominal wall and fixed by four interrupted fascioseromuscular sutures.
- The intestinal lumen is opened.
- The small intestine is everted and fixed by three-point sutures, which take the skin first, then the seromuscular layer of the ileum and finally the seromuscular end of the ileum. This results in an ileostomy everted ca. 2 cm (**Fig. 12.3**).

Creation of a Double-Barreled Ileostomy (Fig. 12.4)

Operative Technique

- An appropriate loop of ileum is pulled through the abdominal wall. The proximal limb must be inferior in position.
- Introduction of the rider and semicircular opening of the distal loop

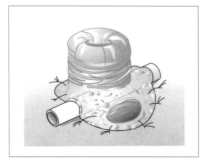

Fig. 12.4   Double-barreled ileostomy

12

- The proximal part of the loop is everted and sutured prominently and the distal limb is anchored at skin level (**Fig. 12.4**).
- The position of the stoma is fixed by a rider for the first week.

Complications after Creation of a Stoma

- Stoma necrosis
- Stoma retraction
- Stoma prolapse
- Parastomal hernia

Re-operation is required in all cases, possibly with refashioning of the stoma.

Continence-Preserving Proctocolectomy (Figs. 12.5, 12.6, 12.7)

Operative Technique

Transanal Proctomucosectomy
- Total abdominal resection of the colon and rectum first, with low division of the rectum (see Chapter 13)
- The rectal stump is brought through the anus with retractors (Parks).
- Inject Parks solution below the rectal mucosa above the dentate line.
- Incise the mucosa with scissors at the dentate line for a distance of 2–3 cm in a cranial direction and dissect the mucosa off the muscle circularly or in strips.
- Transabdominal or transanal division of the rectum wall. A short rectal cuff of 2–3 cm is left.
- Alternatively: mechanical anastomosis, no rectal cuff, direct ileoanal anastomosis

Creation of a Reservoir
- Usually a J-pouch with a limb length of ca. 15 cm is created. A stapling device is usually employed. Tension-free anastomosis is important so mobilization of the ileal mesentery is necessary.
- Mobilization of the ileum: The vasa recta of the corresponding mesentery are divided, preserving the arcade (**Fig. 12.5**). Transillumination is helpful.

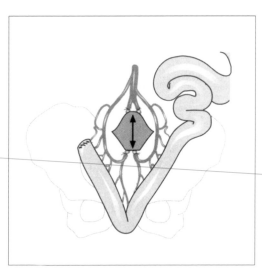

Fig. 12.5 Mobilization of the ileum.

- Creation of J-pouch (**Fig. 12.6**): side-to-side anastomosis with GIA 90 stapler
  - ► The distal loop of ileum is folded to form a "J" and opened transversely at its pole, which is later anastomosed to the anal ring.
  - ► The GIA 90 stapler is introduced through this incision (antimesenteric) and the mechanism is fired.
  - ► To obtain an anastomosis length of 15 cm, the device must be used twice.
  - ► The reservoir should have a capacity of about 160–200 mL.

Anastomosis through the Anus
- The pouch is pulled transanally into the rectal cuff.
- Pouch–anal anastomosis using 12–14 interrupted sutures. The sutures should include the anoderm at the dentate line, the internal sphincter muscle, and all layers of the small intestine (**Fig. 12.7**).
- Protective loop ileostomy ca. 15 cm proximal to the start of the reservoir

Aftercare
- Close the protective ileostomy after ca. 2–3 months, after checking the reservoir with Gastrografin and testing continence.

Complications
- Secondary bleeding
- Ileus
- Local septic processes
- Anastomotic stenosis (endoscopic dilation with bougies usually sufficient)
- Pouchitis

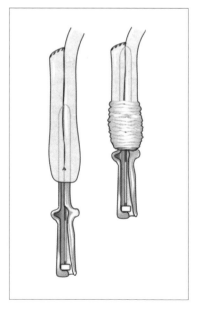

Fig. 12.6 Creation of a J-pouch using a stapler.

12

- In the case of FAP, the first colonoscopy should be performed at the age of 10 years and then annually. If adenomas are found, proctocolectomy is desirable after puberty up to the age of 20 years. Annual pouchoscopy is then indicated. Genetic counseling and screening of the family should be considered.

■ Aftercare

- Regular colonoscopy depending on the histology

- After colonoscopic removal of adenomas, check colonoscopy should be performed depending on the histology. Follow-up colonoscopy is necessary after 3 years in the case of low-grade intraepithelial neoplasia. If this is normal, further colonoscopies should be performed every 5 years.
- If there is high-grade intraepithelial neoplasia or if removal in full is in doubt, short-term follow-up is required (e.g., after a year or less).

■ Colon Cancer

Definition

- Epithelial malignancy between the cecum and the rectosigmoid junction

- Colon cancer is the term for any epithelial malignancy between the cecum and the rectosigmoid junction. The boundary with the rectum is not uniformly established. In Europe it is considered to be 16 cm from the anus measured with a rigid proctoscope.

Epidemiology

- Second commonest malignancy in Western industrialized countries
- Manifestation with increasing age

- In Western industrialized countries, colorectal cancer is the second commonest malignancy. The incidence in the United States is 102 900 cases per year.
- The peak incidence is between the ages of 70 and 75 years.
- Men and women are affected equally often.
- In 2%–7% of cases there are multiple synchronous colorectal cancers.
- 25% of patients have liver metastases when the diagnosis is made.

Etiology

- Multifactorial: age, diet, inflammation, smoking, genetics

- The causes of colon carcinoma are multifactorial. Both genetic predisposition and external influences can induce carcinoma. From 85% to 95% of colon cancers occur sporadically.

Risk Factors
- In 5%–15% of cases, a genetic defect can be found as causal (FAP, hereditary nonpolyposis colon cancer, positive family history).
- Diet: low-fiber, high-fat and high-meat diet, obesity
- Risk diseases: colorectal adenomas, ulcerative colitis, ureterosigmoidostomy, cancer of other organs (breast, uterus, ovary, bladder)
- Age over 40 years
- Tobacco use, alcohol consumption

Protective Factors
- High-fiber, low-fat and low-meat diet
- Rapid stool passage
- Aminosalicylates
- Vitamin C, folic acid

Hereditary Nonpolyposis Colon Cancer (Lynch Syndrome)
- Most common form of hereditary colorectal cancer
- Autosomal dominant inheritance, penetrance not 100%
- Ca. 1%–5% of all colorectal cancers
- Age of manifestation < 45 years
- Increased involvement of the right hemicolon
- Association with cancers of the urogenital tract is possible (Lynch II)
- Cause: germ line mutation or new mutation in a DNA repair gene (various known mutations)
- Diagnostics: evidence of microsatellite instability
- Screening: annual colonoscopy, additional gynecologic/urologic investigation if appropriate, genetic counseling, family screening
- Treatment of cancer: oncological resection
- Prophylactic proctocolectomy not absolutely necessary (20% of mutation carriers do not get cancer)

- Commonest hereditary form
- Usually right hemicolon affected
- Evidence of microsatellite instability

Pathogenesis

- Colorectal cancers arise from epithelial dysplasia, and appear beforehand as adenomas in 90% of cases. In 10% of cases, the cancer occurs de novo without prior signs of adenoma (e.g., when ulcerative colitis has been present for many years). Carcinomatous degeneration of an adenoma occurs due to increasing mutations, usually over years (**adenoma–carcinoma sequence**). In the hereditary forms there are germ line mutations which can lead to obligatory development of cancer, often at a young age.

- 90% adenoma–carcinoma sequence, 10% de-novo cancers

Frequency Distribution
- Ascending colon: 10%
- Transverse colon and descending colon: 10%
- Sigmoid colon: 30%
- Rectum: 50%

Routes of Metastasis
- Lymphatogenous: according to the arterial blood supply initially to the paracolic lymph nodes, then along the feeding arteries as far as the para-aortic lymph nodes and proximally and distally along the marginal artery
- Hematogenous: initially via the portal vein to the liver (75%), then to the lungs (15%) and bone (5%)

- Lymphatogenous to the paracolic lymph nodes
- Hematogenous, especially to the liver

12

Classification (Tables 12.3, 12.4)

Table 12.3   Staging of colorectal cancer (N0: at least 12 examined lymph nodes not involved)

UICC stage	Definition	TNM stage	Dukes stage
0	Carcinoma in situ	Tis, N0, M0	
IA	Infiltration as far as the submucosa	T1, N0, M0	A
IB	Infiltration as far as the muscularis propria	T2, N0, M0	
IIA	Infiltration of all wall layers	T3, N0, M0	B
IIB	Extension beyond the organ	T4, N0, M0	
IIIA	Regional lymph node metastases	T1/2, N1, M0	C
IIIB	N1: 1–3 lymph nodes	T3/4, N1, M0	
IIIC	N2: >3 lymph nodes	Tx, N2, M0	
IV	Distant metastases	Tx, Nx, M1	D

Table 12.4   Histopathological grading

G1	Well differentiated
G2	Moderately differentiated
G3	Poorly differentiated (e.g., mucinous)
G4	Undifferentiated (e.g., small cell, signet ring cell)
Gx	Degree of differentiation not assessable
L0/1	Invading lymphatic vessels
V0/1	Invading veins

Low risk: G1/2, L0, V0, R0.

Symptoms

The symptoms are uncharacteristic. There are no reliable early symptoms.
- Blood mingled with stool
- Change in bowel habits (paradoxical stools, meteorism)
- B-symptoms: fever, night sweats, weight loss
- Reduced energy, fatigue
- Tumor anemia
- Abdominal pains

Complications
- Obstruction
- Tumor perforation (stage T4)
- Fistulas
- Severe bleeding

Diagnostic Approach

- History (especially with hereditary forms)
- Physical examination with digital rectal examination
- Hemoccult test as screening to detect occult blood in the stool
- Laboratory tests: blood count, tumor markers (CEA and Ca 19–9)

- Uncharacteristic: blood in stool, change in bowel habit, B-symptoms, anemia, obstruction, perforation

- History and physical examination
- High colonoscopy with biopsy

12

- Ultrasonography of the abdomen (local lesion, ascites, lymphoma, liver metastases)
- Chest x-ray in two planes
- CT of the abdomen
- High colonoscopy with biopsy

Possible **supplementary investigations:**
- MRI
- Positron emission tomography (PET) / PET-CT
- Urologic investigations (urogram, cystoscopy)
- Gynecologic examination

Recommended preoperative **staging investigations:**
- Digital rectal examination
- High colonoscopy with biopsy
- Ultrasonography of the abdomen
- Chest x-ray in two planes
- CEA measurement

Treatment Approach (Table 12.5)

■ Indications

- Every colon cancer is an indication for surgery in principle. R0 resection should be attempted.
- **Contraindications** to surgery:
  - ▶ Patient's general inoperability
  - ▶ Curative inoperability of the tumor (e.g., diffuse peritoneal metastases, infiltration of the large vessels)
- Resection of metastases or of a second tumor if an R0 situation (curative intent) can be achieved (second operation if necessary)
- Multivisceral resections, if R0 resection is possible (often intraoperative differentiation between inflammatory or tumorous infiltration is not possible, therefore multivisceral resection)
- Oncological procedure even in emergency situations (e.g., obstruction, perforation)
- Adjuvant chemotherapy in UICC stage III
- Palliative measures (resection, local measures, chemotherapy, best supportive care) to prolong life and improve quality of life

- Blood count, markers CEA and Ca 19–9
- Ultrasonography/CT of the abdomen
- Chest x-ray in two planes

- Surgery indicated in principle if no contraindications
- Aim: R0 resection according to oncological criteria (multivisceral resection or resection of metastases if applicable)

Table 12.5   Treatment approach depending on tumor stage

Tumor stage	Treatment
Tis/T1 (low risk)	Local excision
T1 (high risk)/T2–4, N0, M0	Radical operation
Tx, N+, M0	Radical operation and subsequent adjuvant treatment
M1	R0 resection or palliative therapy

12

■ Conservative Treatment

Adjuvant Chemotherapy

- To prolong life after R0 resection in UICC stage III
- For example, FOLFOX regimen

- Aim: prolong life by reducing recurrences
- Indication: after R0 resection of UICC stage III colon cancer
- Postoperative adjuvant chemotherapy after R0 resection of liver or lung metastases is not a general indication. There may possibly be an advantage with regard to overall survival after resection of liver metastases and adjuvant chemotherapy (decision on individual case basis, treatment in study framework).
- Contraindications:
  - ➤ General status less than 2 (WHO)
  - ➤ Uncontrolled infection
  - ➤ Child class B and C cirrhosis
  - ➤ Severe coronary heart disease; heart failure (NYHA III and IV)
  - ➤ Preterminal and terminal renal failure
  - ➤ Impaired bone marrow function
  - ➤ Inability to take part in regular follow-up
- Combined therapy: 5-fluorouracil / folinic acid (Mayo/NSABP regimen), probably survival advantage by combining with oxaliplatin (FOLFOX regimen)
- With liver metastases, no advantage with locoregional chemotherapy (e.g., portal venous infusion or via hepatic artery catheter) compared with systemic chemotherapy

■ Surgical Treatment

General Principles of Cancer Surgery on the Colon

- En-bloc resection with locoregional lymphadenectomy
- Central vessel ligature
- Lateral safety margin at least 10 cm
- No-touch isolation technique

- Prevent intraoperative spread of tumor cells by no-touch isolation technique according to Turnbull et al. 1967, covering the tumor if appropriate.
- Luminal bowel ligature proximal and distal to the tumor with a safety margin of at least 10 cm
- Central vessel ligature
- En-bloc resection with safety margin (three-dimensional) with systematic locoregional lymphadenectomy including the N3 lymph nodes beside the main vessel trunks

Preparation for Surgery

- If reduced general status: preoperative high-calorie parenteral nutrition
- Correction of preoperative anemia
- If appropriate, precautionary marking of a stoma site on the abdominal wall
- Preoperative bowel lavage obsolete, contraindicated with stenosis (laxative if appropriate)
- Perioperative antibiotic prophylaxis (second generation cephalosporin and metronidazole, repeated if necessary during prolonged surgery)
- Intraoperative insertion of a bladder catheter (suprapubic catheter preferable)

Treatment Options with Complete Obstruction, Ileus

- Operation according to oncological criteria, even in an emergency

- The location of the stenosis should be confirmed by preoperative investigations.
- Intraoperative decompression (proximal, distal or through an otomy)

12

- Multistage surgery:
  - ► An emergency prestenotic defunctioning colostomy is fashioned as a cecostomy or transverse colostomy. The tumor is then resected at a second session with restoration of continuity (two-stage). The colostomy can also be left initially to protect the anastomosis and closed later (three-stage).
  - ► Hartmann discontinuity resection is performed especially in the case of obstruction in the left hemicolon. Primary resection of the tumor is performed and a temporary terminal colostomy is fashioned with blind closure of the distal end of the bowel. At a second session, continuity can then be restored after appropriate bowel preparation.
- Primary (single-stage) resection according to oncological criteria depending on tumor location

Procedures with Limited Radicality

- **Indications:**
  - ► Palliative situation to prevent tumor complications such as obstruction or fecal fistula
  - ► Early cancer (T1, N0, L0, V0, G1–2, M0)
- **Procedures:**
  - ► Local therapy:
    - – Endoscopic polypectomy
    - – Local excision (submucous excision or wedge excision)
  - ► Limited resection:
    - – Tubular resection of the segment of bowel containing the tumor without lymphadenectomy
    - – Segmental resection of the bowel segment with limited local lymphadenectomy
  - ► Palliative measures without resection:
    - – Creation of a stoma
    - – Fashioning of an internal anastomosis

Radical Procedures

- **Indication:** standard procedure unless there are contraindications; not early cancer
- **Procedures:**
  - ► Right hemicolectomy
  - ► Left hemicolectomy
  - ► Transverse colectomy
  - ► Sigmoid colectomy
  - ► Extended radical operation (extended hemicolectomy or subtotal colectomy): with tumors located in the region of different lymphatic drainage pathways (e.g., colic flexures, transverse colon), all affected lymph drainage pathways are removed.
  - ► Multivisceral radical resection: radical surgery with removal of infiltrated neighboring organs (R0 resection)
- **General intraoperative procedure:**
  - ► Draping of the abdominal edges to avoid injection metastases
  - ► Exact exploration before starting resection: tumor location, palpation of the colon outline, bimanual palpation of the liver and, if necessary, intraoperative liver ultrasound scan to identify second tumors and metastases)
  - ► Examine operability

12

▶ Establish the resection margins, if appropriate with sealing of the bowel lumen and instillation of a cytostatic irrigation solution into the bowel lumen.

▶ Before open excision of the bowel: placement of draping towels, soft bowel clamps (do not include mesentery in clamps) and disposable clamps

▶ After open excision of the bowel: disinfection of the bowel openings

Right Hemicolectomy
- **Typical extent of resection:**
  ▶ Right hemicolectomy (**Fig. 12.8**): radical excision of the right colic artery and ileocolic artery and clearance of the corresponding lymphatic drainage regions
  ▶ Extended right hemicolectomy (**Fig. 12.9**): additional central ligature of the middle colic artery and clearance of the corresponding lymphatic drainage regions

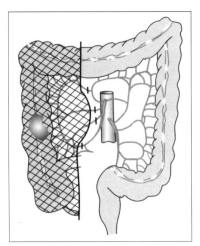

Fig. 12.8 Right hemicolectomy

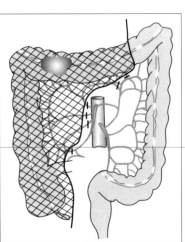

Fig. 12.9 Extended hemicolectomy

- **Indications:**
  - ► Cancer of the cecum and ascending colon: right hemicolectomy
  - ► Cancer of the right colic flexure and proximal transverse colon: extended right hemicolectomy

Operative Technique

- Access: either by midline incision cutting around the left of the umbilicus or by right pararectal/transrectal incision
- Exploration, placing a loop around the intestine at the resection margins. The proximal resection margin is 10–20 cm proximal to the ileocecal valve.
- Mobilize the cecum, ascending colon, and terminal ileum from the lateral aspect by incision of the peritoneum along the "white line"; exposure of the right ureter (**Fig. 12.10**).
- Separate the mesocolon from the Gerota fascia in an avascular plane in the medial direction.
- Mobilize the hepatic flexure, dividing the hepatocolic and duodenocolic ligaments. Ligatures are often required. Cautiously dissect the hepatic flexure from the duodenum and head of the pancreas.
- Divide the gastrocolic ligament, preserving the gastroepiploic vessels as far as the distal resection margin.
- Divide the greater omentum between ligatures at the level of the distal resection margin. The omentum remains attached to the right hemicolon en bloc. The left part of the omentum is left in situ (**Fig. 12.11**).
- V-shaped incision of the serosal layer between the resection margins
- Divide the mesentery between ligatures (**Fig. 12.12**).
- Ligate of the ileocolic artery and vein and right colic artery and vein. The middle colic artery and vein are left (these are ligated during extended hemicolectomy).
- Divide the intestine at the resection margins after a sparing skeletonization. To compensate the difference in lumen diameter, the small intestine is divided obliquely and the large intestine straight across.
- Ileo-transverse end-to-end anastomosis (see p. 197)
- Close the opening in the mesentery with a continuous suture.
- The gastroepiploic vascular arcade is removed in extended resection.

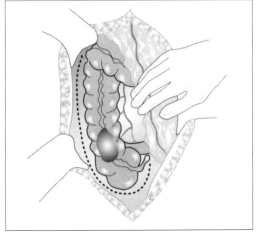

Fig. 12.10 Mobilization of the cecum.

12

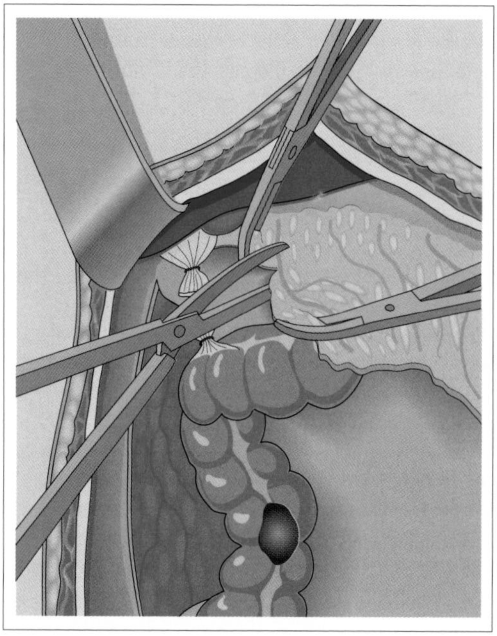

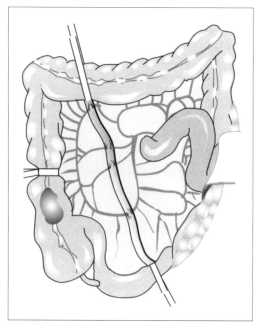

Fig. 12.11 Division of the gastrocolic ligament.

Fig. 12.12 Division of the mesentery.

- **Hazards:**
  - ► Injury of branches of the superior mesenteric artery
  - ► Injury of the right ureter
  - ► Injury of the duodenum
  - ► Tearing of veins on the head of the pancreas

Left Hemicolectomy

- **Typical extent of resection:**
  - ► Right hemicolectomy (**Fig. 12.13**): central ligature of the inferior mesenteric artery
  - ► Extended right hemicolectomy (**Fig. 12.14**): central ligature of the inferior mesenteric artery and middle colic artery
- **Indications:**
  - ► Cancer of the descending colon and proximal sigmoid: left hemicolectomy
  - ► Cancer of the left colic flexure: extended left hemicolectomy

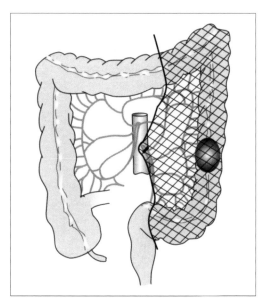

Fig. 12.13 Left hemicolectomy

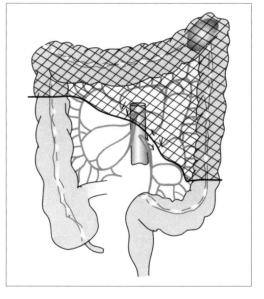

Fig. 12.14 Extended left hemicolectomy

12

Operative Technique

- Access: midline incision cutting around the left of the umbilicus
- Exploration, placing a loop around the intestine at the level of the resection margins (proximally, depends on the tumor site; distally, above the peritoneal reflection).
- Mobilize the descending colon and sigmoid from the lateral aspect by incision of the peritoneum along the "white line"; exposure of the left ureter.
- Separate the mesocolon from the Gerota fascia in an avascular layer in medial direction.
- Divide the greater omentum between ligatures at the level of the proximal resection margin. The omentum remains attached to the left hemicolon en bloc. The right part of the omentum is left in situ.
- Divide the gastrocolic ligament on the left lateral to the proximal resection margin, preserving the gastroepiploic vessel arcade.
- Mobilize the splenic flexure, dividing the splenocolic and phrenocolic ligaments between ligatures.
- V-shaped incision of the serosal layer between the resection margins
- Divide the mesentery between ligatures.
- Divide the inferior mesenteric vein at the lower border of the pancreas. Divide the inferior mesenteric artery and/or left colic artery as centrally as possible (**Fig. 12.15**).
- Divide the intestine at the level of the resection margins after a sparing skeletonization. If necessary, mobilize the hepatic flexure and ascending colon.
- End-to-end anastomosis between the transverse colon and rectum. Good perfusion of the distal bowel end must be ensured, and lower resection may be necessary.
- Close the opening in the mesentery with a continuous suture.
- The gastroepiploic vascular arcade is removed in extended resection.

- **Hazards:**
  - ► Injury of the lower pole of the spleen by traction during mobilization
  - ► Bleeding from the splenocolic ligament
  - ► Injury of the left ureter

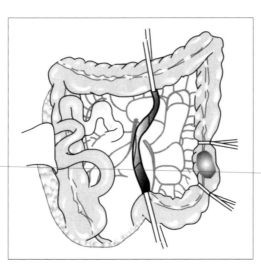

Fig. 12.15   Incision of the mesocolon.

Transverse Colectomy
- **Typical extent of resection:** central ligature of the middle colic artery with clearance of the corresponding lymphatic drainage pathways (**Fig. 12.16**)
- **Indication:** only cancers in the middle of the transverse colon. When located close to a flexure, extended hemicolectomy is standard.

Operative Technique

- Access: midline incision cutting around the left of the umbilicus
- Exploration, placing a loop around the resection margins
- Divide the gastrocolic ligament between ligatures, including the gastroepiploic vessel arcade.
- Mobilize the hepatic flexure and ascending colon (as in right hemicolectomy).
- Mobilize the splenic flexure and descending colon (as in left hemicolectomy).
- Radicular division of the middle colic artery and vein: Reflect the greater omentum upward, incise the mesenteric peritoneum at the origin of the middle colic artery, then carry out central division and ligation of the middle colic artery and vein.
- V-shaped incision of the serosal layer between the resection margins
- Divide the mesentery between ligatures.
- Divide the intestine at the level of the resection margins after a sparing skeletonization with the entire greater omentum.
- End-to-end anastomosis between the ascending and descending colon (see above)
- Close the opening in the mesentery with a continuous suture.

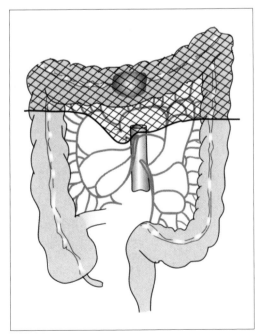

Fig. 12.16   Transverse colectomy

12

Sigmoid Colectomy
- **Typical extent of resection:** ligature of the inferior mesenteric artery distal to the origin of the left colic artery (**Fig. 12.17**)
- **Indication:** cancer in the middle and distal thirds of the sigmoid colon

Operative Technique

- Access: midline lower abdominal laparotomy, cutting around the left of the umbilicus
- Exploration, placing a loop around the proximal resection margin (proximally, junction between the descending colon and sigmoid; distally, rectosigmoid junction above the peritoneal reflection).
- Mobilization from the lateral aspect by incising the peritoneum along the "white line"; exposure of the left ureter.
- Elevate the mesocolon in an avascular plane in medial direction.
- Expose and divide the inferior mesenteric artery, preserving the left colic artery. With tumors in the upper sigmoid colon, perform central ligature of the inferior mesenteric artery if necessary, then check the perfusion of the proximal bowel end, if necessary carry out further resection if perfusion is poor (left hemicolectomy).
- Divide the vein at the level of the arterial ligature.
- Medial incision of the mesenteric peritoneum at its origin along the aorta and blunt dissection from the retroperitoneum, preserving the autonomic nerves. The superior rectal artery is resected also.
- Divide the mesosigmoid between ligatures at the level of the proximal resection margin.
- Mobilization of the proximal rectum (cf. rectal resection):
  - ► U-shaped incision of the pelvic floor peritoneum
  - ► Dissection of the rectum, at first posteriorly in the Waldeyer space, then anteriorly and, finally, laterally in the perirectal region

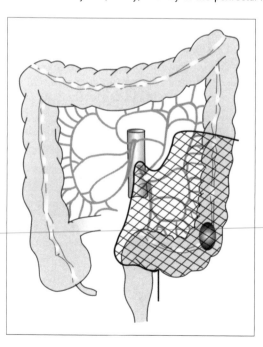

Fig. 12.17 Sigmoid resection

- Divide the upper mesorectum at the level of the distal resection margin (**caution:** no coning), ligating the superior rectal artery.
- Excise the segment of intestine containing the tumor (proximally, open or with a GIA stapler; distally, open or with a TA stapler).
- Approximate the bowel ends. If the tension is too great, mobilization of the splenic flexure can be necessary.
- End-to-end anastomosis between the descending colon and rectum without skeletonizing at the excision margin of the descending colon (p. 197) or mechanical transanal stapled anastomosis
- Close the opening in the mesentery with a continuous suture.

- **Hazards:**
  - ► Injury of the left ureter
  - ► Injury of autonomic nerves
  - ► Inadequate perfusion of the anastomosis, proximally, when the marginal artery is interrupted in the region of the splenic flexure.

■ Palliative Measures

- In the case of a resectable tumor with confirmed distant metastases, the tumor should be removed to ensure bowel passage, for example, in the form of a segmental resection.
- When the primary tumor is inoperable, bypass procedures (e.g., entero-enteric anastomoses) or creation of a stoma may be necessary.
- Stents can be used to ensure bowel passage in the case of stenosing tumors in the rectum, sigmoid, and left hemicolon.
- In patients with advanced cancer in whom curative resection is not possible, palliative chemotherapy should be considered. This can prolong survival time. The treatment of choice currently is 5-fluorouracil / folinic acid alone or in combination with oxaliplatin or irinotecan.
- Radiotherapy is not established in colon cancer.

- Segmental resection
- Bypass by entero-enteric anastomosis
- Creation of a stoma
- Endoscopic stent insertion
- Palliative chemotherapy

■ Aftercare

- Postoperative management after colon resection depends on the patient's condition:
  - ► Avoid drains.
  - ► Remove nasogastric tube directly postoperatively.
  - ► Start early oral feeding.
  - ► Encourage early mobilization.
  - ► Avoid opioid analgesics.

■ Complications

Perioperative Complications

- Bleeding
- Hematoma
- Injury of neighboring organs (e.g., ureter injury → reconstruction)
- Tumor cell dissemination and peritonitis with perforation

12

Late Complications

- Suture leakage
  - ► **Peritonitis** → relaparotomy, irrigation. Bring out proximal colon stump as stoma, with blind closure of distal stump (Hartmann situation); or expose

- Anastomotic leakage
- Recurrence

and close the leak (not usually possible). Further resection may be necessary if wound margins cannot be sutured. Create a protective stoma.

- ► **Abscess** → insertion of a drain (e.g., CT-guided), stoma if necessary
- ► **Fecal fistula** → await spontaneous healing, keep patient fasting or on astronaut diet, otherwise create a stoma
- Secondary bleeding
- Mechanical ileus due to adhesions → relaparotomy and division of the obstruction
- Delayed wound healing (abscesses, seroma, burst abdomen)
- Hernias
- Recurrence

Follow-up Care

- Regular follow-up after R0 resection in UICC stages II and III
- 80% of recurrences are manifested in the first 2 years.

- After curative treatment of a colorectal cancer there is an increased risk for 5 years of **local recurrence** (3%–24%), **distant metastases** (25%), or a metachronous **second tumor** (1.5%–10%). About 80% of recurrences occur in the first two years. Regular cancer follow-up therefore makes sense if recurrence is likely to have therapeutic consequences.
- In UICC stage I, regular follow-up is not necessary because of the favorable prognosis. In this stage, an individual decision should be made regarding follow-up.
- Colonoscopy after 2 and 5 years is reasonable to identify metachronous second tumors.
- After R0 resection of UICC stage II and III colorectal cancers, regular follow-up examinations are indicated (**Table 12.6**).

Table 12.6   Follow-up schedule for colorectal cancer (UICC II and III)

Examination	Months							
	3	6	12	18	24	36	48	60
History, physical examination, CEA		X	X	X	X	X	X	X
Abdominal ultrasonography		X	X	X	X	X	X	X
Colonoscopy		X[a]				X[b]		
Computed tomography	X[c]	X[d]	X[d]	X[d]	X[d]	X[d]	X[d]	X[d]
Chest x-ray in two planes[e]						X		X
Sigmoidoscopy[f]		X	X	X	X			

[a] When a complete preoperative colonoscopy was not performed.
[b] If normal, further colonoscopies every 5 years.
[c] Only for rectal carcinoma 3 months after the conclusion of specific cancer therapy as a baseline.
[d] Optional: useful in young patients for definite identification of local recurrences and liver metastases.
[e] Optional.
[f] Only with rectal carcinoma without neoadjuvant or adjuvant therapy.

Screening

- Annual Hemoccult test and digital rectal examination after the age of 50 years (if positive, colonoscopy is indicated)
- Colonoscopy over the age of 50 years (if normal, repeat every 10 years)
- When there is a hereditary predisposition, screening should start 10 years before the age of manifestation in the affected relative.
- After removal of polyps:
  - ► Low-grade intraepithelial neoplasia: colonoscopy after 3 years
  - ► High-grade intraepithelial neoplasia: colonoscopy in the short term (e.g., after 1 year)

- Colonoscopy and annual Hemoccult test from the age of 50 years
- After polyp removal, colonoscopy monitoring according to the histology

Prognosis

- The cumulative relative 5-year survival rates are ca. 60% for both sexes.
- Five-year survival rates according to UICC stage:
  - ► UICC I: ca. 85%
  - ► UICC II: ca. 50–60%
  - ► UICC III: ca. 30%
  - ► UICC IV: ca. 5%
- 50% of patients develop local recurrence or distant metastases after curative resection, usually as a result of micrometastasis already present at the time of primary surgery. This can be expected especially with node-positive cancers (hepatic metastasis within 5 years: N1 26%, N2 58%).

Further Reading

Andersen HK, Lewis SJ, Thomas S. Early enteral nutrition within 24h of colorectal surgery versus later commencement of feeding for postoperative complications. Cochrane Database Syst Rev 2006 Oct 18; (4): CD004080. Review

Gross V. Aminosalicylates. In: Kruis W, Forbes A, Jauch K-W, Kreis ME, Wexner SD, eds. Diverticular Disease: Emerging Evidence in a Common Condition. Dordrecht, Niederlande: Springer; 2006:175–184

Güenaga KF, Lustosa SA, Saad SS, Saconato H, Matos D. Ileostomy or colostomy for temporary decompression of colorectal anastomosis. Cochrane Database Syst Rev 2007 Jan 24; (1): CD004647. Review

Kornbluth A, Sachar DB and The Practice Parameters Committee of the American College of Gastroenterology. Ulcerative Colitis Practice Guidelines in Adults. American College of Gastroenterology, Practice Parameters Committee. Am J Gastroenterol 2010 Mar; 105(3): 501–523

Kuhry E, Schwenk WF, Gaupset R, Romild U, Bonjer HJ. Long-term results of laparoscopic colorectal cancer resection. Cochrane Database Syst Rev 2008 Apr 16; (2): CD003432. Review

Laurell H, Hansson L-E, Gunnarsson U. Acute diverticulitis—clinical presentation and differential diagnosis. Colrectal Dis 2007; 9: 496–502

Mueller MH, Glatzle J, Kasparek MS, et al. Long-term outcome of conservative treatment in patients with diverticulitis of the sigmoid colon. Eur J Gastroenterol Hepatol 2005; 17: 649–654

National Comprehensive Cancer Network. Clincal Guidelines in Oncology: Colon Cancer V2.2007. www.nccn.org (accessed May 2011)

Reference

Turnbull RB, Kyle K, Watson FR, Spratt J. Cancer of the colon: the influence of the no-touch isolation technic on survival rates. Annals of surgery 1967; 166(3): 420–427

12

13 Rectum

J.M. Mayer

■ Anatomy

- Between the dentate line and 16 cm from the anus, measured with a rigid proctoscope

- The rectum extends from the upper border of the anal canal (dentate line) to 16 cm from the anus, measured with a rigid proctoscope.
- It is divided into three levels:
  - ► Upper third: 12–16 cm from the anus (intraperitoneal)
  - ► Middle third: 6–12 cm from the anus (extraperitoneal)
  - ► Lower third: <6 cm from the anus (extraperitoneal)
- Rectal ampulla: lies against the concavity of the sacrum
- Anal canal: at the level of the pelvic diaphragm, passes in a posterior direction

Fasciae in the Lesser Pelvis

- Anterior and posterior investing fascia
- Lateral: paraproctium forming ligamentous connection with the pelvis

- **Posterior:** The parietal pelvic fascia lines the pelvis posteriorly. It extends from the pelvic ring almost to the tip of the sacrum, meets the pelvic floor, and covers the mesorectum posteriorly as visceral pelvic fascia (investing fascia). Between them is the avascular Waldeyer space.
- **Lateral:** The paraproctium forms a ligamentous connection with the pelvis.
- The Denonvillier fascia is **anterior.** In men, it clothes the posterior wall of the bladder, the seminal vesicles and the posterior wall of the prostate. It is reflected at the urogenital diaphragm and covers the rectum anteriorly as the visceral pelvic fascia (investing fascia).

Arteries (Fig. 13.1)

- Main blood supply: superior rectal artery; no marginal artery
- Middle and inferior rectal arteries: inconstant, supply the distal anterior wall
- After resection, usually adequate blood supply from distally

- Superior rectal artery (unpaired) from the inferior mesenteric artery provides the blood supply to the major part of the rectum. It divides into three terminal branches on the posterior wall of the rectum, which empty into the hemorrhoidal plexus at 3, 7, and 11 o'clock positions.
- Middle rectal arteries (paired, inconstant) from the internal iliac artery run above the levators into the paraproctium and supply a small section of the distal anterior rectal wall together with the inferior rectal arteries (paired, inconstant) from the pudendal arteries, which are branches of the internal iliac artery, running below the levators.
- Blood supply after low anterior rectal resection:
  - ► With ligature close to the trunk of the inferior mesenteric artery, the proximal colon stump is supplied only through the anastomosis of the Riolan and Drummond arcade. It is therefore important to spare the marginal arcade.
  - ► The rectal stump can be supplied only by the inferior rectal arteries and possibly the middle rectal arteries. The longer the rectal stump, the more endangered is its blood supply. Intramural vascular anastomoses usually ensure an adequate blood supply from distally.

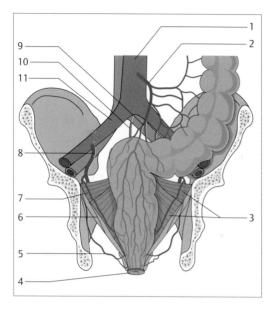

Fig. 13.1 Blood supply of the rectum.
  1: Aorta
  2: Inferior mesenteric artery
  3: Levator ani with pubo-
     rectalis sling
  4: Anal canal
  5. Inferior rectal artery
  6: Levator ani
  7: Middle rectal artery
  8: Internal iliac artery
  9: Superior rectal artery
  10: Middle sacral artery
  11: Common iliac artery

Veins

- The main venous drainage is to the liver through the unpaired superior rectal vein and portal vein system.
- In the lower quarter of the rectum, there may be venous drainage to the lungs via the middle and inferior rectal veins and inferior vena cava (inconstant).

- Main drainage is to the liver through the superior rectal vein.
- Middle and inferior rectal veins usually absent.

Lymphatic Drainage

- The main lymphatic drainage follows the branching of the superior rectal artery to the locoregional lymph nodes in the mesorectum, and from there along the main trunk of the superior rectal artery to the para-aortic lymph nodes.
- Because of the absence of a vascular arcade close to the bowel wall, there are no lymphatic pathways running proximally and distally along the bowel. Malignant cells are usually not found more than 4 cm from the primary tumor. Thus, smaller safety margins are sufficient in rectal surgery.
- The inferior quarter of the rectum has no lymph nodes because of the absence of mesorectum. Lymphatic drainage is intramural in the cranial direction.
- Lymphatic channels along the middle and inferior rectal arteries are present only rarely. Iliac lymph node metastases (lateral pelvic wall) therefore occur rarely, even with supraanal rectal cancer.
- The anal canal also drains to the inguinal lymph nodes.

- Main drainage along the superior rectal artery
- Only slight spread along the bowel because of the absence of a marginal artery
- Drainage to iliac and inguinal lymph nodes usually absent

Innervation

- The distal quarter of the rectum has particularly pronounced innervation.
- This is the site of the procontinence reaction for maintaining the anorectal reflex.
- The epicritic sensibility for distinguishing solid matter, liquid, and gas is located in the anoderm.

13

• Transport occurs only in a distal direction due to the polar arrangement of the rectal musculature.

Anal Canal (Fig. 13.2)

• Between anocutaneous line and dentate line
• Highly sensitive anoderm (epicritic sensibility)

• From the anocutaneous line (junction of keratinized with nonkeratinized squamous epithelium) to the dentate line (junction of nonkeratinized squamous epithelium with rectal mucosa).
• **Anoderm:** highly sensitive to identify the nature of the rectal contents
• Anal crypts open at the level of the dentate line and extend down to the internal sphincter
• **Proctodeal glands:** located between the internal and external sphincters, open posteriorly at 6 o'clock position and anteriorly at 11 to 1 o'clock positions into the anal crypts.
• **Corpus cavernosum of the rectum:** located in submucosal position above the dentate line
• **Closing mechanisms:**
  ► Reservoir function of the rectum
  ► Internal sphincter: smooth muscle, autonomic innervation and permanently contracted
  ► External sphincter: striated muscle, somatic innervation, voluntary contraction
  ► Corpus cavernosum of the rectum—hemorrhoidal plexus, for fine continence
  ► Anorectal angle, about 90° at rest, most important static continence factor
• **Defecation:**
  ► When the ampulla fills with feces: contraction of the rectal muscle and relaxation of the internal sphincter
  ► Defecation occurs with simultaneous voluntary relaxation of the external sphincter and abdominal compression.
  ► If defecation does not take place, there is an increase in the tone of the external sphincter and puborectalis sling with a reduction of the anorectal angle.

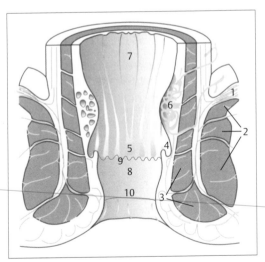

Fig. 13.2 Anatomy of the anal region.
1: Levator ani muscle
2: External sphincter
3: Internal sphincter
4: Anal crypt
5: Rectal columns
6: Corpus cavernosum of the rectum
7: Rectum
8: Anoderm
9: Dentate line
10: Anocutaneous line

■ Rectal Cancer

Definition

- All epithelial malignancies between the dentate line and the rectosigmoid junction 16 cm from the anus (measured with a rigid proctoscope)

- Epithelial malignancies between the dentate line and the rectosigmoid junction 16 cm from the anus

Epidemiology

- See Colon Cancer (p. 214).

Etiology

- See Colon Cancer (p. 214).

Pathogenesis

- See Colon Cancer (p. 215).

Frequency Distribution:
- Upper rectum (12–16 cm): 20.8%
- Middle rectum (6–12 cm): 43.4%
- Lower rectum (< 6 cm): 35.8%

Routes of Metastasis
- **Lymphatogenous:**
  - ► Mesorectal lymph nodes along the superior rectal artery to the para-aortic lymph nodes
  - ► With distal cancers, to the iliac lymph nodes also (rare)
- **Hematogenous:**
  - ► Via the portal vein to the liver
  - ► With distal cancers, to the lung via the vena cava (rare)

- Mainly in cranial direction to para-aortic lymph nodes and to the liver

Classification (Table 13.1)

Table 13.1 **Mason classification of findings on palpation**

Clinical staging	Palpable findings
CS I	Mucosa mobile
CS II	Bowel wall mobile
CS III	Bowel wall partially fixed
CS IV	Bowel wall completely fixed
CS V	Disseminated disease

Symptoms

- See Colon Cancer (p. 216).

13

Diagnostic Approach

- Corresponds to colon cancer
- In addition: proctoscopy with endosonography and CT of the thorax

- The investigations correspond to those for colon cancer (see p. 216).
- The following investigations are performed in addition:
  - ► Rigid proctoscopy with endosonography
  - ► CT of the thorax (particularly with supraanal rectal cancer)
  - ► Sphincter manometry if applicable

Treatment Approach

■ Indications (Table 13.2)

Table 13.2 Treatment approach depending on tumor stage

Tumor stage	Treatment
Tis/T1 (low risk)	Local excision (e.g., transanal resection through entire wall)
T1 (high risk)/T2, N0, M0	Primary surgery
T3/4, N0, M0/Tx, N+, M0	Neoadjuvant therapy, followed by surgery and adjuvant treatment
M1	R0 resection or palliative therapy

■ Conservative Treatment

Neoadjuvant Therapy

- Preoperative chemoradiotherapy in stage T3/4 or N+ stage for downsizing and downstaging, if no distant metastases

- This prior treatment is indicated for locally advanced cancer or cancer with lymphatogenous metastasis. Moreover, neoadjuvant treatment can be considered for supraanal cancers close to the sphincter to achieve a sphincter-preserving operation.
- Preoperative downsizing or downstaging should be achieved so that subsequent R0 resection is possible. In the long-term prognosis, the risk of local recurrence can be significantly reduced, and prolonged overall survival can also be achieved if there is a good response.
- The treatment usually consists of conventionally fractionated radiation (50.4 Gy) or brief radiation (5×5 Gy) accompanied by chemotherapy with 5-fluorouracil as radiosensitizer (alternatively, oxaliplatin, capecitabine or irinotecan).
- Surgery is then performed after 4–5 weeks.

Adjuvant Therapy

- After neoadjuvant chemoradiotherapy: postoperative chemotherapy
- Postoperative stage T3/4 or N+ stage: chemoradiotherapy

- After prior neoadjuvant treatment, postoperative adjuvant chemotherapy with 5-fluorouracil is indicated ca. 4–6 weeks after surgery.
- If an advanced tumor stage (T3/4) or lymph node involvement is found postoperatively, chemoradiotherapy (see above) is necessary. R0 resection and M0 status are always requirements for adjuvant therapy.
- Postoperative chemoradiotherapy should also be given after R1 resection or intraoperative tumor dissemination.
- After R0 resection of liver or lung metastases, adjuvant chemotherapy is not generally indicated (individual case decision).

■ Surgical Treatment

Transanal Full-Thickness Resection

This procedure is feasible for ca. 5% of all rectal cancers.

Indication
- Tis/T1, G1–2, L0, V0, R0, M0
- Diameter ≤3 cm
- Lateral safety margin at least 1 cm

In this situation, lymph node metastases can be expected in fewer than 2% of cases.

Operative Procedure
- **Transanal local excision** after Parks:
  - ► Introduction of an anal retractor, placement of stay sutures, tumor is pulled downward, resection by electrocautery, transverse suture
  - ► Problem: poor vision
  - ► Recurrence rates up to 30%
- **Transanal endoscopic microsurgery** after Buess:
  - ► Wide operating microscope, continuous gas insufflation, use of micro instruments (e.g., UltraCision), transverse suture
  - ► Advantage: better vision; also, lesions within the middle third of the rectum can be reached

Radical Surgery

Operation Principles (Fig. 13.3)
- R0 resection
- Radical division of the inferior mesenteric artery and vein (no prognostic difference between ligature of the inferior mesenteric artery close to the trunk and preservation of the left colic artery)
- **Total mesorectal excision** (TME) of tumors in the middle and lower thirds; **partial mesorectal excision** (PME) of tumors in the upper third (coning, i.e., proximal conical thinning of the mesorectum, must be avoided; **Fig. 13.4**)
- Preservation of investing fascia during dissection
- Observation of safety margins:
  - ► Upper rectum: 5 cm
  - ► Lower rectum with high-grade tumors (G3, G4): 3–4 cm
  - ► Lower rectum with low-grade tumors (G1, G2): 2 cm
- En-bloc resection of organs adherent to tumor (multivisceral resection)
- Sparing of the autonomic pelvic nerves (hypogastric nerves, superior and inferior hypogastric plexus)

- TME or PME, avoiding coning
- Sparing of autonomic pelvic nerves

(Low) Anterior Rectal Resection

Operative Technique

- Lithotomy position
- Access: lower midline laparotomy, cutting to the left of the umbilicus
- Exploration: determine operability and operative procedure (radicality), intraoperative ultrasound scan of the liver
- Mobilize the sigmoid loop from the left by dividing the mesosigmoid from the lateral abdominal wall; exposure of the left ureter. Mobilization of the descending colon is followed by left colon flexure mobilization.

13

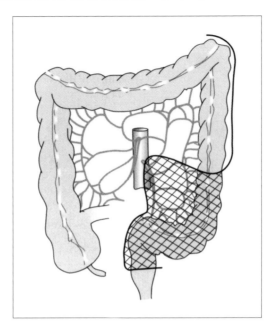

Fig. 13.3 Extent of rectal resection.

- Exposure of the inferior mesenteric artery from the aorta ca. 1–2 cm distal to its origin; incision of the peritoneum from the ligament of Treitz between the aorta and inferior vena cava as far as the pelvis and high ligature of the artery (close to the aorta or preserving the origin of the left colic artery). The inferior mesenteric vein is ligated at the level of the lower border of the pancreas.
- Division of the mesocolon between ligatures at the level of the proximal resection margin. The marginal artery is the only blood supply of the proximal stump still present and must be spared.
- Division of the intestine (e.g., GIA stapler or open division and tying in the anvil of a circular stapler after placing a purse-string suture)
- Division of the mesosigmoid from the retroperitoneum between the ligature of the inferior mesenteric artery and the promontory, sparing the autonomic nerves that run in the retroperitoneum
- Below the promontory a spider's web–like layer (Waldeyer fascia) opens posterior to the rectum between the visceral pelvic fascia (investing fascia of the rectum) and the parietal pelvic fascia. Blunt dissection in the Waldeyer fascia as far as the pelvic floor is often possible (this spares the posteriorly located autonomic nerves and presacral veins and allows complete removal of the mesorectum).
- U-shaped incision of the anterior and lateral peritoneum of the upper rectum (anterior incision ca. 2 cm above the peritoneal reflection)

Mobilization of the Rectum in Men (Fig. 13.4)
- Anterior dissection of the rectum: undermining the peritoneum directly behind the bladder with the index finger and division of the bridge of tissue as far as possible from the rectum to avoid bleeding. Continue from here downward between the visceral pelvic (investing) fascia and the Denonvillier fascia (sparing the autonomic nerves lying anterior to the Denonvillier fascia). If the tumor is in an anterior location, the Denonvillier fascia is removed, exposing the seminal vesicles.

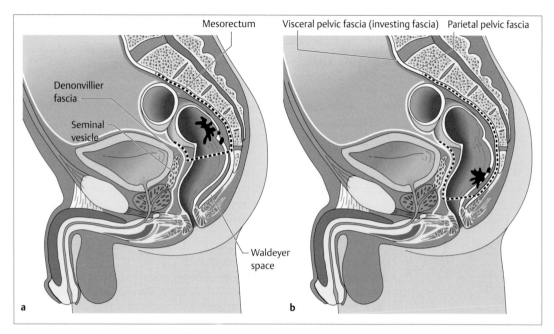

Fig. 13.4 a, b   Rectal resection—fascial relationships in men.
a Partial mesorectal excision.
b Total mesorectal excision.

- Lateral dissection of the rectum: sharp division of the lateral suspensory ligaments (paraproctium); where necessary, ligature of the inconstant middle
  rectal artery
- This means that the rectum has been mobilized as far as the pelvic floor
  formed by the levator ani.

Mobilization of the Rectum in Women
- A groove can be found between the posterior fornix of the vagina and the
  anterior wall of the rectum, through which the anterior incision of the peri-
  toneum is made. The dissection is performed in the obliterated recess of the
  Denonvillier fascia, which surrounds the posterior wall of the vagina down to
  the pelvic floor, the anterior wall of the rectum, and the paraproctium.
- Simultaneous hysterectomy is performed only in the case of tumor infiltration.
  In these cases, removal of the posterior vaginal wall is often also necessary.

Anastomosis
- Restoration of continuity either by open division and end-to-end anastomosis
  (manual suture) or by division using a linear stapler and stapled anastomosis
  using a circular stapler introduced through the anus
- Insertion of an extraperineal Easy Flow drain in the sacral fossa (not obligatory)
- Closure of the pelvic floor peritoneum (not obligatory)
- Consider a protective stoma.

13

Abdominoperineal Intersphincteric Resection

Operative Technique

- Rectal mobilization as for low anterior resection
- Further rectal mobilization in the levator funnel between the external and internal sphincters
- Division at the level of the dentate line in the anal canal
- Anastomosis using a circular stapler
- Consider a protective stoma.

Parks Transanal Anastomosis (1972)
- Very low suprasphincter or intersphincter division of the rectum
- Colon is pulled through distally
- Transanal anastomosis by interrupted sutures through all layers
- Consider a protective stoma.

Colo-anal Pouch Anastomosis (Fig. 13.5)
- Direct sphincter damage or injury of autonomic nerves after low anastomosis can lead to a drop in resting anal pressure. The clinical symptoms can be fecal soiling, high defecation frequency, or imperative urgency. Continence can be improved by creating a pouch anastomosis, without increasing the complication rate.

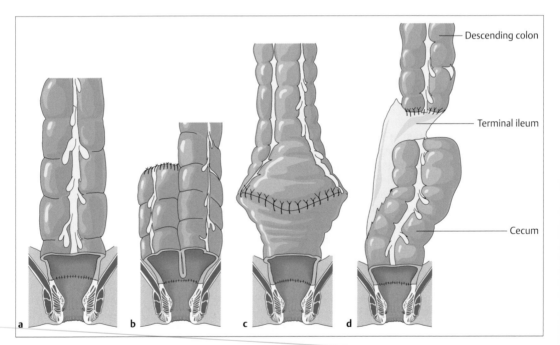

Fig. 13.5 a–d Pouch anastomosis.
a Colo-anal end-to-end anastomosis.
b J-pouch, limb length ca. 6 cm, not possible with a thick mesentery.
c Transverse coloplasty pouch, 4–6 cm proximal to the anastomosis, opening of the free taenia and transverse suture, technically easy.
d Cecal reservoir, interposition of the cecum, technically difficult, no advantage over J-pouch.

13

Abdominoperineal Rectal Amputation

Operative Technique

- Mark the colostomy exit site and insert a transurethral bladder catheter before the start of the operation.
- Rectal mobilization as for low anterior resection
- Closure of the anus by a strong purse-string suture
- Elliptical incision around the anus with a 2-cm margin
- Generous removal of the fat pad in the ischiorectal fossa with removal of its contained lymph nodes
- Division of the anococcygeal ligament at the tip of the coccyx
- Division of the levator ani at its junction with the external sphincter
- During anterior dissection, there is a risk of urethral and prostate injury in men, injury of the posterior vaginal wall in women, and of opening the rectum.
- Primary wound closure after insertion of a Robinson drain into the sacral fossa by suture in layers of muscle, fascia, and skin
- Hemostasis in the sacral fossa; consider insertion of a mesh plug or closure of the pelvic peritoneum.

Fashioning of the Terminal Descending Colostomy
- Excise a circle of skin at the previously determined site.
- Cruciate notching of the rectus sheath, blunt splitting of the rectus muscle, opening of the peritoneum. The correct position of the stoma is at the border of the rectus muscle. The channel in the abdominal wall should just admit two fingers.
- The end of the colon is pulled through the abdominal wall and fixed to the fascia with four interrupted sutures.
- After opening, the proximal stump of the colon is sutured with interrupted seromuscular–intracutaneous sutures.
- Inspection of the abdominal cavity; if necessary, insertion of Easy Flow drains and closure of the abdominal wall.

Other Procedures

Hartmann Discontinuity Resection
- Indications:
  - ► Emergency procedure for tumor perforation and peritonitis
  - ► Palliative procedure to avoid bowel obstruction
  - ► Elderly patients with insufficient sphincter function

Endoscopic Polypectomy
- Indication: polypoid tumors with a base < 3 cm
- Removal by forceps or diathermy loop

■ Palliative Measures

- In the event of general or local inoperability, palliative measures are indicated to halt tumor growth and keep stool passage patent.
- The following can be used locally:
  - ► Electro- or infrared coagulation
  - ► Laser therapy
  - ► Cryotherapy

- Local ablative measures to maintain bowel patency, stent, colostomy, palliative resection, palliative chemotherapy

13

- ► Stents
- ► Proximal colostomy as a last resort
- In the case of nonresectable metastatic cancer, the benefit of palliative chemotherapy to prolong survival and improve quality of life is confirmed. Apart from 5-fluorouracil, irinotecan, oxaliplatin, and specific antibodies are used.
- Palliative resection of the primary tumor can be useful to prevent complications such as obstruction, tumor invasion of neighboring organs, or hemorrhage. Moreover, because of the markedly improved systemic treatment possibilities, secondary resection of metastases may be possible in an attempt at curative treatment; therefore re-evaluation should be considered in the course of therapy.

■ Complications

Perioperative Complications

- Bleeding
- Ureter injury
- Injury of the posterior wall of the bladder or vagina (→ suture)
- Leaking anastomosis:
  - ► Second row of sutures manually (protective stoma)
  - ► New protective stoma
  - ► Hartmann operation
- Urethral injury during rectal amputation

Late Complications

- Secondary bleeding
- Delayed wound healing
- Anastomotic leak: up to 10%, usually on day 4–7
  - ► Intraperitoneal: peritonitis → revision surgery with new anastomosis and protective stoma or Hartmann operation
  - ► Extraperitoneal: abscess → insertion of drain, protective stoma
- Fistulas
- Incontinence
- Impotence and disorder of micturition as a result of injury of autonomic nerves
- Recurrence

Aftercare and Screening

- See Colon Cancer (pp. 228–229).

■ Pelvic Floor Insufficiency

Anatomy

- The pelvic floor forms a functional unit, which closes the abdominal cavity below and prevents prolapse of internal organs (**Fig. 13.6**).
- It consists of muscles, ligaments and connective tissue, which are attached to the bony pelvic ring.

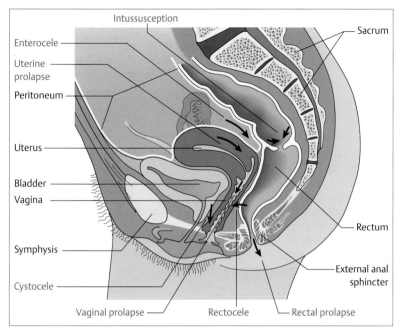

Fig. 13.6 Sagittal section through the female pelvis with pathologies (red labels) due to pelvic floor insufficiency.

- The sphincters ensure competent closure and controlled voiding from the bladder and rectum.
- The female pelvis is wider and less steep, thinner, and less innervated than that of the male.

Epidemiology

- Women are much more often affected than men in a ratio of 9 : 1.

  - Women affected in particular

Etiology

- Complex, multifactorial and dynamic event
- There is often pathology in different compartments (**Table 13.3**), so that different disciplines must be involved in the treatment.
- One-sided treatment approaches can usually only alleviate some of the symptoms and lead more often to recurrence.
- Risk factors:
  - ► Female sex
  - ► Vaginal delivery
  - ► Multiparity
  - ► Excessive straining on defecation with chronic constipation
  - ► Obesity
  - ► Pelvic surgery (e.g., hysterectomy)
  - ► Pudendal nerve neuropathy
  - ► Congenital connective tissue weakness

  - Complex, multifactorial and dynamic event

13

Table 13.3   Compartments of the pelvic floor

Compartment	Pathology
Anterior	Cystocele
Middle	Uterine prolapse, vaginal stump prolapse, enterocele
Posterior	Rectal prolapse

Perineal Descent

- Pelvic floor descent: often fecal and urinary incontinence
- The most frequent disease from the coloproctological aspect
- Two forms of pelvic floor descent:
  - ► Descent present at rest—descending perineum syndrome (DPS)
  - ► Descent provoked by straining
- Multifactorial, including pudendal nerve neuropathy with consequent muscle atrophy
- Continence diminishes due to enlargement of the rectoanal angle and shortening of the anal canal along with muscle fiber atrophy
- Often leads to fecal and urinary incontinence

Rectocele

- Anterior bulging of the rectal wall usually leads to interference with fecal voiding.
- Anterior (most common), lateral, and posterior rectocele
- Arises from stretching of the rectovaginal septum especially due to severe straining
- Large rectoceles interfere with fecal voiding

Enterocele ("Cul de Sac")

- Descent of the small bowel between rectum and vagina may cause constipation.
- Descent of the peritoneum between the anterior rectal wall and vagina in the pouch of Douglas, usually containing small intestine or elongated sigmoid colon
- The cause is divarication of the limbs of the levator (e.g., after hysterectomy)
- Leads to obstruction of the rectum due to anterior impression during defecation
- Often combined with perineal descent and a rectocele

Rectal Prolapse (Table 13.4)

- Valve mechanism due to intussusception leads to incontinence and fecal voiding disorder.
- Telescopic invagination (intussusception) of all layers of the rectum
- Often a sequela of chronic constipation
- Usually combined with an enterocele that presses on the rectum
- Leads to incontinence and interference with fecal voiding (valve mechanism)

Table 13.4   Classification of rectal prolapse

Grade	Definition	Clinical features
1	Internal prolapse, only on proctoscopy	Asymptomatic, fecal voiding disorder
2	Visible on straining	Fecal soiling, incontinence
3	Circular mucosal prolapse at rest outside the anus	Marked incontinence, ulceration, bleeding

13

Symptoms

The symptoms are very varied:
- Incontinence (feces/urine)
- Constipation
- Sensation of incomplete voiding with fecal soiling
- Prolapse of pelvic organs (vagina, uterus, rectum)
- Perineal pain
- Sexual dysfunction, dyspareunia
- Blood and mucus on the stool

- Very varied symptoms: incontinence, constipation, fecal soiling, pain

Diagnostic Approach

- History
- Proctological examination (inspection, palpation)
- Proctoscopy, sphincter manometry
- Gynecological examination
- Urological examination (if necessary including urodynamics)
- Ultrasonography, possibly endosonography
- Radiographic examinations: defecography, colon contrast enema
- Dynamic pelvic floor MRI (imaging of all three compartments)
- Neurological investigations (pelvic floor electromyography, pudendal nerve studies)

- Taking an accurate history is important.

Treatment Approach

■ Conservative Treatment (see also p. 256)

- Stool-regulating measures (dietary fiber, laxatives)
- Pelvic floor exercises
- Active and passive biofeedback

■ Surgical Treatment (Table 13.5)

- There are many different procedures, though no clear evidence-based recommendations can be made.
- The postoperative morbidity is lower after an extra-abdominal approach than after an abdominal approach.
- The risk of recurrence appears to be lower and continence to be better with an abdominal procedure.
- Postoperative constipation appears to be less after resection plus rectopexy than after rectopexy alone.
- With abdominal procedures, laparoscopic surgery is more comfortable for the patient.
- In the more complex pelvic floor insufficiency syndrome—with perineal descent, elongated sigmoid colon, enterocele, or grade 3 rectal prolapse—laparoscopic rectosigmoid resection, possibly with mesh implantation, is standard procedure.

- Complex pelvic floor insufficiency: laparoscopic rectosigmoid resection, possibly with mesh insertion
- Rectal prolapse/rectocele exclusively: transanal tubular resection of all layers of the rectum with stapler

13

Table 13.5   Operative procedures for pelvic floor insufficiency

Operation	Technique
Extra-abdominal	
Delorme	Excision of a transverse strip of mucosa 10–15 cm wide ca. 1 cm above the dentate line Rejoining the mucosal margins with simultaneous duplication of the muscle walls leads to local adhesion
Altemeier	Division of the rectal wall ca. 1 cm above the dentate line Resection of the prolapsed rectum Rejoined by manual suture or staples
Abdominal	
Sudeck	Complete posterior mobilization of the rectum Fixation of the rectum to the presacral fascia
Wells	As Sudeck operation In addition, insertion of a plastic mesh into the concavity of the sacrum, which surrounds two-thirds of the rectum
Ripstein	Mesh sling placed around the rectum from in front and fixed to the sacrum bilaterally
Frykmann and Goldberg	Complete mobilization of the rectum including the rectocele Resection of the rectosigmoid If necessary, rectopexy to the promontory or stabilization by mesh insertion Standard resecting procedure using laparoscopic technique

- Frykmann and Goldberg: standard laparoscopic procedure

New Procedures

- Transanal tubular resection of all layers of the rectum with rectal intussusception/rectocele only

- Transanal tubular full-thickness resection of the rectum:
  - ➤ STARR: stapled transanal rectal resection using PPH stapler/Transtar
  - ➤ Indicated for fecal voiding disorder as a result of obstructive defecation syndrome
  - ➤ The cause is internal rectal prolapse (intussusception), possibly combined with a rectocele.
  - ➤ Not indicated in combination with perineal descent, extensive enterocele, and grade 3 rectal prolapse; functional disorders; or concomitant symptoms of the anterior or middle compartment
  - ➤ Tubular resection of the rectum
  - ➤ The definitive status of this operation method has not yet been adequately evaluated by studies.

Further Reading

Breukink S, Pierie J, Wiggers T. Laparoscopic versus open total mesorectal excision for rectal cancer. Cochrane Database Syst Rev 2006 Oct 18; (4): CD005200. Review
Brown CJ, Fenech DS, McLeod RS. Reconstructive techniques after rectal resection for rectal cancer. Cochrane Database Syst Rev 2008 Apr 16; (2): CD006040. Review
Guenaga KF, Matos D, Castro AA, Atallah AN, Wille-Jørgensen P. Mechanical bowel preparation for elective colorectal surgery. Cochrane Database Syst Rev 2005 Jan 25; (1): CD001544

14 Anus

J.M. Mayer

■ Anatomy

- See Chapter 13.

■ Hemorrhoids

Definition

- Expansion of the corpus cavernosum of the rectum (hemorrhoidal cushions) located above the dentate line, typically at the 3, 7, and 11 o'clock positions
- If symptoms occur, hemorrhoidal disease is present. The classification of hemorrhoidal disease is shown in **Table 14.1**.

- Expansion of the corpus cavernosum of the rectum (hemorrhoidal plexus)

Epidemiology

- Incidence: 40–50 per 100 000 population per year
- Peak incidence between the ages of 45 and 65 years
- One of the most common diseases in industrialized nations
- Ca. 70% of all adults are affected at some time in their life.

- Common disease in industrialized nations, ca. 70% of all adults

Etiology

- Exact etiology unclear
- Impaired defecation is a cause, together with a genetic predisposition.
- Risk factors:
  - ► Chronic constipation associated with severe straining
  - ► Pregnancy
  - ► Obesity
  - ► Chronic diarrhea
  - ► Laxative abuse
  - ► Alcohol abuse

- Genetic predisposition and impaired defecation

Table 14.1 Classification of hemorrhoidal disease

Stage	Description
1	Enlarged corpus cavernosum recti visible on proctoscopy
2	Prolapse on defecation, spontaneous retraction
3	Prolapse on defecation, can be reduced manually
4	Prolapse fixed, thrombosed or fibrosed, irreducible, corresponds to anal prolapse

Symptom

• Bleeding, discharge, pruritus, and pain

The symptoms are independent of size. Grade 1 hemorrhoids are usually asymptomatic.
• Bright red bleeding, dripping or spurting
• Traces of blood on toilet paper
• Pruritus
• Discharge
• Anal eczema
• Anal prolapse with ulcerations
• Disturbance of fine continence with prolapsed hemorrhoids
• Feeling of incomplete evacuation, fecal soiling
• Severe pain with incarceration

Diagnostic Approach

• Inspection, palpation, proctoscopy

• Inspection of the anus with attempted straining
• Palpation of the anal canal
• Proctoscopy: most precise assessment of size and constitution
• Radial cloverleaf wrinkling with anal prolapse
• If there is bleeding, consider high colonoscopy to rule out cancer.

■ Differential Diagnosis

• Anal vein thrombosis (p. 250)
• Skin tag: painless fold of anal skin at the outer margin of the anus
• Hypertrophic anal papilla: proliferative fibrosis because of chronic recurrent inflammation of an anal papilla
• Rectal prolapse: circular mucosal folds (see Chapter 13)
• Prolapsed rectal polyp

Treatment Approach (Table 14.2)

Table 14.2   Treatment of hemorrhoids according to stage

Stage	Treatment
1	Sclerosis
2	Rubber band ligature
3 (isolated nodule)	Milligan–Morgan operation
	Parks operation
	Longo operation
3 (circular prolapse)	Longo operation
	Parks operation
4 (fixed prolapse)	Parks operation
	Fansler–Arnold operation

■ Conservative Treatment

Local Therapy
• Application of ointments and suppositories (e.g., containing steroids) to relieve the symptoms
• No causal therapy

Sclerotherapy
- **Principle:** Stabilization and fixation of the hemorrhoidal convolutions above the dentate line
- High rate of long-term recurrence (up to 70%)
- Blond method: submucous injection of polidocanol into the nodule
- Blanchard/Bensaude method: injection of phenol and almond oil solution into the region of the supplying hemorrhoidal arteries at 3, 7 and 11 o'clock positions

Rubber Band Ligature
- **Principle:** Application of rubber bands using a special ligator, with resulting necrosis and sloughing of the hemorrhoid nodule
- Recurrence rate up to 25%

■ Surgical Treatment

Milligan–Morgan Operation
- **Principle:** Resecting procedure with loss of anoderm (**Fig. 14.1**)
- Resection of up to three nodules, otherwise reconstructive procedure

Operative Technique

- Sphincter stretching (three fingers)
- Clamping of the hemorrhoidal pile at the junction between the skin and anoderm
- Second clamp placed above the dentate line, at the same time clamping the palpable artery
- Transfixion ligature above the proximal clamp
- Incision at the skin–anoderm border with scissors. Division of the anoderm along the pile (bilaterally) as far as the proximal clamp (semicircular incision around the hemorrhoid)
- Dissect the vascular plexus off the internal sphincter.
- Any satellite nodules are divided from the main nodule below the anoderm.
- Remove the proximal clamp and tie again, including the dissected vascular mucosal mass.
- Excise the flap distal to the ligature.

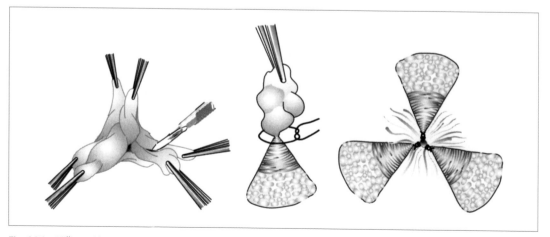

Fig. 14.1 Milligan–Morgan operation

14

- An adequate bridge of skin/mucosa (at least 6 mm) between the piles is important to avoid stenosis.
- Ointment strips
- **Ferguson modification:** continuous suture of the resulting defect

Parks Operation
- **Principle:** Reconstructive procedure with little loss of anoderm (**Fig. 14.2**)

Operative Technique

- Sphincter stretching (three fingers)
- Infiltration of a vasoconstrictor solution in the region of the nodule
- Clamp the nodule.
- Cut just around the nodule, make a longitudinal incision of the anoderm upward as far as the dentate line, and oblique incisions to both sides (Y-shaped).
- Reflect the skin/mucosa and dissect the vascular plexus from the internal sphincter. **Caution:** the anoderm is very sensitive.
- Central ligature of the pile and resection of the nodule
- Suture of the two lateral flaps upward, thus covering the defect and moving the anoderm in a cranial direction

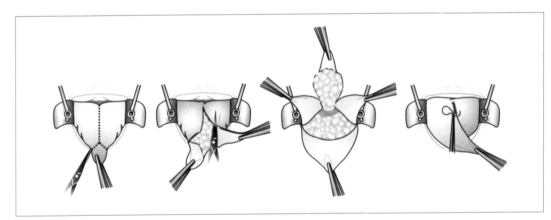

Fig. 14.2   Parks operation

Fansler–Arnold Operation
- **Principle:** Reconstructive procedure without loss of anoderm

Operative Technique

- Resection of the hemorrhoidal tissue with a covering of mucosa from above the dentate line with distal mobilization of a flap of anoderm
- Refixation of the anodermal flap to the rectal mucosa, thus cranial advancement of the anoderm into the anal canal

Stapled Hemorrhoidectomy after Longo (1998) (Fig. 14.3)
- **Advantages:**
  - ► No loss of anoderm
  - ► Little postoperative pain

Operative Technique

- Place a purse-string suture through the rectal mucosa 3 cm proximal to the dentate line.
- Introduce a circular 33 mm stapler (with enlarged housing).
- Tighten the purse-string suture.
- Close the stapler. This divides the mucosa in a circle and separates the mucosa grasped by the stapler with parts of the hemorrhoidal plexus, at the same time joining the proximal and distal mucosa with a double-row of staples ca. 1 cm above the dentate line.
- **Caution:** do not draw the rectovaginal septum into the stapler.

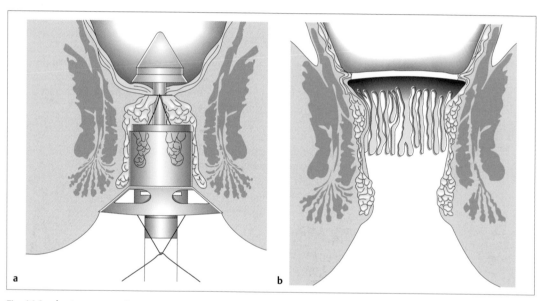

Fig. 14.3 a, b   Longo operation
a Introduced stapler.
b Row of staples after firing the stapler.

Prevention

- High-fiber diet
- Adequate liquids and exercise
- Avoid straining on defecation (read the newspaper!)
- No laxatives, little alcohol
- Weight reduction

■ Perianal Vein Thrombosis

• Very painful thrombosis in the external perianal venous network

- **Definition:** thrombosis in the external perianal venous network
  Synonym: external hemorrhoid
- **Etiology:** unclear, but there are promoting factors (see under hemorrhoids)
- **Symptoms:** very painful

Treatment

Treatment:
• Acute—excision/incision
• Older—ointment/suppositories

- Recent: excision or incision with expression of the thrombus
- Older: ointment or suppositories containing steroid/local anesthetic, cooling

■ Anal Fissure

• Painful ulcer in anoderm, usually at 6 o'clock position
• Associated with sphincter spasm

- **Definition:** longitudinal ulcer in the anoderm
- **Etiology:** unclear, possibly due to breakdown of inflamed crypts
- Promoting factors: passage of hard feces, anal inflammation, manipulation (rectal tube, sexual intercourse)
- Simultaneous sphincter spasm, which causes pain and prevents healing due to reduced perfusion
- Location: 80%–90% are at 6 o'clock position (poorest perfusion), 10%–20% at 12 o'clock position
- Without treatment an acute fissure becomes chronic with formation of an indurated ulcer
- Complication: sphincter sclerosis, stenosis due to scarring (pectenosis)

Symptoms

- Pain on defecation which subsides initially but increases again after minutes to a further severe, cramplike pain.
- Occasionally slight bleeding
- Pain-induced constipation

Diagnostic Approach

- Inspection: skin tag in the posterior commissure, hypertrophic anal papilla at the level of the dentate line
- High sphincter tone, palpation painful

Treatment Approach

■ Indications

• Ointments/suppositories, sphincter dilation, possibly excision, last resort: sphincterotomy

- **Acute fissure**
  - ► Principle: abolish sphincter spasm
  - ► Usually conservative (stool regulation, warm sitz baths, careful dilation, ointments or suppositories containing local anesthetic)
  - ► Surgical only if conservative treatment fails (lateral submucous sphincterotomy)
- **Chronic fissure**
  - ► Attempt conservative treatment initially with topical use of nitrates or calcium antagonists; if unsuccessful try injection of botulinum toxin.
  - ► Operate only if no success: fissurectomy with removal of sentinel pile and hypertrophic anal papilla
  - ► Last resort: lateral submucous sphincterotomy

■ Surgical Treatment

Lateral Submucous Sphincterotomy (Notaras)

Operative Technique

- Perianal incision at 3 o'clock position over the intersphincteric cleft (**Fig. 14.4**)
- Intersphincter stab incision with a lancet-shaped scalpel with the blade parallel to the course of the sphincter
- Advance the scalpel under endoanal digital control as far as the dentate line.
- Rotate the blade toward the anus and divide the internal sphincter along the length of the fissure without injuring the mucosa.
- Close the stab incision.

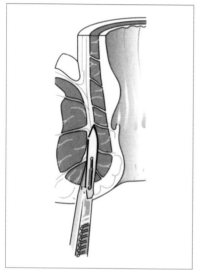

Fig. 14.4   Lateral submucous sphinctero-tomy at 3 or 9 o'clock position.

Complications
- Fistula formation
- Incontinence because of over-extensive sphincterotomy

■ Abscesses and Anal Fistulas (Figs. 14.5, 14.6)

Definition

- Abscess: acute form—either spontaneous perforation or operative opening
- Fistula: chronic form—residue of an abscess (connection between anal canal and skin)
- Goodsall Rule:
  - ► Anterior fistulas run radially.
  - ► Posterior fistulas run in a curve and usually open in the posterior commissure at the 6 o'clock position.
  - ► Anterior second openings that are more than 3 cm distant from the anocutaneous line communicate through a curved track with posteriorly located anal glands.

- Fistulous tracks according to the Goodsall rule

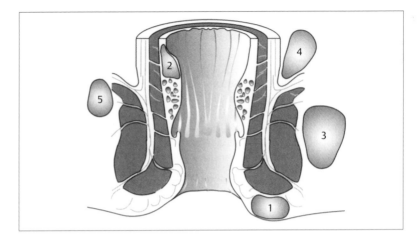

Fig. 14.5 Location of perirectal/perianal abscesses.
1: subcutaneous
2: submucous
3: periproctitic
4: pelvirectal
5: ischiorectal

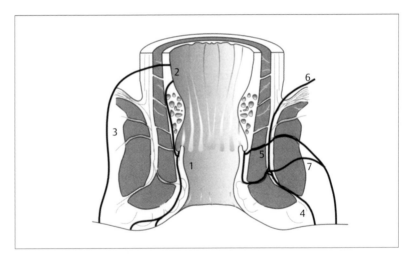

Fig. 14.6 Fistulous tracks
1: subcutaneous
2: submucous
3: extrasphincteric
4, 5: intersphincteric
6: suprasphincteric (intersphincteric)
7: transsphincteric

Etiology

- Principle cause: inflammation of the proctodeal glands located at the level of the dentate line between the internal and external sphincter
- Other causes: Crohn disease, ulcerative colitis, carcinoma, radiation

- Inflammation of the proctodeal glands
- **Caution:** chronic inflammatory bowel disease, carcinoma

Symptoms (Table 14.3)

- **Complication:** Spontaneous closure of a fistula can lead to further abscess and warrenlike fistula tracks with destruction of the sphincter.

Table 14.3 Symptoms of anal abscesses and fistulas

Abscess	Fistula
• Painful swelling and erythema • Possibly pyrexia/leukocytosis • Deep abscesses not visible externally	• Few symptoms • Needle-sized indurated skin opening • Turbid secretion on pressure

Diagnostic Approach

- Inspection (perianal, gluteal, vaginal, including scrotum and labia)
- Palpation (rectal: deep abscesses only palpable transanally/vaginally)
- Fistula probing (injection of methylene blue, contrast imaging)
- Endosonography
- CT/MRI (if deep-seated abscess suspected, MRI provides good imaging of the fistula tracks)
- Proctoscopy (discovery of the internal fistula opening; rule out other diseases)

- Inspection, palpation, proctoscopy with fistula demonstration, possibly MRI/endosonography

Treatment Approach

■ Abscess

- Opening, deroofing and loose packing (at least 3 cm distant from the anal canal to avoid sphincter damage)
- Antibiotic therapy only if concomitant phlegmon or pyrexia
- If applicable, cautious proctoscopy (demonstrate internal fistula opening, rule out concomitant disease)
- Open wound treatment, regular irrigation

- Opening, irrigation, open wound treatment

■ Fistula

- Indication for operation: symptomatic fistula proctoscopy
- Aim: clearance without interfering with continence and recurrence
- Conservative strategies (antibiotics, infliximab) have no place with regard to definitive fistula healing.
- **Caution:** Even splitting the internal sphincter as far as the dentate line can lead to incontinence, and additional division of the external sphincter greatly increases the risk of incontinence.

- Complete removal of the fistula tissue by splitting, possibly with fistula closure by plastic surgery
- **Caution:** incontinence due to sphincter injury

Table 14.4   Treatment depending on course of fistula

Course of fistula	Treatment
• Subcutaneous submucous fistula • Low intersphincteric fistula • Low transsphincteric fistula	Fistula splitting
• High intersphincteric fistula • Transphincteric fistula • Suprasphincteric fistula • Extrasphincteric fistula	Plastic surgical fistula closure
• Complex recurrent fistula system • Severe proctitis	Temporary colostomy

Operative Technique (Table 14.4)

Noncutting Seton Drain
- Draw a double, loosely tied, nonabsorbable suture through the fistula using a probe.
- Produces cleansing of the fistula canal and prevents apparent external healing.
- Acts as preparation for a fistula operation (especially fistula repair). Insertion in the acute inflammatory phase, operative management after consolidation (usually after 2–3 months)
- Cutting seton drain (Hippocratic method) is obsolete.

Fistula Splitting
- Sphincter stretching under anesthesia
- Establish the course of the fistula (Goodsall rule) by
  - ► Palpation
  - ► Probing with a blunt probe and from within with a hooked probe
  - ► If necessary, injection of methylene blue
- Split the fistula over a myrtle leaf probe.
- Excise the fistula tissue (e.g., sharp curette).
- Recurrence rate is up to 10% of cases.
- There is a risk of postoperative incontinence.

Fistula Repair
- Sphincter stretching under anesthesia
- Excision of the outer track as far as the external sphincter
- Transsphincteric cleansing with a sharp curette
- Removal of the anoderm/mucosa at the internal fistulous opening
- Transverse suture of the internal sphincter
- Cover with a flap of anoderm/mucosa.
- Recurrence rate is up to 30% of cases.
- Alternative: complete fistula splitting and secondary sphincter reconstruction

■ Aftercare
- Stool regulation
- Sitz baths

■ Fecal Incontinence

14

Definition

- Continence: capacity for perception, retention and evacuation of bowel content at a time and place of choice
- Incontinence: partial or complete loss of this capacity (**Table 14.5**)

Epidemiology

- Incidence in Europe and the United States: ca. 3%–5% of the population
- Up to 7% in those over the age of 65 years
- A large number of cases go unreported.
- Women are affected more often than men.

- Increased incidence with increasing age, especially in women

Etiology

Causes of Incontinence
- Altered stool consistency:
  - Irritable bowel syndrome
  - Inflammatory bowel disease
  - Diarrhea
  - Radiation enteritis
  - Malabsorption syndrome
- Disordered reservoir function:
  - Altered rectal reservoir (following rectal resection, pouch etc.)
  - Chronic inflammatory bowel disease
  - Collagenoses
  - Rectal tumors
  - External compression of the rectum
- Pelvic floor dysfunction:
  - Disordered pelvic floor innervation (descending perineum syndrome, pudendal nerve neuropathy)
  - Congenital lesions (anal atresia, spina bifida, myelomeningocele)
  - Other (rectal prolapse, dyscoordination, chronic constipation)
- Disordered sphincter function:
  - Sphincter defect (obstetric trauma, anorectal surgery, trauma)
  - Sphincter degeneration
  - Tumor
  - Inflammation
- Disordered sensation:
  - Neurological causes (dementia, neuropathy)
  - Overflow incontinence (medication, encopresis, constipation)
- Combined conditions

Symptoms (Table 14.5)

Table 14.5   Classification of fecal incontinence

Classification	Symptoms
Grade 1	Incontinence for gas
Grade 2	Incontinence for liquid feces, soiling
Grade 3	Incontinence for solid feces, gross incontinence

Diagnostic Approach

- Depends on the suspected genesis
- The history is important.

- History (stool diary)
- Inspection (skin changes, scars)
- Digital rectal examination (resting sphincter pressure, squeeze pressure, length of the anal canal, rectocele) (**Fig. 14.7**)
- Examination of anocutaneous reflex (afferent: sensitive anoderm, efferent: sphincter contraction)
- Endosonography (imaging of sphincter, fistulas, abscesses)
- Sphincter manometry (poor comparability of the different measuring systems) (**Fig. 14.7**)
- Neurological examination (pelvic floor electromyography, pudendal nerve latency measurement—prolonged with nerve overstretching as a result of perineal descent)
- Defecography/dynamic MRI (intussusception, prolapse, enterocele)
- CT/MRI (morphological imaging of the pelvic floor and sphincter apparatus)
- Proctoscopy ([post-] inflammatory changes, intussusception)

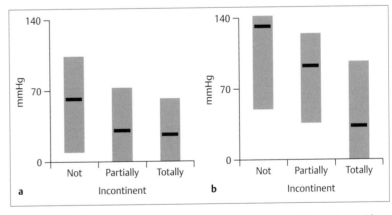

Fig. 14.7 a, b   Resting pressure (**a**) and maximum voluntary pressure (**b**) in patients without and with partial and complete incontinence.

Treatment Approach

■ Conservative Treatment

- Treatment of first choice except when the cause or extent of a lesion makes success unlikely (**Table 14.6**)

Table 14.6   **Conservative treatment measures for fecal incontinence**

Treatment measure	Effect
Local measures (anal hygiene, skin protection, anal tampons)	Prevents perianal eczema
Targeted defecation (enemas, suppositories)	Prevents incontinence events
Influencing stool consistency (low-fiber diet, stool thickeners, e.g., loperamide)	Delays transit, increases stool consistency
Sphincter training, pelvic floor exercises	Increases voluntary activity of the external sphincter
Biofeedback training	Operant conditioning to improve the coordination of pelvic floor activity
Passive anal electrostimulation	Increases sphincter force

- Very varied methods, the scientifically proven evidence for which is often low
- Additional treatment of the underlying disorder (if possible)

■ Surgical Treatment

Sphincter Reconstruction
- **Indication:** sphincter defect after trauma, perineal tear, fistula operation
- Up to 50% loss of substance possible
- **Operative technique**: exposure of the ends and overlapping suture or end-to-end

Preanal, Postanal, and Total Pelvic Floor Repair
- **Indication:** Neurogenic incontinence, complete pelvic floor insufficiency without sphincter defect
- **Principle:** Lengthening of the anal canal, elevation of the pelvic peritoneum, correction of the anorectal angle
- **Operative technique:** Tightening of muscular structure of the pelvic floor (sphincter muscle, levator ani)

Sacral Nerve Stimulation
- **Indication:** Severe treatment-refractory incontinence with an intact sphincter
- **Principle:** Stimulation of the sacral nerves (S2/S3) by a pulse generator and electrodes

Dynamic Gracilis Repair
- **Indication:** Extensive sphincter defects that cannot be reconstructed, absence of muscle activity
- **Operative technique:** Muscle transposition and electrostimulation by pacemaker via electrodes
- Complications: relatively frequent (infection, disorder of evacuation)

Artificial Sphincter
- **Indication:** Extensive sphincter defects that cannot be reconstructed
- **Operative Technique:** Implantation of a fluid-filled cuff (around the anal canal below the levator), which can be emptied through a pump prior to defecation
- Complications: infection, erosion

Colostomy
- Last resort: terminal colostomy with a short rectal stump
- Full social activity, which is less likely with diapers use.

■ Anal Carcinoma

Definition (Table 14.7)

Table 14.7 Comparison between anal canal and anal verge carcinoma

Parameter	Anal canal carcinoma	Anal verge carcinoma
Location	Between the dentate line and anocutaneous line	In a circle within 5 cm of the anocutaneous line
Frequency	80%	20%
Histology	Ca. 75% squamous epithelial carcinoma 15–20% adenocarcinoma	Predominantly squamous epithelial carcinoma
Sex distribution (m : f)	1 : 1.2	1 : 1

Epidemiology

- Incidence: 1 per 100 000 population per year
- Ca. 1%–2% of all gastrointestinal cancers
- Peak incidence between the ages of 60 and 70 years

Etiology

- Unclear
- Risk factors:
  - ➤ Chronic inflammation (e.g., Crohn disease)
  - ➤ Infection with the human pathogenic papilloma viruses (HPV; especially types 16, 18 and 58)
  - ➤ Infection with the herpes simplex virus (HSV; type 2)
  - ➤ Immunosuppression

Classification (Table 14.8)

Table 14.8 TNM Classification

	Anal canal carcinoma	Anal verge carcinoma
Tis	Carcinoma in situ	Carcinoma in situ
T1	≤2 cm	≤2 cm
T2	2–5 cm	2–5 cm
T3	>5 cm	>5 cm
T4	Any size with infiltration of neighboring organs	Any size with infiltration of deep extradermal structures
N0	No lymph node metastases	No lymph node metastases
N1	Metastasis in perirectal lymph nodes	Regional lymph node metastases
N2	Metastasis in inguinal/iliac lymph nodes unilaterally	
N3	Perirectal/iliac/inguinal metastasis bilaterally	
M0	No distant metastases	No distant metastases
M1	Distant metastases	Distant metastases

Symptoms

- Usually nonspecific
- Bleeding
- Pain
- Discharge
- Pruritus
- Continence disorders / stool irregularity
- Inguinal lymph node enlargement
- **Caution:** can be associated with benign disease

- Usually nonspecific

Diagnostic Approach

- Inspection
- Digital rectal examination
- Proctoscopy with endosonography
- Biopsy: small lesions can be removed in full
- **Caution:** all tissue removed in the anal region must be regarded as potentially malignant and must be examined histologically
- CT/MRI of the pelvis and abdomen
- Colonoscopy
- Chest x-ray in two planes
- Gynecological or urological examination if appropriate with advanced tumor

- Inspection, palpation, endoscopy with biopsy, endosonography, CT/MRI

Treatment Approach

Before initiating treatment, histological confirmation of malignancy and differentiation between squamous epithelial and adenocarcinoma are necessary (**Fig. 14.8**).

14

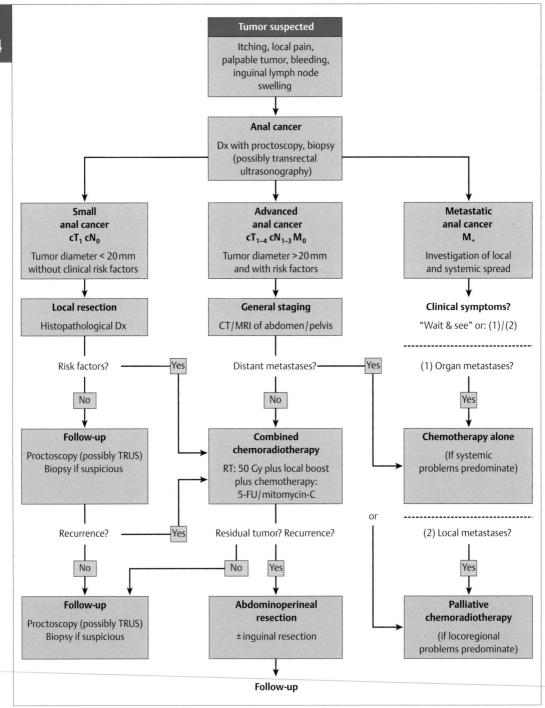

Fig. 14.8 Diagnostic and treatment approach to squamous epithelial carcinoma of the anus. Risk factors: G3/G4 differentiation, invasion of lymphatics or veins, R1 resection, lymph node metastases. 5-FU, 5-fluorouracil; RT, radiotherapy; TRUS, transrectal ultrasonography. (From Seegenschmiedt and Betzler 2001, see p. 413.)

Squamous Epithelial Carcinoma
- Chemoradiotherapy is the "gold standard" for advanced disease; it achieves high cure rates with preservation of sphincter function.
- Persistent or locally recurrent carcinoma after chemoradiotherapy can still be cured in 50% of cases by rectal amputation.
- Chemotherapy: 5-fluorouracil as radiosensitizer, possibly combined with mitomycin or cisplatin
- Radiation: split-course concept with 50–59 Gy, possibly increasing the dose by means of brachytherapy
- Primary surgical excision of T1 cancers, only if sphincter apparatus is undamaged
- For solitary metastases in lung or liver, consider surgery of the metastases.
- Palliative measures: colostomy if obstruction, palliative chemo(radio)therapy

Adenocarcinoma
- Radical abdominoperineal amputation of the rectum, possibly after neoadjuvant chemoradiotherapy
- High risk of recurrence and metastases, so poor prognosis

- Chemoradiotherapy is the "gold standard": high chance of cure with sphincter preservation
- Rectal amputation if tumor persists after chemoradiotherapy
- Primary surgical excision for T1 carcinoma preserving the sphincter

- Rectal amputation, possibly after neoadjuvant chemoradiotherapy

Aftercare

- Diagnosis and treatment of complications such as stenosis, incontinence, pain, bleeding, or perianal eczema (**Table 14.9**)

Table 14.9   Follow-up of squamous epithelial carcinoma of the anus

Examination	Weeks[a]	Months[a]								
	6	3	6	9	12	18	24	36	48	60
History, physical examination	X	X	X	X	X	X		X	X	X
Abdominal ultrasound			X		X	X	X	X	X	
Chest x-ray in 2 planes					X			X		X
Proctoscopy, endosonography if appropriate	X	X	X	X	X	X	X			
MRI or spiral CT of the pelvis			X		X	X	X			

[a] After the conclusion of chemoradiotherapy.
Source: From Anal carcinoma—Interdisciplinary guidelines of the German Cancer Society and the German Society for Surgery. Coloproctology 2000; 22: 231–235.

14

Prognosis

- After primary chemoradiotherapy:
  - ► Five-year survival rates up to 90%
  - ► Local recurrence rate 19%
  - ► Up to 20% secondary sphincter loss due to late sequelae
- Five-year survival rate ca. 50% with persisting or locally recurrent carcinoma after chemoradiotherapy and subsequent rectal amputation

Further Reading

Heitland W. Diagnostik und Therapie des Analkarzinoms. Chirurg 2008; 79: 183–192
Heitland W. Fisteln und Fissuren. Chirurg 2008; 79: 439–443
Longo A. Treatment of haemorrhoidal disease by reduction of mucosa and haemorrhoidal prolapse with a circular stapling device: a new procedure – 6th World Congress of Endoscopic Surgery. Mundozzi Editore. 1998; 777–784
Nelson RL. Operative procedures for fissure in ano. Cochrane Database Syst Rev 2010 Jan 20; (1): CD002199. Review
Ruppert R, Kirchdorfer B. Chirurgische Therapie des Hämorrhoidalleidens. Viszeralchirurgie 2006; 41: 388–393
Schiedeck THK. Diagnostik und Therapie der Stuhlinkontinenz. Chirurg 2008; 79: 379–389

15 Intestinal Obstruction

H. Brunn

Definition

- Ileus is a collective term for the most varied forms of interference with downward passage of bowel contents. A distinction is made between complete and incomplete (sub-) ileus depending on the degree of obstruction.

Classification

- A distinction is made between primary mechanical and primary functional disorders: **mechanical obstruction** versus **paralytic ileus.**
- Mixed forms occur: mechanical obstruction can result in bowel paralysis so that paralytic aspects are then also present.
- Mechanical obstruction is classified, according to the site of obstruction and the part of the intestine affected as a result, into **large bowel** and **small bowel obstruction.**
- Differentiation of small bowel obstruction into **high** (duodenum and jejunum) and **low** (ileum)
- **Strangulated obstruction:** involvement of the vascular supply also (e.g., volvulus)
- Distinction between acute life-threatening (e.g., volvulus) and chronic ileus (e.g., chronic adhesions)

- Distinguish between mechanical and paralytic ileus.

Etiology and Physiology

■ Mechanical Obstruction

- Causes of bowel obstruction (**Table 15.1**):
  - ► Compression from without (**extraluminal** cause)
  - ► Pathological changes in the wall (**intramural** cause)
  - ► Obstruction of the lumen (**intraluminal** cause)
- A combination of several causes is possible.

- Adhesions are the commonest cause of intestinal obstruction in surgical patients.

Table 15.1 Causes of mechanical obstruction.

Extraluminal cause	Intramural cause	Intraluminal cause
• Adhesions/bands • Hernias • Peritoneal carcinomatosis • Volvulus • Torsion	• Inflammatory bowel disease • Stenosing tumor • Vascular lesions • Strictures, e.g., after radiation • Hirschsprung disease • Malformations	• Foreign body / bezoar • Gallstones • Meconium • Intussusception • Coprostasis

15

Mechanical obstruction is present in the majority of patients referred to a surgical clinic because of ileus:

- Two-thirds of obstructions involve the small bowel and a third involve the large bowel.
- **Causes of small bowel obstruction:**
  - ► Adhesions and bands (60%)
  - ► Malignant tumors (mainly peritoneal carcinomatosis; 20%)
  - ► Hernias (10%)
- **Causes of large bowel obstruction:**
  - ► Colon cancer (70%)
  - ► Stenosis due to diverticulitis
  - ► Stenosis due to chronic inflammatory bowel disease
  - ► Hernias and volvulus
- The frequency of the cause of obstruction varies depending on age:
  - ► In neonates, apart from meconium ileus, a malformation is most often the underlying cause.
  - ► In childhood, the causes are mainly malformations, hernias, intussusception and foreign bodies.
  - ► In younger adults, bands and adhesions, incarcerated hernias, volvulus and Crohn disease are the main causes.
  - ► In older people, malignant tumors, inflammatory stenosis, and tumors along with hernias and adhesions/bands predominate. Gallstone ileus, sigmoid volvulus, and fecal impaction are rarer causes.

Large Bowel Obstruction

- Special feature: competent ileocecal valve

- In mechanical large bowel obstruction, the ileocecal valve remains competent in ca. 90% of cases.
- The disease remains limited to the colon (initially).
- With increasing passive filling with gas and feces there is increasing pressure on the bowel wall, interfering with the intramural circulation.
- Especially in the cecum, ischemic perforation of the wall can then occur, followed by fecal peritonitis.
- Hypovolemia, liberation of mediators and bacterial translocation are lesser problems in large bowel obstruction compared with small bowel obstruction (no microvilli and thus its surface area is 200 times smaller than that of the small bowel mucosa, and there is no hypersecretion).

■ Paralytic Ileus

- Postoperative ileus is the most common form of paralytic ileus in surgical patients.

- Paralytic ileus can be produced by metabolic, reflex, and toxic drug-induced causes (**Table 15.2**).
- Every untreated mechanical obstruction progresses secondarily to bowel paralysis.
- Paralytic ileus represents the most frequent form of ileus overall, though not in surgical patients.

■ Advanced Ileus Disease

- Interruption of the vicious circle is the sine qua non in the treatment of advanced ileus

- Advanced ileus disease is a result of untreated intestinal obstruction and affects the entire body.
- The critical pathophysiological parameter is distension of the bowel wall (mainly the small bowel), due to accumulation of gas and fluid proximal to the obstructed part of the bowel.

Table 15.2   Causes of paralytic ileus

Metabolic	Reflex	Toxic drug-induced
• Electrolyte disorders (e.g., hyper-/hypokalemia, hypercalcemia) • Myopathies • Neuropathies • Interference with intestinal perfusion/mesenteric infarction • Protein, vitamin B and thyroxin deficiency	• Postoperative • Peritonitis (e.g., perforation of a hollow organ) • Other inflammation (e.g., pancreatitis) • Retroperitoneal processes (vertebral fractures, hematomas, bleeding, pyelonephritis) • Other peritoneal irritation (biliary colic, adnexal torsion, ureter colic, overfull bladder)	• Opiates, antidepressants, narcotics, anti-Parkinson drugs • Catecholamines • Laxative abuse • Uremia

15

- Massive fluid and electrolyte loss into the bowel lumen (hypovolemia, hypokalemia and hyponatremia) occurs, which is further increased by vomiting.
- Disorders of the microcirculation with hypoxia (including sequestration of fluid in the edematous bowel wall) have various consequences (**vicious circle**) (**Fig. 15.1**):
  - ► Increase in bowel wall distension
  - ► Increased bacterial overgrowth with bacterial dislocation, systemic endotoxin absorption, and migratory peritonitis
  - ► Elevation of the diaphragm with respiratory insufficiency and atelectasis
  - ► Increasing accumulation of fluid in the intestinal lumen and intestinal wall leads to a reduction of venous return, culminating in hemorrhagic infarction of the bowel wall and passage of blood into the lumen.

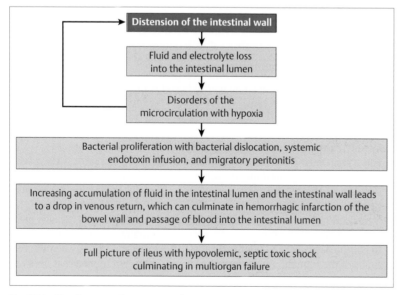

Fig. 15.1   Development of a vicious circle.

15

Special Forms of Obstruction

■ Incarcerated Hernia

- A common cause of obstruction with primary circulatory dysfunction is **hernial incarceration**, and incarceration of internal hernias (e.g., retrocecal, Treitz hernia, hernia through the foramen of Winslow) should be considered.
- A painful hernia with symptoms of obstruction should always be regarded as strangulated. Irreducibility of a hernia, however, is not always synonymous with incarceration.
- With retrograde incarceration on the other hand, two non-incarcerated loops of bowel are present in the hernial sac while the strangulated segment between them remains in the abdominal cavity.

■ Adhesions/Bands

- Adhesions/bands due to previous operations are the most common cause of small bowel obstruction.

- Damage to the peritoneum results in exudation and formation of fibrin and disturbance of peritoneal fibrinolysis. Fibrinoid adhesions that are present for some time become organized after a few days with the formation of stringlike and extensive adhesions.
- Reintervention is required within months to years after ca. 4% of all abdominal or pelvic operations due to small bowel obstruction, particularly small bowel adhesions in the pelvis.
- Bands are further causes of strangulation.

■ Obstruction Due to Peritoneal Carcinomatosis

- Recurrent obstruction due to known advanced gastrointestinal or gynecological tumor
- Obstruction is often incomplete when the patient presents; therefore there is often sufficient time with conservative management to inform the patient of the prospects of an operation and find out his/her wishes.

■ Volvulus

- Danger of bowel wall gangrene and perforation

- Twisting of a segment of bowel leads to obstruction of the bowel at two sites.
- The blood supply of the obstructed loop of bowel is impaired by the torsion of the vessels.
- There is an increase in intraluminal pressure.
- The patient is in immediate danger of bowel wall gangrene and perforation with consequent peritonitis.

Sigmoid Volvulus
- Usually occurs with an elongated sigmoid colon
- Often associated with long-standing neurological or psychiatric disease with corresponding psychotropic medication (interferes with colon motility)
- Chronic laxative abuse, which is often present in chronically constipated bed-bound patients
- "Overloading" of the sigmoid colon is assumed in pathogenesis. Usually there are subacute, self-limiting episodes of torsion initially, which lead to narrowing of the base of the mesosigmoid due to adhesive strands between the two limbs of the sigmoid, thus promoting the occurrence of torsion that does not resolve spontaneously.

Small Bowel Volvulus
- In adults this condition is usually associated with bands, adhesions, Meckel diverticulum, or internal hernias.

■ Intussusception

- This involves invagination of a segment of bowel (intussusceptum) caused by peristalsis into the distal bowel lumen (intussuscipiens). It occurs most commonly at junctions between freely mobile and relatively fixed segments of bowel (typical: ileocecal intussusception).
- In infancy and early childhood, intussusception is the second most frequent cause of an acute abdomen after appendicitis; the cause remains unclear in 90% of cases.
- The disease is rare in adults (maximum of 5% of intestinal obstructions), but in three-quarters of these cases there is a defined cause. The small intestine is affected predominantly and the causes in the majority of cases are benign conditions (e.g., Meckel diverticulum, polyps), whereas malignant tumors predominate in the large bowel.

• Typical: ileocecal intussusception

■ Gallstone Ileus

- Caused by incarceration of a large gallstone
- The causal biliary enteric fistula usually arises as a result of acute cholecystitis or pressure necrosis over an impacted gallstone with migration of the gallstone from the gallbladder into the gastrointestinal tract through a closed perforation, which is often clinically silent; this is usually into the duodenum, more seldom into the colon or stomach. In the intestine, the stone can become wedged anywhere but usually in the relatively narrow lumen of the ileum.
- The stone often causes reversible spasm of the intestinal muscle with repeated wedging.

■ Acute Pseudo-obstruction of the Colon

- Ill-defined condition, also known as Ogilvie syndrome, represents a form of idiopathic ileus with massive dilatation of the colon without an identifiable cause.

• Ogilvie syndrome

■ Postoperative Ileus

- After abdominal procedures involving opening of the abdomen, there is a more or less pronounced paralysis of the stomach and intestine with accumulation of gas and fluid together with delayed passage.
- The time to resumption of motility differs in the various segments:
  - ► Small intestine after 5–24 hours
  - ► Stomach after 1–3 days
  - ► Colon after 2–5 days
- Resumption of colon activity proceeds from proximal to distal.
- Duration of atony is dependent especially on the motility of the left hemicolon.
- With excessive postoperative ileus the prolonged paralysis (inhibition of local, intrinsic and contractile systems) leads to overgrowth of the physiological bacterial intestinal flora with a risk of bacterial translocation, endotoxin absorption and the clinical picture of sepsis.

• The severity of postoperative ileus can be influenced pre- and intraoperatively.

15

- The electrophysiological activity of the intestine is under neural control (central nervous system, enteric neural plexus) and is modulated by local factors and hormones.
- The development of postoperative ileus is characterized by a change in these regulatory mechanisms.
- These disorders are reactions to the surgical procedure and concomitant drug treatment.

- Important factors:
  - ► Direct surgical trauma
  - ► Manipulation of the intestine (local secretion of neurotransmitters and inflammatory mediators, e.g., nitrogen monoxide (NO), vasoactive intestinal peptide (VIP), substance P, direct activation of the sympathetic nerve plexus) and the internal organs
  - ► Administration of opioids
  - ► Medications used in anesthesia
  - ► Electrolyte disturbances and possibly fluid imbalance as a result of excessive intra- and perioperative fluid replacement

Symptoms

- Clinical picture often unclear

- An abrupt onset with severe, constant or colicky pains is typical of strangulation (e.g., due to an adhesive band), with initial vomiting and localized tenderness over the strangulated segment of bowel.
- With proximal occlusion of the small intestine, depending on the location, hyperperistaltic cramps can be expected at brief intervals but may not occur at all. There is always early copious bilious vomiting and rapid dehydration. Meteorism is largely absent or is limited to the epigastrium.
- Distal small intestinal occlusion is characterized by colicky pains (periumbilical or epigastric) at somewhat longer intervals. Vomiting is delayed for 1–2 days, is bilious initially, later feculent. Meteorism increases and is located in the center of the abdomen.
- An insidious onset is typical of large bowel obstruction, often over weeks, with marked meteorism, often more pronounced in the flanks, with pain on extension, failure to pass gas or feces, and vomiting occurring late.
- The clinical picture of primary paralytic ileus is usually determined by the underlying disease; pain is usually absent. Overflow vomiting can occur; on the other hand, some patients still have an appetite. Bowel sounds are absent.
- Overall, according to the different underlying causes, the clinical picture of intestinal obstruction is often vague and confusing. The classical symptoms (vomiting, pain, meteorism, failure to pass gas and feces) vary in severity and sometimes only occur late. Often an acute abdomen is not present initially.

Diagnostic Approach

- Early diagnostic investigation required

- Early investigation is critical as all forms of obstruction, after varying latency, ultimately end up as ileus disease, which is difficult to treat.

15

■ History

- Note the duration and nature of current symptoms.
- Is the pain colicky? Where is it located and how long is the painfree interval?
- Nausea, hiccuping, kind of vomiting?
- Is there a change in bowel habit, blood in the stool, or failure to pass gas and feces?
- Ask about previous abdominal surgery (including laparoscopic and vaginal procedures) or inflammation (cholecystitis, pancreatitis, adnexitis).
- Was there a previous tumor?
- Any chronic inflammatory bowel disease (diarrhea, pain, fever)?
- Is there a hernia?

■ Clinical Examination

Inspection
- Overall impression, dry mouth, tongue brown, cracked, diminished skin turgor, neck veins collapsed, (orthostatic) hypotension (dehydration)
- Vomiting: Clear gastric juice, bilious, or fecal vomiting? Occasionally, blood or "coffee grounds" may show because of gastric dilatation with mucosal hemorrhage. Feculent vomit looks and smells like liquid feces as a result of bacterial overgrowth. However, true fecal vomiting requires a short circuit, as with a gastrocolic fistula.
- Scars from previous surgery
- Distension of the abdominal wall due to meteorism is minimal with high obstruction, but is more marked with more distal and more prolonged obstruction culminating in a "tympanitic abdomen" with effaced umbilicus. Occasionally it is possible to distinguish whether central small bowel meteorism or distension of the outline of the large bowel in the flanks predominates. In a thin abdomen there may be visible peristalsis (late sign of small bowel obstruction).

Auscultation
- Hyperperistalsis of increased volume and frequency is typical of the early phase of mechanical ileus, and can also occur with enteritis. Borborygmi, that is, gurgling, growling, rumbling bowel sounds, are audible without a stethoscope.

  • Uninterrupted auscultation for at least 2 minutes

- Squirting noises can occur when peristalsis overcomes intestinal stenosis.
- With increasing bowel distension, the sounds become more high-pitched, tinkling, and metallic.
- Since waves of peristalsis often only occur intermittently at intervals of several minutes, auscultation must be sufficiently prolonged or be done during an attack of pain.
- To establish the absence of bowel sounds ("dead silence"), uninterrupted auscultation for at least 2 minutes is necessary and the bowel sounds should not be elicited by tapping on the abdominal wall.
- Are there vascular sounds?

Palpation
- Palpation of all hernial orifices (including scars). Small incarcerated femoral hernias in obese women in particular are easily overlooked. An incarcerated obturator hernia is rarer and likewise difficult to diagnose (usually in undernourished elderly women); anterolateral guarding on rectal examination,

  • The presence of local or generalized signs of peritonitis is crucial when planning management.

15

pain on the inner surface of the thigh, especially on moving the adductors (Howship–Romberg sign).
- Other findings on abdominal palpation that can help to clarify the situation include, for instance, an enlarged metastatic liver, an inflammatory or neoplastic mass, occasionally an intussuscepted loop or an isolated distended bowel loop in strangulated obstruction (Wahl sign).
- Rectal examination (or palpation of a colostomy): ampulla empty? Fecal impaction? Stenosing tumor? Bloody mucus as evidence of intussusception?

■ Laboratory Tests

- Contribute little to direct diagnosis of obstruction
- Measurement of lactate when ischemia is suspected is not reliable.
- Laboratory tests are important for estimating dehydration/electrolyte shift and generally in preparation for surgery.

■ Diagnostic Imaging

Plain Abdominal X-ray

• Standard investigation

- Standard investigation to assess the extent and location of the obstruction (erect and left lateral decubitus views)
- Shows mechanical small bowel obstruction (not located too high) in the majority of cases: dilated small bowel loops with preserved Kerckring folds and with fluid levels
- With complete small bowel obstruction, gas-free colon after more than 24 hours ("empty colon frame")
- A closed strangulated loop can escape detection on plain abdominal x-ray due to the absence of gas filling.
- In large bowel obstruction, prestenotic distension of the haustrated colon (and of the small bowel in the event of an incompetent ileocecal valve) can be identified.
- Exact localization of the obstruction on the basis of the gas shadow is not always possible.
- In paralytic ileus, fluid levels are seen in the small and large bowel; because of the muscle relaxation, the circular mucosal folds of the jejunum are effaced.
- Occasionally there are indicative concomitant findings—for example, a loop of intestine leading to a hernial orifice, intramural gas bubbles as evidence of gangrene of the bowel wall, a ureter stone or dislocated gallstone, aerobilia, or free air.

Ultrasonography
- Can provide important information in addition to the plain abdominal radiograph
- More sensitive than radiography in the early phase
- Fluid-filled dilated bowel loops with erect mucosal folds ("piano keyboard appearance" in the jejunum)
- Intestinal wall edema and nonpropulsive peristalsis
- Collapsed bowel beyond the stenosis
- Absence of peristalsis in the entire bowel in paralytic ileus
- A dilated akinetic loop and increased peristalsis proximal to it are highly suspicious for strangulation
- Often free fluid between the intestinal loops also

- Reactive thickening of the bowel wall in chronic obstruction
- Occasional evidence of a tumor or diverticulitis (pathological cockade), intussusception as double cockade, an obstructing gallstone
- Doppler or duplex ultrasonographic imaging of mesenteric artery occlusion

Important **limitations** of ultrasonography:
- Luminal gas interferes with imaging
- Operator dependent
- Inferior to CT in demonstrating and localizing intestinal obstruction

Computed Tomography
- CT provides the most information of all imaging methods and is therefore the method of choice. Conventional investigations with contrast agents are becoming less important.
- Intravenous, rectal and, if appropriate, oral administration of contrast agent
- Clarification of uncertain complex situations in the presence of tumors or abscesses
- Localization of small bowel obstructions (e.g., strangulated loops, intestinal wall hemorrhage, and intussusception)
- Assessment of vascular situation possible

• CT is method of choice.

Investigations Employing Contrast Agents
- Water-soluble contrast agent (Gastrografin)
- Localization of an obstruction in complete obstruction (not always reliable because of dilution)
- Incomplete obstruction can be demonstrated by passage of contrast.
- Due to the hyperosmolarity of the contrast agent, fluid influx into the bowel lumen, stimulation of peristalsis, electrolyte shifts, and severe colic are possible.
- Oral passage of contrast is potentially dangerous in large bowel obstruction (increase in risk of perforation).
- Aspiration of Gastrografin must absolutely be avoided because of the risk of severe lung damage.
- Obstruction of the colon can be localized by Gastrografin enema.

Angiography
- To assess vessels when mesenteric artery occlusion is suspected

Endoscopy
- Depending on the clinical situation, to investigate large bowel obstruction (biopsy)

Treatment Approach

Initial Measures
- Volume administration through a large-bore peripheral venous line to counteract impending or overt dehydration.
- Bladder catheter to monitor fluid balance
- Placement of as large a nasogastric tube as possible to relieve abdominal pressure, eliminate nausea and vomiting; often relieves pain, improves respiration.

• Treat dehydration and electrolyte imbalance before surgery
• Early antibiotic treatment with strangulation

Other measures depending on the clinical picture:
- Correction of electrolyte shifts and acid–base balance
- Intensive therapy
- If strangulation is suspected, early antibiotic treatment is indicated.

■ Indications

- Complete mechanical obstruction is always an absolute indication for urgent operation.
- If a severe perfusion disorder of the bowel is suspected (e.g., strangulation or gangrene) and in peritonitis, the operation must be performed immediately as an emergency.
- In large bowel obstruction, the situation is usually less urgent than with small bowel obstruction, so that there is sufficient time for specific preoperative investigations.
- With paralytic ileus, surgery is indicated when a surgically treatable disease is the cause (e.g., organ perforation, peritonitis, abscess, prolonged mechanical obstruction).
- Surgery is also indicated when large bowel rupture due to massive overdistension is imminent.

■ Conservative Treatment

- If there are no indications for surgery, conservative treatment can be attempted.
- Important components include:
  - ► Fluid replacement
  - ► Correction of electrolyte disturbances
  - ► Insertion of a bladder catheter and nasogastric tube (see above)
  - ► Patient kept fasting
  - ► Parenteral nutrition
- An attempt can be made with enemas and use of prokinetic agents to reestablish bowel motility.
- In paralytic ileus that is not caused by a surgically treatable disease, the cause (medications, metabolic disturbances) should be sought and treated consistently.
- In pseudo-obstruction of the colon, intravenous administration of prostigmine and colonoscopic aspiration (decompression) have proved effective.
- However, a crucial component of conservative treatment is close monitoring and reassessment of the need for surgery. If in doubt, surgery should always be performed.

Postoperative Ileus

- With physiological bowel paresis and the absence of other pathological findings, spontaneous bowel voiding can be awaited for 3–6 days without special measures.
- Criteria for instituting treatment:
  - ► Increasing abdominal distension
  - ► Increasing reflux
  - ► Worsening of general condition (pulmonary and renal failure, metabolic decompensation)
- However, there are few therapeutic concepts available for treating postoperative ileus reliably and with few side effects.

15

- Complete mechanical obstruction: absolute indication for emergency surgery

- In case of doubt, always operate.

- Few possible treatments, so preventive measures are important.

- Administration of prokinetic agents is possible when the indication for re-laparotomy has been ruled out beforehand.
- Decompressing measures (e.g., intestinal tube, enema) are also possible if there are no contraindications (e.g., anastomosis).
- However, avoidance of extended postoperative ileus by preventive measures is the "treatment" of choice.

Preventive Measures
- Minimally traumatic surgery (atraumatic dissection and handling of organs)
- Sympathetic block by thoracic epidural anesthesia for 2–3 days is effective for both prevention and treatment, especially when it is started intraoperatively.
- Routine use of a nasogastric tube (**caution:** atelectasis, pneumonia) has not been proved to have a positive effect on postoperative bowel motility.
- Early postoperative enteral nutrition has predominantly positive effects (can be used in the absence of hiccups, nausea, and vomiting).
- Early postoperative mobilization makes it easier for the patient to pass gas and have a bowel movement. It also represents a positive signal for the patient and reduces postoperative complications (thromboembolism, pneumonia).
- Use of nonsteroidal anti-inflammatory drugs (on the one hand, by cutting down use of opioids and, on the other hand, they may possibly have a direct anti-inflammatory effect in the intestinal wall).

■ Surgical Treatment

- Corresponding to the variety of possible causes of obstruction, almost the entire range of abdominal surgery is employed in its treatment.
- When obtaining the patient's informed consent, the uncertainty regarding the extent of the surgery that often exists preoperatively must be pointed out (resections, short bowel syndrome, colostomy).
- Draping of the operation field must be accordingly liberal.
- Perioperative antibiotic prophylaxis is indicated.
- The standard approach is a midline lower or middle laparotomy, which is extended if necessary.
- Existing midline or paramedian scars can be used as access; however, it must be anticipated that the distended vulnerable bowel may be adherent to the scar.
- Once access to the free abdominal cavity is achieved, any ascites is assessed (bloody and serous with strangulated obstruction).
- Depending on the extent of existing adhesions, the small bowel must first be dissected from the anterior and lateral abdominal wall, and adhesions between loops of bowel may also need to be divided.
- As a guide to the site of the obstruction, it is first established whether the cecum is distended or if the terminal ileum appears collapsed.
- Decompression of the bowel by massaging it should be performed very gently, or if possible not at all, as this may result in problems (endotoxin absorption, serosal injury, prolonged postoperative atony).
- When there are extensive adhesions or large bowel obstruction, open decompression can often be performed with a bowel aspirator through an enterotomy, if possible in the region of a bowel segment to be resected. This facilitates the eventration of the small bowel that is necessary for further exploration and finally abdominal wall closure.
- If small bowel resection becomes necessary because of a pathological condition causing the ileus or because of impaired perfusion, this can usually be

- Entire range of abdominal surgery

done in a single stage with primary anastomosis. Existing incongruence of the bowel lumen is corrected by different distances between sutures on either side or by an antimesenteric incision of the nondistended limb of bowel.

- The vitality of a bowel loop is assessed from its color, peristalsis triggered by tapping it, and the presence of arterial pulsation. In case of doubt, the loop is wrapped in moist warm towels for 10 minutes: **recovery of motility** is particularly important (reliable results have also been reported by assessing fluorescence after intravenous injection of fluorescein).
- If the need to resect larger segments of small bowel remains doubtful, preservation of the distal segments being more important because of the absorption capacity, a second-look operation after 24 or 38 hours should be planned.

Large Bowel Obstruction

- Observe principles of oncological surgery.
- A one- or two-stage procedure is possible

- When large bowel obstruction is due to malignant occlusion, the principles of oncological surgery must be followed.
- When there is obstruction of the right hemicolon with peritonitis, the procedure of choice is (extended) right hemicolectomy with primary ileo-transverse colostomy.
- If the left hemicolon is obstructed, the problem is anastomosis to the proximally distended and edematous colon.
- The three-stage procedure, which was standard in the past—with creation of a stoma for primary decompression, resection of the tumor in a second session, and finally closure of the colostomy and restoration of continuity—has largely been abandoned because of the relatively high mortality, of even the primary procedure (ca. 10%–15%), long hospitalization, and ultimately low resection rate (permanent colostomy in 20%–40% of cases). It is now performed only as an exception when the patient's general condition is very poor (or the colostomy is left as definitive palliation when the tumor is unresectable).
- Surgery is often performed in two stages, usually as a Hartmann discontinuity resection with terminal colostomy and closure of the distal stump. (With sufficient length, the distal stump can be brought out as a Miculicz mucous fistula.)
- An alternative is resection with primary anastomosis and protective colostomy or ileostomy (however, continuity is finally restored in only ca. 60% of patients).
- Two-stage procedures are recommended especially with perforation and peritonitis, poor general condition of the patient, or limited surgeon experience; otherwise, a single-stage procedure is increasingly advised.
- When an emergency single-stage procedure is performed, subtotal colectomy with ileosigmoidostomy/-rectostomy competes with segmental resection (left hemicolectomy, sigmoid resection, anterior resection of the rectum).
- Advantages of subtotal colectomy:
  - High anastomotic safety due to complete removal of the dilated part of the large bowel
  - Avoidance of time-consuming and complex lavage, so less fecal contamination and consequent wound infection
  - With malignant disease, which is not always certain intraoperatively, subtotal colectomy is more radical oncologically; synchronous second cancers

and adenomas are removed, metachronous tumors are prevented and follow-up is easier
  ► Subtotal colectomy is recommended particularly with cecal perforation or a palpable second tumor.
- Compared with segmental resection, the major disadvantage is postoperative diarrhea, which is problematic especially in elderly patients with impaired continence. It may be increased by possible subsequent chemotherapy but can also be influenced pharmacologically. As prevention, only a few centimeters of terminal ileum should be resected and 10–20 cm of colon should be preserved, if possible.

Incarcerated Hernia
- If there are local signs of inflammation or obvious obstruction, or if reduction fails, an inguinal or femoral hernia is treated surgically locally as an emergency and the incarcerated loop including the constricting groove is inspected, if necessary after splitting the hernial ring. If resection is necessary and cannot be performed safely through the existing access, this is followed by a midline lower abdominal laparotomy.

Adhesions/Bands
- In obstruction due to adhesions, the causative band or area of adhesions must be divided. The collapsed and dilated bowel can be used as a guide. The cause must be found at the junction of the two. If chronic adhesions are the cause and surgery becomes necessary, all adhesions should be divided as far as possible.

Obstruction Due to Peritoneal Carcinomatosis
- Surgical treatment options are, in particular, bypass anastomosis or a colostomy.

Volvulus
- In emergency surgery because of volvulus, resection of the affected segment of bowel is often necessary and useful (e.g., small bowel for prevention).

Intussusception
- In adults, generally a laparotomy is performed to eliminate the cause. The small intestine should usually be disinvaginated manually at operation to limit the extent of resection depending on its appearance; intussusception of the colon should be resected according to oncological principles without further manipulation.

- In general, laparotomy is performed.

Gallstone Ileus
- The gallstone is extracted through an enterolithotomy (in bowel wall not damaged by pressure). Treatment of the biliary enteric fistula is desirable in principle to prevent recurrent cholecystitis and cholangitis. When there is an inflammatory mass in the right upper abdomen and the patients, who are usually elderly, are in poor general condition, this part of the operation may be delayed or omitted completely.

■ Aftercare

- The aftercare depends on the cause and the operation.
- After surgical therapy of obstruction, further attention should be paid to the correction of still-persisting fluid and electrolyte shifts.
- Depending on the patient's clinical condition, mobilization and increasing diet can then follow.

■ Complications

- The possible complications are varied, depending on the chosen operation method and the cause of the obstruction.

Further Reading

Köninger J, Gutt CN, Wente MN et al. Postoperativer Ileus. Pathophysiologie und Prävention. Chirurg 2006; 77: 904–912

Kreis ME, Jauch KW. Ileus aus chirurgischer Sicht. Differenzialdiagnose und therapeutische Konsequenzen. Chirurg 2006; 77: 883–888

Plusczyk T, Bolli M, Schilling M. Ileuskrankheit. Chirurg 2006; 77, 898–903

16 Spleen

H. Brunn

■ Anatomy

- The adult spleen is about 11 × 7 × 4 cm in size and weighs 100–200 g.
- The spleen is located at the level of the left 9th to 11th ribs in the posterior axillary line. The longitudinal axis follows the line of the 10th rib. Under physiological conditions, the spleen does not project beyond the costal margin.
- It is related anatomically to the left dome of the diaphragm, the gastric fundus, the left colic flexure, the left kidney and the tail of the pancreas.
- The spleen is surrounded by an easily damaged connective tissue capsule, 0.1 mm in thickness, which is connected to the suspensory ligaments (splenocolic ligament, phrenicosplenic ligament, splenorenal ligament, gastrosplenic ligament).
- Accessory spleens are observed in up to 30% of people, often in the vicinity of the splenic hilum.
- The splenic artery arises from the celiac trunk and passes along the upper border of the pancreas, initially accompanied by the splenic vein. At the splenic hilum, it divides into several branches, leading to the segmental blood supply of the spleen.
- Venous drainage is through the splenic vein, which combines with the superior mesenteric vein to form the portal vein.

■ Physiology

- Removal and destruction of old and pathologically fragile erythrocytes and other diseased or aged cell forms of the red blood cell series (including platelets)
- Elimination of cellular inclusions such as Howell–Jolly bodies (chromatin residues) and Heinz bodies (denatured hemoglobin). After splenectomy, the liver takes over this function.
- Immunological:
  - ► Filtering and processing of antigens
  - ► Main source of IgM antibody production
- After splenectomy, the phagocytosis of pathogenic microorganisms falls mainly to the liver. However, clearance of encapsulated bacteria (e.g., pneumococci) then becomes a problem.

- After splenectomy, the liver takes over some of its functions.

■ Hypersplenism Syndrome

- This is a qualitative and quantitative increase of some or all functions of the spleen.
- Splenomegaly is possible.
- As a result there is a reduction in one or more classes of blood cells.

16

- Hypersplenism syndrome may also be a secondary result of other diseases. The most frequent cause is hepatic cirrhosis with portal hypertension.

Diagnostic Approach

■ Clinical Examination

- Normal-sized spleen not usually palpable

- The enlarged spleen may be palpated bimanually with the patient in supine or right lateral decubitus position, one hand palpating and the other hand fixed.
- A palpable impulse on deep palpation indicates splenic enlargement.

■ Laboratory Tests

- In hematological disorders with splenic involvement:
  - ► Differential blood count
  - ► Bone marrow aspiration

■ Diagnostic Imaging

Ultrasonography
- The spleen and its size are readily imaged with ultrasonography.
- Free fluid around the spleen or nonhomogeneity of the parenchyma (splenic rupture/trauma) can also be identified.

Computed Tomography
- Should the ultrasound examination not be diagnostic, CT can be used as a further diagnostic imaging method (e.g., polytrauma CT).

Treatment Approach

■ Indications for Splenectomy

- Individual indication necessary

- Hereditary spherocytosis with marked anemia and severe hemolytic crises
- Werlhof disease (idiopathic thrombocytopenic purpura) if conservative therapy has failed
- Other hematological diseases associated with hypersplenism; in this case, it is even more important to decide on the indication in conjunction with hematology colleagues
- As part of abdominal tumor surgery
- Splenic injury (traumatic/iatrogenic)
- Other rare indications (ruptured splenic artery aneurysm, in portal hypertension)

■ Surgical Treatment

Special Preoperative Measures
- Pneumococcal vaccination prior to splenectomy

- Prior to elective splenectomy, pneumococcal vaccination up to 10 days before operation

Open Splenectomy

Operative Technique

- Supine position
- Incision along the left costal margin, midline incision if appropriate for a very large spleen
- Opening of the omental bursa
- Find and ligate the splenic artery at the upper border of the pancreas.
- Divide the suspensory ligaments (**caution:** treat short gastric vessels running in the gastrosplenic ligament).
- After complete eventration of the spleen, the vessels at the splenic hilum are divided gradually and removal of the organ is then possible.
- Remove any accessory spleens in the region of the hilum.
- If necessary, place a drain in the splenic bed.

- In the case of traumatic splenic injury, primary midline incision may be appropriate: if splenectomy is necessary, this allows prompt mobilization and dislocation of the spleen with manual compression of the vessels, and primary dissection of the hilum with division of the vessels if necessary.

Laparoscopic Splenectomy

Operative Technique

- Supine position, tilted to the right
- Infraumbilical optical trocar, 5-mm trocar in the right upper abdomen and epigastrium, 12-mm trocar in left lower abdomen
- If necessary, manually assisted laparoscopic operation, then infraumbilical optical trocar, epigastric hand port, and 12-mm trocar in left mid-abdomen
- Division of the suspensory ligaments, for example with ultrasonic scissors
- Exposure of the splenic hilum and division, for example with a linear stapler
- Removal of the spleen using a specimen bag through the hand port or extension of a trocar port. If histological examination of the entire organ is not required, it can be divided in the specimen bag within the abdomen.
- If necessary, place a drain in the splenic bed.

Spleen-Preserving Surgical Options

Segmental Resection
- Find and clamp the segmental arteries at the splenic hilum.
- With appropriate demarcation, perform segmental resection along the demarcation line:
    ► If necessary, after prior transfixion of the parenchyma
    ► If necessary, subsequent infrared coagulation of the resection surface
- Application of fibrin glue and/or fleece

Hemostasis without Resection
- Management of superficial bleeding with infrared coagulator/fibrin glue/fibrin fleece
- Direct capsule suture if appropriate
- Place an absorbable mesh around the spleen and tighten the mesh until hemostasis is achieved (full mobilization of the spleen is required for this).

16

left hepatic artery from the celiac trunk (or left gastric artery). The cystic artery arises from the right hepatic artery.

- **Portal vein:** This arises from the junction of the superior mesenteric vein and the splenic vein. It is joined in the hepatoduodenal ligament by the left gastric vein and cystic vein, then divides at the liver hilum into right and left branches to supply the corresponding liver lobes.
- **Veins:** Venous drainage is into the inferior vena cava through hepatic veins, which do not have a connective tissue sheath (so are easy to distinguish from branches of the portal vein by intraoperative ultrasonography). Hepatic veins are located between the hepatic segments but do not follow their boundaries and receive branches from neighboring segments; their intrahepatic course can be followed with ultrasound imaging.
- Most frequent variant: three large hepatic veins (right, left, middle); the middle hepatic vein runs on the boundary between the right and left liver lobes.
- The liver, like other glands, is made up of **lobules**. The blood flows radially from the interlobar portal vein and arterial branches through the liver sinusoids to the central vein located in the center of the lobule. The bile canaliculi are intracellular and open into the interlobular bile ducts. The **"Glisson triads"** are located at the boundaries of adjacent lobules, each containing an interlobular portal vein, artery, and bile duct branch. Branching of the Glisson triad means that each segment is independent of the other segments with regard to blood supply and biliary drainage, and can be removed surgically without endangering the function of the remainder of the liver.
- Intrahepatic **lymph channels** are located within the Glisson capsules; daily lymph production is 1–3 L; it increases up to 10 L in hepatic cirrhosis.

■ Benign Liver Tumors

Focal Nodular Hyperplasia (FNH)

- FNH frequent in middle-aged women taking contraceptives
- Not precancerous

- Mainly in middle-aged women, usually solitary and found in subcapsular location
- Causal association with long-term use of **contraceptives**
- More frequent than hepatocellular adenoma, but not precancerous

Symptoms

- None, often discovered by diagnostic imaging of other conditions

Diagnostic Approach

- Important: distinguish with certainty from adenoma and other diagnoses for further treatment.

- On **ultrasound scan,** usually visible as a hypoechoic focal lesion
- **Contrast ultrasonography:** method of choice for secure diagnosis
- **CT** and **MRI:** diagnosis with great certainty because of the typical behavior of the contrast agent
- In case of doubt, confirmation by **biopsy** or laparoscopic **resection in full** (e.g., if there is a prior history of malignancy)

Treatment Approach

- **Observation:** Regression is possible after contraceptives are discontinued.
- If in favorable position and diagnosis unclear, **laparoscopic resection** of the lesion in full is preferable to biopsy from the oncological aspect.

Hepatocellular Adenoma

- Mainly in middle-aged women; association with long-term use of **contraceptives** likely
- Malignant degeneration possible, therefore distinction from FNH particularly important

• Malignant degeneration possible, operation obligatory

Symptoms

- Rarely, can cause symptoms due to bleeding or rupture; usually an incidental finding during other diagnostic imaging

17

Diagnostic Approach

- Ultrasonography
- Contrast ultrasonography
- CT
- MRI

Treatment Approach

- **Resection in full** (R0 resection) because of the risk of degeneration

Hepatic Hemangioma

- The most common benign primary tumors of the liver, with a prevalence of 5%–7%

• Most common benign tumor

Symptoms

- Usually an incidental finding on ultrasound imaging
- Larger hemangiomas can be a cause of **abdominal pain** as a result of partial infarction or due to pressure on surrounding tissue
- Can also rupture or form abscesses

• Usually an incidental finding

Diagnostic Approach

- **Ultrasonography:** nearly diagnostic with hyperechoic, smoothly demarcated lesion without a halo
- **CT** and **MRI:** also give typical appearance; usually inferior to ultrasonography for diagnosis

• Hyperechoic lesion on ultrasonography

Treatment Approach

- Operation indicated if painful, complications or diagnosis uncertain
- Treatment is then resection of the lesion in full.

Hepatic Cysts

- Isolated cysts are a frequent incidental finding without clinical significance.
- With **polycystic organ degeneration** (usually combined with cystic kidneys), there is progressive cystic remodeling of the entire organ.

Symptoms

- Pain due to pressure on the remainder of the liver or other organs. Large cysts can cause considerable **upper abdominal symptoms.**
- Occasionally acute pain due to spontaneous rupture of a cyst

Treatment Approach

- **Laparoscopic deroofing** is accomplished by resecting in full the wall of the cyst facing toward the free abdomen.

▪ Malignant Liver Tumors

Primary Hepatic Carcinoma

- HCC: increasing incidence
- Risk factors: liver cirrhosis, hepatitis B and C

- This occurs especially in a liver previously damaged by hepatitis or cirrhosis; can be solitary or multiple.
- A distinction is made between **hepatocellular carcinoma** (HCC), **cholangiocarcinoma** and mixed types. The incidence of HCC is increasing as a result of increasing hepatitis C infections.
- Patients with **liver cirrhosis** and chronic **hepatitis C**, chronic **hepatitis B,** or hemochromatosis have the greatest risk. In addition, **aflatoxin** (a mycotoxin in food) is also held responsible for the development of liver cancer.

Metastasis
- Often in the vicinity of the primary tumor (**satellite metastases**)
- **Lymphatogenous metastasis** to the hilar, perigastric, peripancreatic and para-aortic lymph nodes
- Hematogenous, predominantly **lung metastases**

Classification (Table 17.1)

Table 17.1   TNM classification

T—primary tumor	
Tx	Primary tumor not assessable
T0	No evidence of primary tumor
T1	Solitary tumor without vascular invasion
T2	Solitary tumor with vascular invasion or multiple tumors, ≤ 5 cm
T3	Multiple tumors, solitary tumor > 5 cm or with involvement of a major branch of the portal vein or hepatic vein
T4	Tumor directly invading neighboring organs with the exception of the gall-bladder or tumors perforating the visceral peritoneum
N—regional lymph nodes	
Nx	Regional lymph nodes not assessable
N0	No regional lymph node metastases
N1	Regional lymph node metastases
M—distant metastases	
M0	No distant metastases
M1	Distant metastases

17

Symptoms

- Nonspecific upper abdominal symptoms
- Palpable guarding, icterus, and ascites are late symptoms.

Diagnostic Approach

- **Laboratory test:** alpha-fetoprotein (AFP) as specific tumor marker
- **Ultrasonography** and contrast ultrasonography
- **CT** (triphasic): arterial, portal venous, and venous phase. This investigation usually suffices for reconstruction of the arterial vascular anatomy.
- Additional **MRI** is rarely necessary
- **Positron emission tomography (PET)-CT:** rarely necessary as a primary investigation, possibly for diagnosis of recurrence (distinguishes scar tissue from tumor tissue)
- If cholangiocarcinoma is suspected, endoscopic retrograde cholangiography (ERC) with brush cytology

Treatment Approach

■ Indications

- **Resection** of small hepatocellular carcinomas, as well as **liver transplantation** in selected cases, are potentially curative procedures but possible in only a few patients. The cirrhosis which is usually present considerably limits the prospect of surviving a major liver resection. These procedures are usually not possible in Child B and Child C patients (**Table 17.2**). With Child A patients, liver cirrhosis likewise markedly increases the operation risk as the functional reserve is already greatly impaired. However, in patients in good general condition, resections up to hemihepatectomy are possible.

- Resection often not possible because of liver cirrhosis; transplantation rarely indicated and possible

Table 17.2 Child classification of liver cirrhosis

Parameter	Child A	Child B	Child C
Bilirubin	< 2 mg/dL	2–3 mg/dL	> 3 mg/dL
Albumin	> 35 g/L	30–35 g/L	< 30 g/L
Ascites	No	Treatable	Refractory to treatment
Neurological symptoms	No	Slight	Severe
INR	< 1.7	1.7–2.3	> 2.3

INR: international normalized ratio.

- The Child score requires precise knowledge of the severity of the hepatic encephalopathy.
- The **serum** level is a good parameter of prognosis, and is often markedly reduced as a sign of diminished organ function. There is a clear inverse correlation between cholinesterase level and average life expectancy.
- Where tumors are greater than 5 cm in size and resection is not possible or contraindicated, local interventional procedures are indictated, including:
  - ► Ultrasound-guided percutaneous alcohol injection
  - ► Radiofrequency thermoablation
  - ► Cryotherapy
  - ► Laser ablation
  - ► Transarterial chemoembolization, also possible with larger tumors
- **Chemotherapy** and **immunotherapy:** not firmly established. Suitable patients in good general condition should be included in studies. Both chemoembolization (lipiodol) and regional arterial chemotherapy and intravenous chemotherapy are employed. Additional immunotherapy with interleukin 2 and anti-CD3 activated autologous lymphocytes is under investigation.

Prognosis
- Despite progress in surgical therapy, local ablative procedures, and arterial chemoembolization, the **recurrence rate** is high, especially because of the untreatable underlying disease and the occurrence of new tumors due to the persisting risk factors.
- Five-year survival rate is 20%–30%.
- Whether specific tumor follow-up improves prognosis remains doubtful; in patients in good general condition, regular ultrasonography, CT, and measurement of AFP are employed to discover recurrences early.

Liver Metastases

Treatment Approach

■ Indications

- Liver metastases from **colorectal carcinoma** are the most frequent indication for surgery of metastases.
- Because of improved surgical techniques and adjuvant or neoadjuvant chemotherapy concepts, the 5-year survival rate and thus the cure rate is between 40% and 50%. In individual series the 5-year survival rates are over 70%, though the exclusion criteria also have considerable importance for the end result of such studies.
- All the limits usually given in the past for the size and number of metastases that could be regarded as resectable are no longer relevant. The only factor

Sidebar notes:

- Child classification and cholinesterase are important indicators for deciding on surgery.
- Consider ethanol injection and thermoablation if inoperable, consider chemoembolization for large lesions.

- Good prognosis for resectable liver metastases from colorectal carcinoma

17

relevant for prognosis is R0 resection and the absence of lymph node metastases and other distant metastases.

- Limiting factor: Circa 20% of healthy liver tissue must be preserved for adequate liver function. The liver is the only parenchymal organ that preserves the capacity for regeneration by hypertrophy. The residual liver usually reaches 70% of its initial size after a few weeks.
- **Resection of recurrences** is also possible but is technically demanding because of altered hepatic anatomy and scarring. Provided the tumor biology within the liver or other distant metastasis does not outstrip regeneration, even repeated surgery of recurrences may be promising in isolated cases.
- Additional use of locally ablative procedures (radiofrequency thermoablation) can produce R0 situations, which would not have been achievable with resection alone.
- In some patients in a supposed palliative situation with extensive hepatic metastases, a marked reduction in tumor mass was achieved by "palliative chemotherapy," so that successful liver resection was possible secondarily. In this way, the concept of **neoadjuvant chemotherapy** became established in the treatment of liver metastases.
- Morbidity and mortality after liver resection have fallen considerably because of improved surgical techniques and perioperative anesthesiological management (mortality < 2% in many studies). The indication for resection of **non-colorectal metastases** should therefore be decided generously, even when benefit is doubtful.
- The benefit of surgery of liver metastases has not been proved for any malignant disease apart from colorectal carcinoma.
- Rule of thumb for establishing indication: The longer the interval between the occurrence of the primary tumor and the occurrence of the metastases, the more the benefit of surgical treatment can be assumed. Provided the patient is not injured by the surgery in itself, therapeutic benefit can be assumed due to the reduction of tumor burden even if long-term cure is not achieved.
- If primary R0 resection is not possible, the following options can be considered to achieve a secondary R0 situation, especially for young patients and those in good general condition:
  - ► Conditioning of the liver by **ligature of a portal vein branch** or interventional radiological **embolization.** Unilateral occlusion of the portal circulation region induces hypertrophy of the other side. A possibility mostly when there is extensive right-sided liver metastasis and a small anatomical left hepatic lobe (segments 2 + 3), if an extended right hemihepatectomy (and possibly local excision/thermoablation on the left) would lead to a R0 situation.
  - ► **Neoadjuvant chemotherapy.** If there is a good response with an often obvious reduction of the tumor mass, an initially nonresectable situation may become resectable.
  - ► **Two-stage procedure:** for example, primary hemihepatectomy of the side with the greater tumor burden, possibly with additional atypical resection and thermoablation of metastases on the opposite side, leaving poorly accessible lesions. Further assessment of resectability may be undertaken after several more cycles of chemotherapy, if applicable. Primary resection also causes hypertrophy of healthy liver tissue, so that further resection can be performed at a later time to achieve an R0 situation.

17

- Other procedures that can be employed alone or in combination with resection:
  - ▶ **Radiofrequency thermoablation:** because of the ease of handling, particularly established for intraoperative use
  - ▶ **Cryoablation** and **laser ablation:** technically complex equipment, results are similar to those of radiofrequency thermoablation
  - ▶ Regional **chemotherapy** through an arterial port: does not exhibit better results than intravenous chemotherapy with modern drug combinations (oxaliplatin/5-fluorouracil, irinotecan/5-fluorouracil)

■ Surgical Treatment

Liver Resection

- Anatomical if possible
- 20% healthy, well-perfused, and drained hepatic tissue should remain.
- Atypical resection and thermoablation extend the spectrum.

- Anatomical resection as far as possible. Resection margins according to the anatomy of the afferent and efferent blood vessels, which divides the liver into eight segments (see **Fig. 17.1**). Parenchymal dissection along the segment boundaries is more avascular and necrosis due to absence of blood supply or drainage is avoided (not so important, as necrotic liver tissue has little influence on the postoperative course provided infection does not occur).
- It is important that at least 20% healthy liver tissue remains after resection, with a good arterial and portal venous supply and intact venous drainage.
- Along with hemihepatectomy, segmental resection, wedge resection, and atypical resection, every combination of resecting procedures is feasible in principle, as is the combination of resection and ablative procedures (radiofrequency thermoablation).
- Three-phase CT is sufficient for planning the operative strategy. Further angiographic imaging is not usually necessary, and intraoperative ultrasound imaging provides the surgeon with the best orientation.
- The following **operative procedures** can be performed singly or in combination:
  - ▶ Right hemihepatectomy (segments V–VIII)
  - ▶ Extended right hemihepatectomy (segments IV–VIII; right trisegmentectomy)
  - ▶ Left hemihepatectomy (segments II-IV)
  - ▶ Extended left hemihepatectomy (segments II, III, IV, V, VIII; left trisegmentectomy)
  - ▶ Left lobectomy (segments II/III)
  - ▶ Central liver resection (segment IV or segments IV, V, VIII)
  - ▶ Segmental resection or bisegmental resection
  - ▶ Wedge resection
  - ▶ Atypical resection
  - ▶ Thermoablation

General Liver Resection Technique

Operative Technique

General Remarks
- Anesthesia: low volume administration and low central venous pressure (CVP) results in less blood loss.
- The start of every resection is basically the same. This refers both to the special anesthesiological requirements and to positioning, incision, dissection of the liver hilum, and exposure/ligation of the large vessels.

- **Anesthesia:** Very important as the intraoperative management considerably co-determines the amount of blood loss and therefore the morbidity and mortality. Epidural catheter, large-volume central venous access and arterial blood pressure measurement are preconditions. Restrictive volume administration, anesthesia with low CVP, and low arterial pressure are important, especially during parenchymal dissection. Venous congestion in the hepatic veins is reduced in particular, so that the tendency to bleeding from the liver parenchyma is considerably reduced. This alone often allows avoidance of a Pringle maneuver (clamping the portal venous and arterial blood supply of the liver).
- **Positioning:** The patient is in supine position with a pad under the back (gel bolster) at the level of the tip of the sternum to displace the liver anteriorly.

Incision
- For all liver resections an extended right costal margin incision is sufficient. It is started just to the left of the tip of the sternum at the left costal arch and continued along the right costal arch as far as the right flank.
- Alternatively, upper transverse laparotomy with midline extension into the epigastrium, but incisional hernia is more frequent and there is greater operation trauma.

17

Intraoperative Ultrasonography
- Obligatory after inspection and palpation (extent of the malignant disease, assessment of the liver with regard to fatty change and cirrhosis; important for the possible extent of the resection)
- Intraoperative ultrasonography not infrequently yields new findings that will change the operative strategy (establishment of the resection margins with regard to the vascular anatomy, discovery of new lesions); most sensitive method for detecting focal hepatic lesions
- The liver parenchyma is examined systematically with regard to tumor extent, assignment to hepatic vascular anatomy and presence of further, hitherto unidentified foci.

- Intraoperative ultrasonography is crucial for operative strategy.

Dissection of the Liver Hilum
- **Establishment of the operative strategy:** From the results now available, a decision is made on what strategy to employ to achieve R0 resection. Large resections at the start, followed by any additionally required smaller resections and thermoablation.
- Involvement of the lymph nodes in the liver hilum can influence the decision for or against resection (**Fig. 17.2**).
- Use of bipolar electric scissors and forceps. First, the connective tissue layer in the hepatoduodenal ligament is divided anteriorly with its contained lymph nodes. Then the lymph nodes in the angle between the duodenum, pancreas head, and hepatoduodenal ligament are dissected.
- Further dissection on the posterior side of the hepatoduodenal ligament. Then dissection of the lymph nodes proceeds along the common hepatic artery as far as the celiac trunk. All lymph nodes are sent for frozen section.

- Lymph node involvement in the hepatoduodenal ligament influences the resection decision.

Cholecystectomy
- Obligatory in the event of major liver resection
- If the gallbladder is not included with the main specimen, it is removed anterograde with bipolar electric scissors in the connective tissue plane between the muscularis and the gallbladder bed. As long a section as possible of

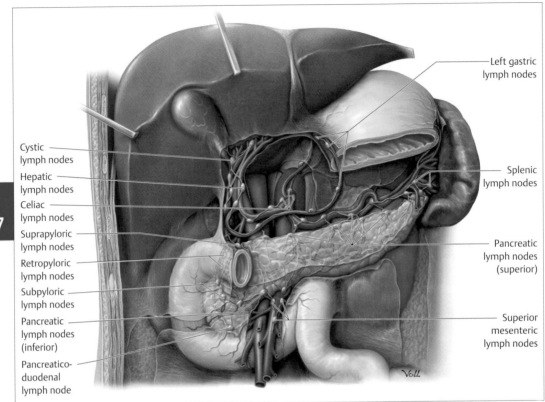

Cystic
lymph nodes

Hepatic
lymph nodes

Celiac
lymph nodes

Suprapyloric
lymph nodes

Retropyloric
lymph nodes

Subpyloric
lymph nodes

Pancreatic
lymph nodes
(inferior)

Pancreatico-
duodenal
lymph node

Left gastric
lymph nodes

Splenic
lymph nodes

Pancreatic
lymph nodes
(superior)

Superior
mesenteric
lymph nodes

Fig. 17.2   Lymph nodes in the liver hilum. (Illustration: M. Voll; from Schünke et al. 2005, see p. 413.)

the cystic duct is left and divided and left open, and an angiography catheter is then tied in for later filling of the bile duct system with diluted blue solution.
- The gallbladder and any attached lymph nodes can be sent for frozen section.

Mobilization of the Liver
- While waiting for the frozen section result the liver is mobilized according to the anticipated extent of resection.
- Incise the falciform ligament on the liver surface and divide the right or left triangular ligament, that is, complete mobilization of the corresponding half of the liver.

Exposure and Ligation of the Large Vessels
- Before hemihepatectomy, central or difficult segment resection, dissect free and ligate the large vessels; these include:
    - The portal vein in the liver hilum, hepatic artery proper, and both of its branches in the liver hilum
    - The entire liver hilum (so-called Pringle maneuver)
    - The vena cava immediately above the entry of the renal veins
    - The vena cava above the entry of the hepatic vein
- For ligating the portal vein and vena cava, use Mersylene tape with previously placed tourniquet.

Parenchymal Dissection

- In the case of major anatomical resections, start by dividing the afferent arterial and portal venous branches and the efferent hepatic veins. Endo-GIA vascular staplers can be used to divide hepatic veins and main portal vein branches—staples save space, avoid narrowing of the remaining vessels, and are quick and safe to use.
- The part of the liver that is no longer perfused is now demarcated. If the extent of the tumor allows this, it is desirable to establish the resection margin ca. 0.5 cm in the now under-perfused area, as blood loss during resection is then lower.
- In the case of segmental resection or atypical resection without prior division of the blood supply, the resection line is established from the tumor extent found on ultrasound imaging and from the vascular anatomy.
- The planned resection line is traced on the liver surface with the electrocautery.
- Numerous methods have been described for parenchymal dissection and are employed depending on the institution and availability of equipment.
  - ▶ **Ultrasonic dissection:** The probe sets cells oscillating and heats them until they burst. Since cells with a high water content burst faster, structures with a greater connective tissue content (vessels) withstand this and are more accessible to targeted surgical management (bipolar electrocoagulation, clip ligature, transfixion ligature). The devices allow simultaneous use of monopolar electrocoagulation, so that the surgeon can coagulate minor bleeds immediately.
  - ▶ **Water jet dissection:** Different physical principle; here, too, the softer hepatocytes are destroyed faster than the connective tissue structures.
  - ▶ **Ultrasonic scissors and "LigaSure":** These take small portions of tissue in their entirety and vessels are sealed by the simultaneous use of pressure and heat. (Disadvantage: poorer exposure of anatomical structures in the vicinity of large vessels.)
  - ▶ **Coagulation and mechanical division:** By using bipolar scissors or special devices with a thermoablative effect, the tissue is coagulated gradually along the resection line, including the smaller and medium-sized vessels contained therein and is then divided mechanically. The disadvantage again is the poorer anatomical view in the vicinity of large vessels.
  - ▶ **Endo-GIA stapler:** The tissue is divided gradually along the planned resection line with Endo-GIA stapler magazines. Particularly time-saving and expensive, the disadvantage is likewise the poor anatomical view it affords.
  - ▶ **Finger fracture method:** The liver tissue is squashed between the fingers, the remaining vessels are divided between clamps and ligated (relatively crude procedure, hardly in use any longer).
- **Pringle maneuver:** If there is a greater tendency to bleeding during the dissection, either the entire liver hilum is clamped, or the portal vein and the hepatic artery and their branches are clamped individually. Overall, this has a detrimental effect on postoperative liver function so it is preferable to omit it. However, clamping for ca. 20 minutes does not lead to any significant damage. Clamping for up to 60 minutes is regarded as still possible. So-called conditioning is better than clamping; this involves releasing the blood flow for a few minutes after clamping for ca. 5 minutes, and this is then followed by a period of longer clamping.

17

- Pringle maneuver reduces blood loss during parenchymal dissection.

17

- **Hanging maneuver:** In hemihepatectomy, the liver can be elevated in the planned resection line by careful tunneling under the liver and over the vena cava as far as the entry of the middle hepatic vein, followed by passage of a wide tape (tape cut off an abdominal drape). This facilitates correct maintenance of the resection line, especially when the right liver lobe cannot be readily mobilized because of the size of the tumor (if necessary, the hepatic vein(s) is (are) divided only after the parenchymal dissection).

Biliary-Enteric Anastomosis
- If the size of the tumor necessitates resection of bile duct structures at the same time, a biliary-enteric anastomosis can be constructed between the unilateral main bile duct or its branches to an excluded Roux-en-Y loop after the resection.
- If the ducts are too delicate for direct anastomosis, the loop can also be sutured directly to the liver parenchyma.

Conclusion of the Operation
- **Hemostasis:** After 3–5 minutes compression of the resection surface with a hot abdominal sponge, oozing usually ceases spontaneously. Persistent bleeding is managed with targeted transfixion sutures. To prevent the residual tendency to oozing, the resection line is cauterized (electrocautery, infrared coagulator, laser).
- **Inspection for bile leaks:** Injection of dilute blue solution into the angiography catheter (cystic duct), bile duct clamped with bulldog clamp. The bile duct system is thus filled retrogradely and bile duct leaks (leakage of blue) on the resection surface can now be transfixed and ligated.
- **Sealing of the liver surface** with fibrin glue or other hemostatics is optional.
- **Wound draining with silicone drains**, closure of the abdomen in layers with continuous absorbable sutures.

Right Hemihepatectomy (Fig. 17.3)

Operative Technique

- Division of the right triangular ligament and exposure of the right hepatic vein
- Division of the right hepatic artery and right hepatic duct
- Division of the right branch of the portal vein
- Division of the right hepatic vein
- Division of the parenchyma from the gallbladder bed to the hepatic vein triangle
- Division of the vein branches from the right lobe of the liver draining directly into the vena cava

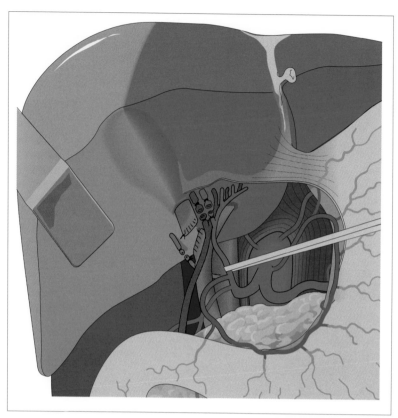

Fig. 17.3   Vascular management at the liver hilum in right hemihepatectomy (light blue liver parts to be removed).

Extended Right Hemihepatectomy

Operative Technique

- Identical procedure to right hemihepatectomy but the resection line runs in the region of the falciform ligament
- Additional division of the middle hepatic vein and portal vein and arterial branches for segment IV
- Depending on tumor growth, the left hepatic duct is also resected if necessary and a biliary-enteric anastomosis to a Roux-en-Y loop is fashioned.

Left Hemihepatectomy (Figs. 17.4, 17.5)

Operative Technique

- Division of the left triangular ligament and exposure of the opening of the hepatic vein
- Division of the left hepatic duct and left hepatic artery
- Division of the left branch of the portal vein
- Division of the left hepatic vein
- Depending on extent of the tumor, resection of the caudate lobe also

17

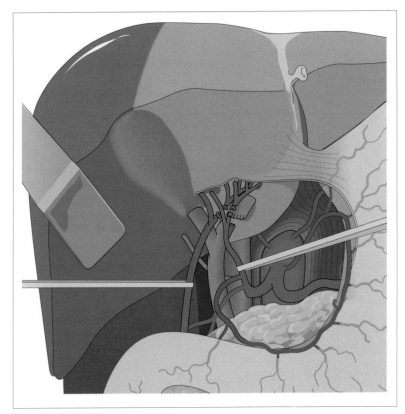

Fig. 17.4   Liver hilum in left hemihepatectomy (light blue liver parts to be removed).

Extended Left Hemihepatectomy

Operative Technique

- Same steps as in left hemihepatectomy; in addition, ligation of the middle hepatic vein is obligatory
- After starting parenchymal dissection, ligation of the segmental branch of the portal vein for segments V and VIII (**Fig. 17.5**).
- Resection line in the liver parenchyma shifted to the right according to the segment boundaries

Central Liver Resection

- Targeted ligature of the segmental bile ducts and arterial branches
- Management of the segmental portal vein branches and **middle hepatic vein** in the course of the parenchymal dissection

Bisegmental Resection

- The most frequent bisegmental resection is left-sided lobectomy (segments II and III). The parenchymal bridge to the left of the falciform ligament is relatively narrow, and the left hepatic vein can usually be exposed readily and divided. The portal vein branch and bile duct for segments II and III are exposed and divided within the parenchyma in the resection line.

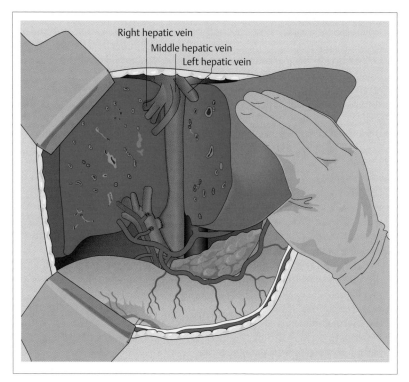

Fig. 17.5   Parenchymal division in left hemihepatectomy.

- Other bisegmental resections (e.g., segments V/VI) are more complex technically because of the large resection surface. The aim is exposure of the segmental vessels, especially the portal vein branches supplying the segments.

Segmental Resection
- The principle is as described above. The resection line is guided by the respective segment border, and the central vascular trunk with portal vein branch and bile duct can be exposed and ligated only after the start of the parenchymal dissection (the same applies for the arterial supply but this plays no part in orientation).

Wedge Resection of the Liver
- Suitable for superficial lesions located at the edge
- The wedge-shaped resection line is traced on the parenchyma around the lesion.
- When the liver parenchyma is soft, a soft bowel clamp can be applied laterally on both sides.
- The wedge is excised in healthy tissue with the bipolar electric scissors and any vessels still bleeding are ligated or cauterized.

Atypical Liver Resection

- When wedge excision is not possible because of the unfavorable position of a lesion. A spherical or cylindrical area is removed in healthy tissue.
- Ensure by ultrasonography that no major vessels are involved; in that case, anatomical resection would be necessary.
- After incision of the liver surface, elevate the part to be resected by stay sutures at the edge, if appropriate; this makes the vascular structures more visible.
- Ultrasonic dissection is more suitable as major vessel branches often run deeply, which are more difficult to control after "bloody division."

Thermoablation

- Lesions up to ca. 3 cm in diameter. Ablation of lesions up to 5 cm in size is technically possible. The heating zones form a maplike relief, so the probability of destroying all tumor tissue is lower with increasing lesion diameter.
- An open surgical procedure has the advantage that neighboring organs can be specifically protected from the harmful thermal effect.
- Portal vein branches can also be specifically clamped for the duration of the thermoablation; this prevents cooling by blood flowing at the edge of the metastasis.
- Targeted cooling of bile ducts is possible, to avoid bile duct strictures due to the thermal effects.
- Depending on the size of the metastasis, a suitable probe is selected and placed in the center of the metastasis.
- The procedure requires experience in interventional ultrasonography; aspiration aids and acoustic transducers are available with simultaneous imaging of a lesion in two planes.
- There are different manufacturers and probes: different techniques have been developed to increase the depth of penetration and extent of the thermoablation:
  - ► Unfolding of a fanlike probe with several arms that spread out in the metastasis
  - ► Cooling of the inside of the probe to prevent carbonization of the tissue close to the probe (leads to an increase in tissue resistance and therefore prevents the spread of current)
  - ► Instillation of saline into the tumor to increase tissue conduction
- Thermoablation is then performed according to the equipment manufacturer's instructions.

Laparoscopic Liver Resection

- Laparoscopic liver resection, possible with smaller lesions

- Procedure identical to the open procedure
- Suitable especially for resection of small marginal lesions up to segmental and bisegmental resection. Larger anatomical liver resections are also possible laparoscopically, but risk/benefit assessment usually decides in favor of an open surgical procedure.
- In the case of vessel injury, large volumes of blood are released within a short time, and vision and control of the bleeding are then difficult.
- **Caution:** to avoid air embolism, the intraperitoneal pressure should be lower than the CVP.
- Use narrow ultrasonic scissors or Ligashure device for parenchymal dissection.
- Divide bigger vessels with the Endo-GIA stapler.
- Electrocoagulation or infrared coagulation for hemostasis in the parenchyma
- Removal of the specimen in a specimen bag

■ Complications

- Serious complications are rare due to improvements in operative surgical technique and perioperative management.
- Major bile leaks have become very rare owing to the techniques described above; surgical revision is occasionally necessary after biliary-enteric anastomosis.
- Minor bile leaks through the silicone drains are observed more often and usually seal off spontaneously within a few days.
- Right-sided pleural effusion, especially after right hemihepatectomy, usually resolves spontaneously; intensive respiratory therapy may be required to avoid atelectasis if extensive, pleural aspiration is required initially; if flow is rapid, insert a chest drain for a few days.
- Subphrenic or perihepatic abscess: treatment with ultrasonically or CT-guided aspiration and drainage

• Bile leakage, pleural effusion, abscess

17

■ Hydatid Disease of the Liver (Echinococcosis)

Etiology

- **Zoonosis** due to tapeworms (cestodes). In contrast to other tapeworms, humans are only an intermediate host in the development cycle of the echinococci and the pathogens only reach the larval stage. Adult echinococci are not found in humans so it is not possible to find eggs in the stool.
- Two types of pathogen can be distinguished morphologically in humans:
  - ➤ The dog tapeworm *Echinococcus cysticus* (*granulosus*) is distributed worldwide. The most important final host is the dog; the tapeworm eggs are found in the feces and as a result in the fur also. Apart from humans, hoofed animals such as sheep, cattle and horses also act as intermediate hosts.
  - ➤ Dogs, foxes, and cats are end hosts of *E. alveolaris*. The main intermediate hosts apart from humans are field mice. Transmission to humans is mainly via contaminated woodland berries.
- The chorion of the larva is digested in the stomach. The larva then reaches the portal vein system through the duodenal mucosa and from there it reaches the liver. In 20%–30%, *E. cysticus* affects the lungs in addition to the liver and also other organs in a smaller percentage of those affected.
- The two types show different growth patterns in the intermediate host:
  - ➤ *Echinococcus cysticus* grows by compression and develops into a large hydatitid cyst with a three-layer structure from without inward. The boundary with the compressed liver tissue is formed by the pericyst, a reactive fibrous membrane that can become calcified. This is followed by a delicate intermediate layer containing chitin. The inner wall of the cyst consists of a germinative membrane, where the brood capsules originate with scolices, the heads of the later tapeworms. Millions of these then enter the fluid-filled cavity of the cyst.
  - ➤ *Echinococcus alveolaris* grows by infiltration, forming numerous small cysts, which increase by exogenous budding. The appearance in the organ can be mistaken for hepatic carcinoma.

Symptoms

- In **cystic echinococcosis,** there are usually no symptoms for many years or only nonspecific upper abdominal symptoms. With increasing growth of the hydatids, a palpable mass in the right upper abdomen or hepatomegaly may develop. Sometimes, a chest or abdominal x-ray shows an abnormal elevation of the right diaphragm or calcifications in the right hypochondrium.
- **Alveolar form:** often progressive, painless liver enlargement with a nodular surface and early icterus. Abdominal x-ray can show diffuse clumps of calcification in the liver region.

Diagnostic Approach

- **Fine-needle biopsy is contraindicated.**

- **Serological methods** are based on detection of antibodies. The *E. cysticus* antibody titer can fluctuate depending on the affected organ (for instance, it is lower when the lung is involved), the thickness, and calcification of the cysts. Cross-reactions with other worm diseases are possible. Antibody detection should therefore be confirmed by a second serological test.
- Routine laboratory tests are not very useful; in isolated cases there is elevation of C-reactive protein, leukocytosis, eosinophilia, and raised cholestasis parameters.
- The most important screening method is **ultrasonography,** which shows the typical multilayered structure of solitary cysts. The sonographic appearance of alveolar echinococcosis is less typical and difficult to distinguish from neoplastic disease.
- **CT** has the greatest diagnostic reliability for preoperative planning; it provides information about the size, shape, and position of the cysts.
- If material is obtained at surgery, microscopic evidence is readily adduced. With lung involvement invading the bronchial system, sputum can be used for **microscopic** evidence.
- Fine-needle biopsy is contraindicated if echinococcosis is suspected.

Treatment Approach

■ Conservative Therapy

- Nonoperable forms require drug treatment.
- Drugs such as mebendazole and albendazole are effective with both types of *echinococcus,* even if they are only parasitostatic. They are used as sole or adjuvant chemotherapy, especially when incomplete resection of the affected tissue is anticipated.

■ Surgical Treatment

- **Surgical clearance:** The operation tactic depends on the number, size, and location of the cysts.
  - ▶ In **cystectomy** (hydatectomy), cysts projecting from the surface of the liver are punctured and the content is aspirated. The cyst is then filled with 20% saline. The solution must be left for at least 5 minutes to achieve complete killing of the parasites. The parasite cysts are shelled out leaving the fibrous host capsule behind. After ligature of opened bile ducts, the residual cavity may be plugged with greater omentum.

▸ In **pericystectomy**, the entire cyst including host capsule is dissected in full from the surrounding liver tissue. It can then be plugged with omentum. Technically more difficult.
▸ **Liver resection**
▸ Ultrasound-guided **injection of alcohol** into the cyst
• Surgery is indicated for *E. alveolaris* only when radical removal of the affected organ structures is technically possible.
• Resection procedures correspond to those for liver tumors.

■ Portal Hypertension

Definition

• Results from the vascular resistance and blood flow in the portal circulation, defined as a constant elevation of the pressure gradient between the portal vein and the inferior vena cava of over 7 mmHg.
• Portal vein pressure can be measured by direct (intraoperative pressure measurement, cannulation of the umbilical vein, percutaneous transhepatic puncture of portal vein branches) and indirect methods (measurement of the hepatic vein closing pressure).

17

Etiology

• Raised resistance to outflow from the portal vein and splenic vein is usually due to hepatic cirrhosis; more rarely, it is caused by outflow obstruction in the region of the large hepatic veins (Budd–Chiari syndrome), portal vein thrombosis, or segmental stenoses in the course of the splenic vein.

• Pre-, intra- and posthepatic forms

• Leads to the development of portosystemic collaterals. Submucosal and subepithelial esophageal and fundal varices are clinically important. They can lead to life-threatening hemorrhage.
• **Prehepatic** portal hypertension: most frequent cause is **thrombosis** of the portal vein or splenic vein.
• **Intrahepatic** portal hypertension: most frequent cause is **hepatic cirrhosis.**
• **Posthepatic** portal hypertension: caused by **obstruction** of the hepatic veins (Budd–Chiari syndrome) or of the inferior vena cava just above the entry of the hepatic veins, for example with constrictive pericarditis.

Consequences of Portal Hypertension
• Collaterals in the esophagus and mediastinum, which convey blood from the splenic and gastric veins to the azygos and hemiazygos veins
• Rupture of thin-walled collateral vessels in the mucosa and submucosa of the esophagus and stomach, which is the most dangerous complication

• Rupture of thin-walled collateral vessels, esophageal varices bleeding, ascites, encephalopathy, renal failure

• The risk of bleeding from esophageal varices is much greater than from varices in the gastric fundus. The structure of the wall of the varices, liver function, and the degree of coagulation disorder play a part.
• Collaterals in the submucosa of the rectum, which convey blood from the mesenteric veins to the inferior hemorrhoidal veins
• Collaterals in the retroperitoneum, especially between the splenic vein and the left renal vein

- Due to collaterals between the portal and the systemic circulation, substances that are normally extracted by the liver pass from the bowel into the circulation.
- Apart from ammonia, a variety of other substances are involved in the development of portosystemic encephalopathy.
- The rise in hydrostatic pressure in the hepatic sinusoids causes increased production of hepatic lymph. If the capacity of the hepatic lymph drainage is exhausted, exudation of lymph into the peritoneal cavity occurs, thus producing ascites.
- Other factors in the development of ascites: albumin deficiency with reduced oncotic pressure, functional changes in the renal tubule and increased sodium absorption
- Reduction in renal blood flow, redistribution of renal perfusion and functional renal failure (so-called hepatorenal syndrome)

Symptoms

- Clinical picture: symptoms of liver cirrhosis (spider nevi, ascites, palmar erythema, encephalopathy, icterus, splenomegaly, anemia)
- Esophageal variceal hemorrhage is often the first symptom.

Esophageal Variceal Hemorrhage
- Triggering factors are not known; the bleeding usually happens spontaneously and acutely.
- The main symptoms are **hematemesis** and/or **melena**
- Circulatory reactions culminating in irreversible **hemorrhagic shock**
- Ceases spontaneously in 40%–50% of cases
- High tendency to **recurrent bleeding** with conservative treatment only
- The crucial factor in mortality is the extent of the hepatic dysfunction.

Diagnostic Approach

- **Laboratory tests:** blood count, total protein, albumin, bilirubin, cholinesterase, liver enzymes
- **Ultrasonography:** dilatation of the portal vein, splenic vein, mesenteric veins; ascites, splenomegaly, changes in the liver parenchyma
- **Computed tomography:** as three-phase CT, the most reliable investigation with regard to both vessels and parenchymatous organs and ascites
- **Splenoportography** (if adequate assessment not possible by CT)
- **Gastroscopy:** assessment of esophageal and fundal varices
- **Laparoscopy** and **liver biopsy** (puncture with coagulation of the puncture site): preferable to blind puncture in the presence of ascites

Treatment Approach

■ Conservative Treatment

- Acute treatment of bleeding esophageal varices: EC, FFP, emergency gastroscopy with sclerotherapy, ligature or embolization

- After admission with suspected variceal bleeding, intensive medical treatment immediately with administration of **erythrocyte concentrate** (EC) and **fresh frozen plasma** (FFP)
- Then rapid **emergency gastroscopy**. If possible, sclerotherapy, ligation or embolization of the varices. Emergency sclerotherapy leads more often to definitive hemostasis than treatment with tubes or drugs.

- Repeat sclerotherapy, if necessary, to prevent recurrent bleeding
- Rapid hemostasis is also possible by means of a Sengstaken–Blakemore or Linton tube.
- Possibly, medical reduction of the portal vein pressure

■ Surgical Treatment

- If liver function is adequate, consider **shunt operation** after two or three recurrent bleeds. Preferably **P**ercutaneous **T**ransjugular **I**ntrahepatic **P**ortosystemic **S**hunt (TIPS), especially in patients with a high risk of bleeding for whom liver transplantation is planned. It does not interfere with the transplantation operation site. The disadvantage is an increased rate of occlusion or stenosis compared with surgical shunts.
- If transplantation is not indicated, surgical shunts can be justified in patients with bleeding esophageal varices that cannot be controlled endoscopically, provided the patient's general condition or encephalopathy do not preclude this.

- Emergency shunt rarely indicated

17

Pressure-Lowering Shunt Operation

- **Portocaval end-to-side anastomosis** is the simplest, fastest, and most effective method with the lowest thrombosis rate.
- **Mesentericocaval anastomosis** has a high occlusion rate (15%–30%, synthetic interposition graft). Both methods lead to complete diversion and interruption of portal hepatic perfusion.
- **Distal spleno-renal anastomosis** (Warren shunt) is more difficult technically but preserves mesenterico-portal liver perfusion for a time.
- With a view to later liver transplantation, the distal splenorenal anastomosis and mesenterico-caval shunt should be the preferred surgical shunt procedures.

- Shunt operations to reduce the pressure in the portal vein circulation

Devascularization Operations

- Esophageal and gastric devascularization with splenectomy
- Mechanical devascularization with circular staplers
- These procedures do not eliminate the portal hypertension and are therefore encumbered with a high rate of recurrent bleeding. Their advantage is that hepatic perfusion is preserved.

Timing of Operation

- **Emergency surgery**, performed during acute hemorrhage that cannot be controlled by conservative means; the aim is immediate and definitive hemostasis; with the exception of patients in hepatic coma or with general contraindications such as massive pneumonia requiring ventilation, uncontrollable alcoholic delirium, or decompensated heart failure
- **Early elective** operation within 24–48 hours after the initial arrest of bleeding to prevent early recurrence
- **Elective** operation in a bleeding-free interval ca. 2–3 weeks after a hemorrhage; potential patients are those with recurrent bleeding despite long-term sclerotherapy
- Patients with decompensated liver failure are not candidates for an elective shunt operation.
- Because of the high complication rates due to the liver cirrhosis and the poor prognosis of the underlying disease, restraint is warranted when deciding whether shunt surgery is indicated.

■ Liver Trauma

Definition

- Involvement of the liver in 5%–30% of patients with blunt abdominal trauma
- **Parenchymal injuries** with or without tear of the organ capsule. The latter can lead to a delayed "two-stage" rupture.

Classification (Table 17.3)

Table 17.3   Classification of traumatic liver injuries (after Moore)

Grade	Description
Grade I	Liver capsule injury
Grade II	Nonbleeding liver tear up to 1 cm deep, nonbleeding perforation, subcapsular hematoma
Grade III	Slightly bleeding parenchymal tears, subsegmental tissue destruction
Grade IV	Large parenchymal tears, tissue destruction limited to one liver lobe
Grade V	Extensive bilateral liver parenchymal destruction, injury of the hepatic veins or retrohepatic caval tear

Treatment Approach

■ Indications

- In blunt abdominal trauma with stable circulation, trial of conservative treatment is permissible with close ultrasound monitoring.
- Operation is indicated in every case of penetrating abdominal trauma; if necessary, do initial diagnostic laparoscopy.
- Ensure provision of adequate blood transfusion units, especially in the event of urgent operative revision.

■ Surgical Treatment

- Primary hemostasis by tamponade
- Suture methods for controlling hemorrhage are obsolete.

Operative Technique

- Midline laparotomy or transverse upper abdominal laparotomy for **access**, depending on which other organs might also be involved.
- After inspection of the extent of the organ injury and examination of the abdominal cavity for other injuries, the main focus is on secure and lasting **hemostasis**.
- The most effective and simplest form of primary hemostasis consists of tamponading (packing) the liver.
- Suture methods to control hemorrhage are obsolete.
- In rare cases, resection is necessary in the emergency situation. Tears of the large vessels outside the liver (portal vein, vena cava, opening of the hepatic veins) should be managed surgically as far as possible.
- Larger vascular tears in the region of parenchymal tears should, if possible, also be selectively transfixed and ligated.
- To get a better overview of the injury situation, a Pringle maneuver (clamping the liver hilum) can be performed without problems in the case of severe injuries for up to about 60 minutes.

- All unclear bleeding situations, including uncontrollable bleeding from tears of the vena cava or hepatic veins, can be controlled by firm packing with abdominal sponges when the patient's circulatory status is unstable. Firm packing with abdominal sponges is placed around the entire liver. About 15 abdominal sponges are required.
- The best time for surgical revision with removal of the abdominal packs and then specific hemostasis, as necessary, is the second postoperative day when circulatory conditions are better.

■ Postoperative Complications

- Secondary bleeding
- Bile fistulas
- Infections, especially subphrenic and subhepatic abscesses

Further Reading

Adam R, Avisar E, Ariche A et al. Five-year survival following hepatic resection after neoadjuvant therapy for nonresectable colorectal (liver) metastases. Ann Surg Oncol. 2001; 8: 347–353

Beal IK, Anthony S, Papadopoulou A, et al. Portal vein embolisation prior to hepatic resection for colorectal liver metastases and the effects of periprocedure chemotherapy. Br J Radiol. 2006; 79: 473–478

Gurusamy KS, Ramamoorthy R, Imber C, Davidson BR. Surgical resection versus nonsurgical treatment for hepatic node positive patients with colorectal liver metastases. Cochrane Database Syst Rev 2010 Jan 20; (1): CD006797. Review

National Cancer Institute. Adult Primary Liver Cancer Treatment (PDQ). Im Internet: http://www.cancer.gov/cancertopics/pdq/treatment/adult-primary-liver/healthprofessional; Stand: 03.03.2008

Portier G, Elias D, Bouche O et al. Multicenter randomized trial of adjuvant fluorouracil and folonic acid compared with surgery alone after resection of colorectal liver metastases. J Clin Oncol. 2006; 24: 4976–4982

18 Gallbladder and Biliary Tract

M. Voelz

■ Anatomy

Gallbladder
- Located below the right lobe of the liver (laterally under the quadrate lobe, corresponding to the anterior part of segment IV)
- Related to the right colic flexure, descending part of the duodenum, and the portal vein

Bile ducts (Fig. 18.1)
- Parallel to the branches of the portal vein, the right and left hepatic ducts combine to form the common hepatic duct.
- From the opening of the cystic duct, it is called the **common bile duct** (divided into supraduodenal, retroduodenal, intrapancreatic, and intramural sections) (**Fig. 18.2**).

- The anatomy of the junction and opening of the common bile duct and pancreatic duct is variable.

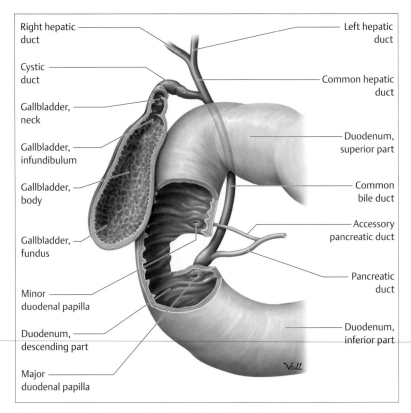

Fig. 18.1 Division of the extrahepatic bile ducts. (Illustration: M. Voll; from Schünke et al. 2005, see p. 413.)

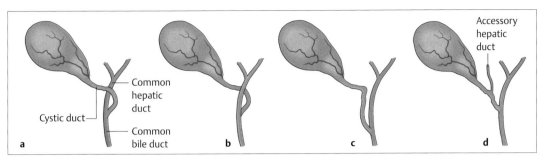

Fig. 18.2 a–d   Some variations of the cystic duct.

- It opens into the duodenum with the pancreatic duct (Wirsung duct) at the papilla of Vater (major duodenal papilla). An accessory pancreatic duct is also called the Santorini duct.
- **Type I** (common, Y-type): the two ducts unite and open together through the hepatopancreatic ampulla into the major duodenal papilla.
- **Type II** (rare, V-type): the two ducts open together in the major duodenal papilla without prior confluence.
- **Type III** (rare, U-type): separate opening of the two ducts
- Important for gallbladder dissection:
  - ► **Calot triangle,** bounded by the cystic duct, hepatic duct, and undersurface of the liver
  - ► **Cystic duct** with different possible openings into the common bile duct
  - ► An accessory hepatic duct is occasionally present and is easily overlooked during dissection, which leads postoperatively to biliary secretion.
  - ► **Foramen of Winslow** (omental foramen, epiploic foramen), below the hepatoduodenal ligament, access to the omental bursa

Arterial Supply and Venous Drainage
- Common hepatic artery from the celiac trunk
- Variant: absence of the common hepatic artery; the arterial supply to the liver arises from the superior mesenteric artery.
- All imaginable variants are possible for the course of the hepatic artery proper and its branching into the right and left hepatic arteries (crossing above and below the bile ducts).
- Of particular note: the right hepatic artery runs toward the infundibulum of the gallbladder and then kinks sharply to run again toward the liver (**caution:** can be mistaken for the cystic artery during dissection).
- Cystic artery from the right hepatic artery. All conceivable variations are possible. The three most frequent are shown in **Fig. 18.3.**
- Venous drainage is into the portal vein.

- Variable anatomy of the hepatic arteries
- Variable anatomy of the cystic artery

18

Diagnostic Approach

■ Clinical Examination

- **Tenderness** in the right upper abdomen; possibly a palpable mass with gallbladder hydrops or empyema
- **Murphy sign:** interruption of breath due to pain with pressure on the right upper abdomen on deep inspiration
- **Icteric sclerae** if the biliary tract is occluded

■ Laboratory Tests

- Raised **parameters of cholestasis:** bilirubin, alkaline phosphatase (AP), γ-glutamyl transferase (γGT); transaminases (GOT and GPT) to a lesser degree
- Lipase and amylase elevation with concomitant pancreatitis

■ Diagnostic Imaging

- Ultrasonography is the most important investigation

- **Ultrasonography:** the most important diagnostic method. The following are assessed:
  - ► Gallbladder stones (acoustic shadows)
  - ► Sediment level in the gallbladder (differential diagnosis: empyema or sludge with parenteral nutrition)
  - ► Wall structure: triple-layered and thickened in acute cholecystitis
  - ► Caliber of the common bile duct: normally up to 7 mm
  - ► Free fluid especially around the gallbladder and liver
  - ► Congestion of intrahepatic bile ducts (double-barrel phenomenon)
  - ► Presence of liver abscesses
  - ► Head of pancreas: detection of a prepapillary calculus is difficult
- **Upper abdominal CT:**
  - ► With complicated disease course and poor ultrasonographic conditions
  - ► For differential diagnosis when **tumor** in the gallbladder, bile ducts, or head of pancreas **is suspected**
- **MRCP** (magnetic resonance cholangiopancreatography): further investigation, especially when tumor is suspected
- **Hepatobiliary sequence scintigraphy:** rarely, to differentiate an intra- or extrahepatic cause of jaundice
- **PTC** (percutaneous transhepatic cholangiography): very rarely required when endoscopic retrograde cholangiopancreatography (ERCP) is not possible
- **Intravenous cholangiography:** hardly ever indicated because of use of ERCP and MRCP

■ Invasive Investigations

- ERCP: method of choice for diagnosis and treatment when bile duct stones are suspected

- **ERCP:**
  - ► When choledocholithiasis is suspected
  - ► Usually with retrograde **papillotomy** when calculi are found
  - ► Allows assessment of the esophagus, stomach, and duodenum at the same time
- **Gastroscopy:** for differential diagnosis to rule out a gastric ulcer

Treatment Approach

■ Indications

- **Cholecystectomy:**
  - ► For all symptomatic and complicated forms of cholecystolithiasis.
  - ► Clinically silent gallstones are a relative indication for operation; they cause complications in up to 30% of patients.
  - ► Since nearly all gallstones form in the gallbladder, cholecystectomy eliminates the cause of the stones. Recurrent gallstones in the bile ducts occur in only 2% of cases. There is therefore hardly any indication for medical stone dissolution or lithotripsy.
- **ERCP:**
  - ► Clearance of the bile duct system in the case of choledocholithiasis, where possible, before cholecystectomy
  - ► After endoscopic stone removal, cholecystectomy is indicated even without evidence of cholecystolithiasis.
- **Common bile duct exploration:**
  - ► After a failed attempt at endoscopic stone removal
  - ► When endoscopic stone removal is impossible due to altered anatomy (e.g., Roux-en-Y situation after gastrectomy)
- Secondary complications of gallstone disease (fistulas to the intestinal tract, liver abscesses, peritonitis, gallstone ileus) require operative treatment.

- Cholecystectomy when gallstones are found with or without complications

18

■ Conservative Treatment

Drug Therapy
- Medical gallstone dissolution is possible only with pure **cholesterol stones** (10% of all gallstones).
- As the cause is not eliminated, this is hardly ever indicated.
- The drugs employed are oral ursodeoxycholic acid or quinodeoxycholic acid; possible side effects include diarrhea and elevated transaminases.
- Alternative: irrigation with *tert*-butylmethyl ether through a percutaneous transhepatic catheter (rapid action, hardly any side effects)

- Hardly any indication for ESWL and medical stone dissolution

Lithotripsy
- As the cause is not treated, this is hardly ever indicated.
- **Extracorporeal shock wave lithotripsy** (ESWL) is possible only for small stones; the gallbladder must contract and the stones are then dispelled with colic. There is a high recurrence rate.

■ Surgical Treatment

Endoscopic Retrograde Cholangiopancreatography

- ERCP is the primary treatment procedure for choledocholithiasis.
- Following papillotomy, the stone either passes spontaneously or it is removed at the same session, for example, with a Dormia basket.

- ERCP is the treatment of choice for choledocholithiasis

Laparoscopic Cholecystectomy

- Standard procedure for (symptomatic) cholecystolithiasis and recent acute cholecystitis without further complications.
- Recent developments are intended to avoid an incision through the abdominal wall to remove the gallbladder (NOTES = natural orifice transluminal endoscopic surgery). That is, an attempt is made to remove the gallbladder

through natural body orifices (transvaginal or transgastric). The advantages are doubtful. There is further potential for complications due to unsterile access or involvement of otherwise unaffected regions of the abdomen (e.g., abscess in the pouch of Douglas after transvaginal cholecystectomy).

- **Contraindications** to laparoscopic procedure: portal hypertension, advanced pregnancy, possibly severe pulmonary obstruction, suspected gallbladder carcinoma.
- Adhesions after previous operations can be divided laparoscopically if necessary. There should be a balance between effort and benefit.

Operative Technique

Positioning (Fig. 18.4)
- Flat lithotomy position with stirrups, monitor at the right of the patient's head
- The surgeon stands between the patient's legs (alternatively on the patient's left)
- Alternatively, the patient lies flat, the camera assistant sits on the right beside the patient, and the surgeon stands on the left.

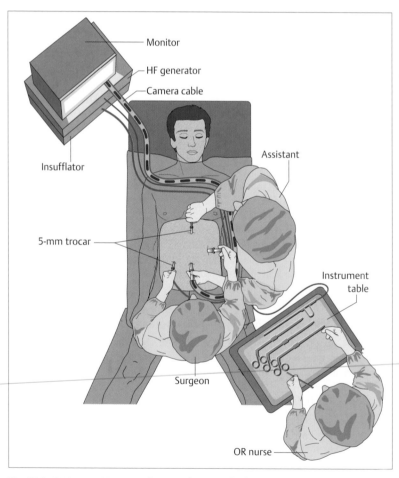

Monitor

HF generator

Camera cable

Insufflator

Assistant

5-mm trocar

Instrument table

Surgeon

OR nurse

Fig. 18.4   Patient positioning and trocar placement for laparoscopic cholecystectomy.

Creation of Pneumoperitoneum

- **Caution:** blind entry is particularly dangerous—safety steps must be followed carefully
- Transverse subumbilical incision ca. 2–3 cm long (later used for removal of the gallbladder)
- By means of towel clamps inserted to the left and right of the wound, the abdominal wall is lifted firmly by the assistant. **Caution:** the patient must not strain; good relaxation is required.
- The Veress needle is inserted in a slightly oblique direction toward the upper abdomen. The needle triggers the safety mechanism when the fascia is penetrated and does so a second time when it enters the peritoneum.
- Safety test:
  - ► Flush the cannula with 0.9% NaCl.
  - ► Rule out aspiration of blood.
  - ► Drip 0.9% NaCl onto the needle. This must disappear spontaneously because of the negative intraperitoneal pressure.
- The peritoneal cavity is filled with CO_2. The pressure in the abdominal cavity (and thus the pressure display) alters as the abdominal wall is elevated and lowered as an indirect sign of correct position.
- A rapid rise in pressure indicates an incorrect position. Remove the needle and repeat the entire procedure.
- Check that the abdominal cavity is filled evenly, by percussion and inspection. Pay meticulous attention to the vital signs (extremely rare: air embolism due to puncture of the vena cava).
- If all of the safety tests according to the above procedure are not successful, a minilaparotomy is performed.

- Vital: safety tests when creating the pneumoperitoneum

Alternative: Minilaparotomy

- Generally employed procedure in some clinics. The fascia is demonstrated through the incision described above and elevated with two sharp clamps. The incision is made between the clamps and dissection is continued down to the peritoneum. The incision is extended if necessary until the adhesions beneath it can be divided and the optical trocar can be inserted. If the fascial incision has become too large, it can be made smaller by interrupted sutures until airtight closure is obtained.
- The optical trocar is then inserted.
- A further 10-mm operating trocar and two other 5-mm operating trocars are then placed depending on the surgeon's position.

Cholecystectomy

- The gallbladder is elevated toward the diaphragm and the infundibulum is drawn laterally to the right to expose the Calot triangle.
- The cystic duct and cystic artery are dissected free and the gallbladder serosa is incised anteriorly and posteriorly, from the infundibulum as far as the liver bed (**Fig. 18.5**).
- To be certain that it is the cystic duct, the openings into both the gallbladder and common bile duct should be demonstrated.
- The cystic duct is clipped and divided, with two clips centrally and one clip peripherally (metal or absorbable plastic).
- Division of the cystic artery, likewise with two clips centrally and one clip peripherally. Ensure that it is the cystic artery, which is confirmed only by verifying that it opens into the gallbladder. **Caution:** the right hepatic artery can easily be mistaken for the cystic artery when it runs close to the gallbladder infundibulum and curves away toward the liver only after that.

18

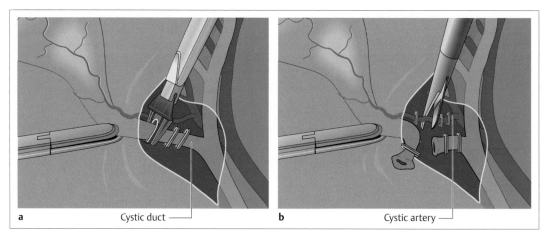

Fig. 18.5 a, b   Exposure and division of the cystic duct (**a**) and cystic artery (**b**).

- Subserosal division of the gallbladder from the liver bed with electrocautery hook
- Hemostasis in the liver bed by electrocoagulation
- Switch the optical trocar to the second 10-mm trocar.
- Remove the gallbladder through the infraumbilical incision with a spreader.
- If the gallbladder is inflamed or has been opened or tumor is suspected, remove it in a specimen bag.

Conclusion of the Operation
- Elevate the fascia at the subumbilical incision using single-pronged hooks and close it with 2–3 interrupted fascial sutures.
- Create the pneumoperitoneum again and inspect the operative field for leakage of blood or bile.
- Irrigate the operative field, if necessary bringing out a 6-mm Easy-Flow drain through the right-sided trocar (rendezvous technique).
- Remove the trocars under direct vision. Skin closure with intracutaneous sutures

Conventional (Open Surgical) Cholecystectomy

Operative Technique

- Right costal margin incision (alternative: transrectal incision)
- Identification of the common bile duct and common hepatic duct, cystic duct, and cystic artery in the Calot triangle
- Ligature and division of the cystic artery
- Ligature and division of the cystic duct
- Subserous excision of the gallbladder (bipolar electric scissors)

Alternative: Anterograde Cholecystectomy
- Particularly when the anatomy is unclear due to severe inflammation
- Start with subserous excision of the gallbladder.
- Divide the structures from their immediate connection to the gallbladder.

Common Bile Duct Exploration

Operative Technique

- Choledochotomy on the anterior wall between stay sutures
- Stone extraction (**Fig. 18.6**) with forceps, basket, Fogarty catheter, or stone curette
- After mobilizing the duodenum (Kocher maneuver) and passing the hand beneath it, check the patency of the papilla with a biliary probe.
- Choledochoscopy with a flexible choledochoscope: inspect distally as far as the papilla, if possible into the duodenum; centrally as far as the branching into segmental bile ducts.
- If necessary, localization of further calculi and removal under vision with Fogarty catheter, forceps, or Dormia basket (**Fig. 18.7**)
- If necessary, dilation of the papilla with bougies of increasing size
- Cut a T-tube to size and place it in the bile duct.
- Close the choledochotomy and test for water-tightness.
- Finally, contrast radiographic imaging of the bile duct system and its outlet into the duodenum through the T-tube

18

■ Aftercare

Laparoscopic and Conventional Cholecystectomy
- Clinical review and blood count on postoperative day 1
- Blood count, C-reactive protein (CRP) and bilirubin on postoperative day 3
- Discharge on postoperative day 4 if asymptomatic and laboratory parameters are normal, otherwise do ultrasonography and institute further diagnostic measures as appropriate.

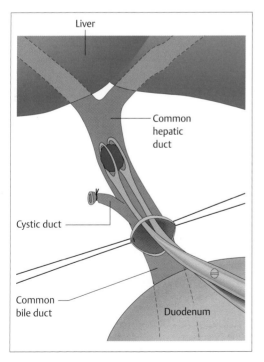

Liver

Common hepatic duct

Cystic duct

Common bile duct

Duodenum

Fig. 18.6 Choledochotomy and stone extraction.

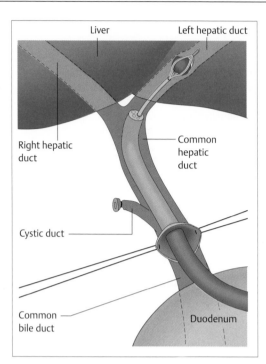

Fig. 18.7 Choledochoscopy and stone extraction with Dormia basket.

Common Bile Duct Exploration
- Check cholestasis parameters.
- After normal bilirubin is obtained, elevate the drainage bag.
- Final contrast imaging through the T-tube
- Removal of the T-tube 1 week postoperatively at the earliest

■ **Complications**

Perioperative Complications

Laparoscopic and Conventional Cholecystectomy
- Bowel injury
- Bile duct injuries (often unnoticed)
- Bleeding from the cystic artery and right hepatic artery
- Bleeding from a hepatic vein running behind the gallbladder bed
- Narrowing of the common bile duct by an incorrectly placed clip (due to lateral tension on the gallbladder infundibulum)
- Division of the main bile duct or a main branch of it by mistaking it for the cystic duct

Common Bile Duct Exploration
- Perforation of the retroduodenal common bile duct:
  - ► Due to intraoperative probe manipulation
  - ► Due to failed endoscopic attempt at stent insertion
- **Treatment:**
  - ► Duodenotomy and transduodenal papillotomy
  - ► Insertion of a T-tube, the distal limb of which extends into the duodenum
  - ► Alternative: decompress the bile duct with a Völcker drain, which passes through the duodenum to the exterior via a Witzel channel.

Late Complications

Laparoscopic and Conventional Cholecystectomy
- Secondary hemorrhage due to slippage of a clip or diffuse bleeding from the gallbladder bed
- Bile peritonitis due to slippage of a clip from the cystic duct
- Bile peritonitis due to unnoticed opening of accessory bile ducts
- Subhepatic abscess, infected hematoma
- Obstructive jaundice due to residual bile duct calculi

■ Acute Cholecystitis

Etiology

- Painful tense filling of the gallbladder due to impaction of a stone in the cystic duct or gallbladder infundibulum and subsequent inflammation, initially abacterial; possible development of gallbladder hydrops
- Subsequent secondary bacterial infection (ascending from the duodenum, hematogenous spread, lymphatogenous spread)
- Initially phlegmonous and fibrinous, which may progress to gallbladder empyema and/or an ulcerated phlegmonous or necrotic gallbladder

18

Symptoms

- Signs of right-sided upper abdominal peritonitis with guarding
- Concomitant or preceding colic
- Pyrexia, possibly septic temperature pattern with chills
- Nausea and vomiting
- Resistance to palpation in the right upper abdomen

- Fever
- Guarding in the right upper abdomen

Diagnostic Approach

■ Laboratory Tests

- Raised inflammatory parameters (leukocytosis, CRP elevation)
- AP, γGT with concomitant cholangitis or when caused by choledocholithiasis

■ Diagnostic Imaging

- **Ultrasonography**
  - ► Tenderness, due to the transducer, correlates with ultrasonographic signs
  - ► Thickened gallbladder wall with triple-layer phenomenon
  - ► Dense echo pattern, possible fluid level with empyema (differential diagnosis: sludge)
  - ► Free fluid around the gallbladder wall (pericholecystitis)
  - ► Inflammatory infiltration of the liver bed, possibly with abscess

- Ultrasonography is the method of choice to confirm the diagnosis.

■ Differential Diagnosis

- Duodenal/gastric ulcer
- Acute pancreatitis
- Neoplasm or inflammatory processes involving the right colic flexure
- Irritable colon
- Renal colic

- Appendicitis (especially when in retrocecal location)
- Right-sided pneumonia
- Myocardial infarction
- Right-sided pyelonephritis

Treatment Approach

■ Indications

Conservative Treatment
- If no perforation or gallbladder empyema, clinically and on ultrasonography
- If the clinical signs and symptoms have been present for over 3 days
- If severe concomitant disease contraindicates early surgery

Indications for Operation (p. 309 ff)
- Immediate operation: suspected perforation, local/advancing peritonitis
- Early operation: within 72 hours after the onset of symptoms
- Interval operation: ca. 6 weeks after the conclusion of conservative treatment

■ Conservative Treatment

- **Intravenous antibiotics** (e.g., ceftriaxone) and **fasting** until the patient is symptom-free

■ Surgical Treatment

- Open cholecystectomy is fast and safe

- **Open cholecystectomy:** faster than laparoscopic with acute inflammation, all complications are controlled safely; anterograde procedure preferable because of unclear situation in the inflamed hepatoduodenal ligament
- **Laparoscopic cholecystectomy:** often technically possible but more time-consuming, indicated with recent disease without evidence of complications, also of benefit in severely obese patients; if necessary early conversion to open cholecystectomy

■ Gallbladder Carcinoma

Epidemiology

- Fifth most common tumor of the gastrointestinal tract
- Peak incidence in 6th to 7th decade
- Women : men = 2 : 1
- Cholecystolithiasis is a predisposing factor (risk of degeneration 1%–3%).
- Increased risk with chronic calcifying cholecystitis (porcelain gallbladder)

Classification (Tables 18.1, 18.2)

Table 18.1 TNM classification of gallbladder carcinoma

T—primary tumor	
Tx	Primary tumor not assessable
T0	No evidence of primary tumor
Tis	Carcinoma in situ
T1	Tumor infiltrates lamina propria or muscularis
	T1a: tumor infiltrates lamina propria
	T1b: tumor infiltrates muscularis
T2	Tumor infiltrates perimuscular connective tissue, no infiltration of serosa or liver
T3	Tumor infiltrates the serosa (visceral peritoneum) and/or infiltrates the liver directly and/or another adjacent structure (stomach, duodenum, colon, pancreas, omentum or extrahepatic bile ducts)
T4	Tumor infiltrates the portal vein or hepatic artery or multiple extrahepatic organs or structures
N—regional lymph nodes	
Nx	Regional lymph nodes not assessable
N0	No regional lymph node metastases
N1	Regional lymph node metastases
M—distant metastases	
M0	No distant metastases
M1	Distant metastases

18

Table 18.2 Stage classification (AJCC)

Stage	TNM classification
0	Tis, N0, M0
1a	T1, N0, M0
1b	T2, N0, M0
2a	T3, N0, M0
2b	T1–3, N1, M0
3	T4, any N, M0
4	any Tm, any N, M1

Symptoms

- Usually asymptomatic
- Courvoisier sign: painless gallbladder enlargement
- Late symptoms: jaundice, weight loss, cachexia

Diagnostic Approach

- **Ultrasonography:** parietal tumor in the gallbladder lumen (differential diagnosis: parietal calculus not casting an acoustic shadow); possibly infiltration of the liver bed
- **ERCP:** to assess the intra- and extrahepatic bile ducts
- **CT:** for differential diagnosis, liver metastases
- **Magnetic resonance cholangiography:** if necessary, as supplementary bile duct investigation
- **Diagnostic laparoscopy:** if necessary, to assess operability, with intraoperative laparoscopic ultrasonography

Treatment Approach

■ Indications

Chemotherapy
- Efficacy of adjuvant therapy not proven, and the same applies for attempts at neoadjuvant therapy

Surgical Treatment with Curative Intent
- **Cholecystectomy:** adequate in tumor stages Tis, T1a, and T1b
- Additional resection of the gallbladder bed with a ca. 3-cm margin or anatomical liver resection (segments IVb and V) (**Fig. 17.1**) with lymphadenectomy in the hepatoduodenal ligament for tumors more than stage T2
- Resection of the common bile duct if infiltrated
- Extended right hemihepatectomy with central bile duct resection and biliary-enteric anastomosis rarely possible or useful

Palliative Therapy
- Endoscopic or interventional radiology biliary diversion to treat jaundice
- If patient is in good general condition, chemotherapy may be attempted

Aftercare

- Purely symptomatic; the prognosis is not improved by identifying recurrence
- Palliative treatment measures as required

Prognosis

- Cure is possible in the early stages without lymph node involvement.
- No cure is possible in advanced stages apart from isolated cases.

■ Extrahepatic Bile Duct Carcinoma

Classification (Tables 18.3, 18.4)

- For AJCC stage classification, see **Table 18.2.**

Table 18.3   TNM classification of extrahepatic bile duct carcinoma

Distal extrahepatic bile ducts (from cystic duct insertion into common hepatic duct)		Proximal extrahepatic bile ducts (right, left, and common hepatic ducts)	
T—primary tumor		**T—primary tumor**	
Tx	Primary tumor not assessable	Tx	Primary tumor not assessable
T0	No evidence of primary tumor	T0	No evidence of primary tumor
Tis	Carcinoma in situ	Tis	Carcinoma in situ
T1	Tumor limited to bile duct	T1	Tumor limited to bile duct with extension up to the muscle layer or fibrous tissue
T2	Tumor penetrates bile duct wall	T2a	Tumor invades beyond wall of bile duct to surrounding adipose tissue
		T2b	Tumor invades adjacent hepatic parenchyma
T3	Tumor infiltrates gallbladder, liver, pancreas, duodenum, or other adjacent organs	T3	Tumor invades unilateral branches of the portal vein or hepatic artery
T4	Tumor involves the celiac axis or the superior mesenteric artery	T4	Tumor invades the main portal vein or its branches bilaterally; or the common hepatic artery; or the second-order biliary radicals bilaterally; or unilateral second-order biliary radicals with contralateral portal vein or hepatic artery involvement
N—regional lymph nodes (RLN)		**N—regional lymph nodes (RLN)**	
Nx	RLN not assessable	Nx	RLN not assessable
N0	No RLN metastasis	N0	No RLN metastasis
N1	Regional lymph node metastasis	N1	RLN metastasis including nodes along cystic duct, common bile duct, common hepatic artery and portal vein
M—distant metastases		**M—distant metastases**	
M0	No distant metastasis	M0	No distant metastasis
M1	Distant metastasis	M1	Distant metastasis

Table 18.4   Bismuth–Corlette classification of Klatskin tumors

Type	Description
I	Proximal common bile duct tumors not involving the hepatic bifurcation
II	Obstruction of both hepatic ducts without involvement of segmental bile ducts
III	Obstruction of both hepatic ducts, involvement of segmental bile ducts on one side
IIIa	Involvement of segmental bile ducts on the right
IIIb	Involvement of segmental bile ducts on the left
IV	Obstruction of both hepatic ducts, involvement of segmental bile ducts bilaterally

• Bismuth classification is critically important for planning surgical treatment.

Symptoms

• Lead symptom is painless jaundice

18

Diagnostic Approach

- **Ultrasonography:** assessment of bile ducts, tumor extent, liver metastases
- **ERCP:** imaging of the bile duct system, brush cytology; with Klatskin tumors, determination of type
- **CT:** assessment of upper abdominal organs and tumor extent
- **Magnetic resonance cholangiography:** when ERCP is unclear
- **Laboratory tests:** tumor markers CA 19–9 and CEA, inflammatory parameters, liver function tests
- The diagnosis can often be made only **at operation.**
- **Differential diagnosis:** inflammatory conditions, sclerosing cholangitis, Mirizzi syndrome

Treatment Approach

■ Indications

Surgical Treatment with Curative Intent

- If the patient is in good general condition and tumor is resectable, the surgical procedure should be as radical as possible.
- **Distal bile duct cancers:** partial duodenopancreatectomy (Whipple OP)
- **Bile duct cancers in the middle third:** surgery rarely indicated as the tumor extends either proximally or distally. If indicated, complete resection of the extrahepatic bile ducts, cholecystectomy, and lymphadenectomy of the hepatoduodenal ligament, if necessary with resection of the adjacent part of the portal vein or a hepatic artery. Always resect the tumor en bloc; dissection through the tumor is futile. Reconstruction by hepaticojejunostomy.
- **Proximal bile duct cancers:** extended right hemihepatectomy is the standard operation as the left hepatic duct is much longer, so that a tumor-free end is more likely to be found for biliary-enteric anastomosis; resection of adherent portal vein if necessary, reanastomosis by direct suture. Hepaticojejunostomy to the proximal part of the left hepatic duct. In rare cases (Bismuth type IIIb), left hemihepatectomy is indicated.

Palliative Therapy

- Usually endoscopic stent placement (ERCP)
- If not possible, transhepatic bile diversion

Chemotherapy

- Benefit of adjuvant or neoadjuvant chemotherapy not proven
- Palliative chemotherapy can be tried if patient's general condition is good.

Aftercare and Prognosis

- Symptomatic aftercare; prognosis is not improved by detecting recurrence. Palliative treatment as needed. Prognosis poor even with radical surgery.

Further Reading

National Cancer Institute. Extrahepatic Bile Duct Cancer Treatment. In Internet: http://www.cancer.gov/cancertopics/pdq/treatment/gallbladder/healthprofessional; accessed: 16.05.2008
National Cancer Institute. Gallbladder Cancer: Treatment. In Internet: http://www.cancer.gov/cancertopics/pdq/treatment/bileduct/healthprofessional; accessed: 16.05.2008.

18

- In spite of poor prognosis, if tumor is resectable, surgery should be as radical as possible.

19 Pancreas

N.T. Schwarz

■ Anatomy

- The pancreas is a retroperitoneal organ located at the level of the 1st to 3rd lumbar vertebrae. It is divided anatomically into the head (with uncinate process), neck, body, and tail.
- The mesenteric vessels run at the lower border of the neck of the pancreas, and the portal vein begins at the confluence of the superior mesenteric and splenic veins, behind the junction of the head and neck of the pancreas.
- The distal common bile duct passes to the duodenum posteriorly within the parenchyma of the head of the pancreas.
- The head is fixed and is enclosed by the "C" of the duodenum. This allows only slight mobility.
- The pancreas can be accessed abdominally through three routes:
  - ► Through the lesser omentum
  - ► Through the gastrocolic ligament
  - ► By division of the ligament of Treitz in combination with the Kocher maneuver (mobilization of the duodenum; see Chapter 9); this allows full mobilization of the head

Excretory Ducts
- Two excretory pancreatic ducts are distinguished:
  - ► Wirsung duct is the main excretory outlet
  - ► Santorini duct, which drains only the superior part of the head of the pancreas; it often opens separately into the duodenum
- The Wirsung duct and the common bile duct nearly always open together into the duodenum in the papilla of Vater.

Arteries
- The arterial supply of the pancreas (**Fig. 19.1**) is through the superior pancreaticoduodenal artery, which arises from the common hepatic artery.
- The head of the pancreas is also supplied by the inferior pancreaticoduodenal artery, which arises from the superior mesenteric artery.
- While the arterial blood supply of the head of the pancreas is relatively constant, the vascular supply of the body and tail of the pancreas is variable, usually through short arteries arising from the splenic artery and through branches of the transverse pancreatic artery, which runs horizontally.

Veins
- The venous drainage from the head of the pancreas is through the superior mesenteric vein.
- The body and tail are drained by the splenic vein.

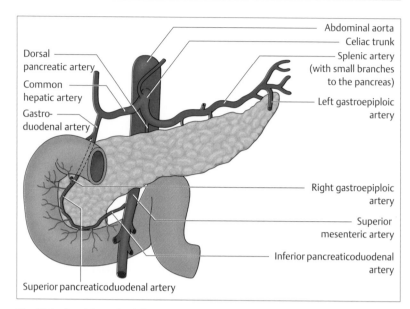

Fig. 19.1   Arterial supply of the pancreas.

Lymphatic Drainage
- The lymphatic drainage is via peripancreatic and so-called "collecting" lymph nodes (**Fig. 19.2**).
- N1 or **peripancreatic lymph nodes:**
  ► 1: anterior pancreatoduodenal lymph nodes
  ► 2: posterior pancreatoduodenal lymph nodes (not shown in **Fig. 19.2**, posterior to 1)

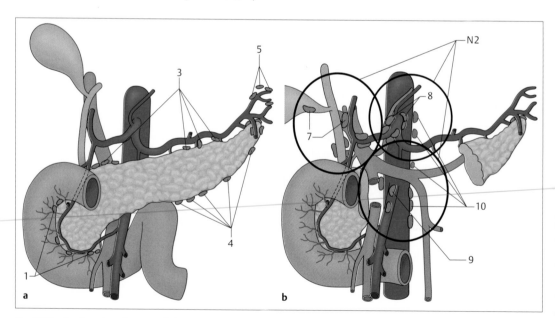

Fig. 19.2 a, b   Lymph nodes around the pancreas.

► 3: suprapancreatic lymph nodes (a, head region; b, body and tail, **Fig. 19.2**)
► 4: infrapancreatic lymph nodes (a, head region; b. body and tail, **Fig. 19.2**)
► 5: splenic lymph nodes
► 6: subpyloric lymph nodes (not drawn in **Fig. 19.2**)
- N2 or **collecting lymph nodes:**
► 7: lymph nodes at the liver hilum
► 8: celiac lymph nodes
► 9: lymph nodes at the origin of the superior mesenteric artery
► 10: upper para-aortic lymph nodes

■ Physiology

- The pancreas is divided histologically into exocrine and endocrine tissue.
- The islets of Langerhans produce the hormones insulin, glucagon, and somatostatin.
- About 1500 mL of alkaline pancreatic secretion are produced daily, containing, in addition to electrolytes, enzymes for splitting carbohydrates (amylase), fats (lipase, phospholipases), nucleic acids (ribo- and deoxyribonucleases), and proteins (trypsin, chymotrypsin). The proteases are present as inactive proenzymes and are converted into active enzymes by enterokinases in the duodenum to protect the organ from autodigestion.
- The exocrine and endocrine potency of the pancreas is so great that overt insufficiency (diabetes mellitus, malabsorption) only occurs with loss of ca. 80% of the parenchyma.

- Overt insufficiency only after loss of ca. 80% of the parenchyma

19

■ Acute Pancreatitis

Definition

- Inflammation of the pancreas
- Can arise primarily in the organ or occur as concomitant pancreatitis in association with other diseases
- A distinction is made between acute and chronic pancreatitis.

Epidemiology

- Approximately two or three new cases of the disease per 100 000 population in Europe annually

Etiology

- The most frequent causes are biliary tract disease (50% due to cholelithiasis), alcohol abuse (20%–25%), and endoscopic retrograde cholangiopancreatography (ERCP).
- Rarer causes are periampullary duodenal diverticula, duodenal compression by the superior mesenteric artery, pancreatic trauma, medications and toxic effects, primary hyperparathyroidism, hyperlipoproteinemias, and pancreatitis in association with mumps, infectious mononucleosis, and viral hepatitis. Pancreatitis is idiopathic in 15% of cases.
- In the majority of cases there is acute edematous pancreatitis, which can also be associated with peripancreatic fat necrosis.

- In 80% of all cases, acute pancreatitis is caused by alcohol or gallstones.

Classification

- It can be difficult to differentiate between mild (edematous) and severe (hemorrhagic necrosing) forms of acute pancreatitis. This has been superseded by the Atlanta classification (**Table 19.1**).
- Pancreatic failure, which is reversible within 24 hours, should not necessarily be regarded as severe pancreatitis.

Table 19.1 Atlanta classification of acute pancreatitis

Severe acute pancreatitis	Organ failure and/or local complications (necrosis, pseudocyst, abscess)
Mild pancreatitis	Minimal organ dysfunction, uncomplicated course
Acute fluid collection	In the early phase, in or around the pancreas
Acute pseudocyst	Collection of secretion surrounded by a wall of granulation tissue. About 4 weeks after the onset of the pancreatitis
Pancreatic necrosis	Focal or diffuse area of necrotic pancreatic tissue with fat necrosis

Source: From Bradley EL, 3rd. A clinically based classification system for acute pancreatitis. Summary of the International Symposium on Acute Pancreatitis, Atlanta, Ga; September 11 through 13, 1992. Arch Surg 1993; 128: 586–590.

Symptoms

- Upper abdominal pain, possibly with radiation to the back
- Nausea, vomiting, meteorism, bowel atony, elastic guarding, possibly jaundice, fever, oliguria

Diagnostic Approach (Table 19.2)

- Physical examination
- Measurement of laboratory parameters

- Detailed physical examination on diagnosis and in the course of the acute pancreatitis for early detection of complications
- Measurement of lipase is more important than amylase as it has a longer half-life: specificity 97%, sensitivity 67%.
- When acute pancreatitis is suspected, **transabdominal ultrasonography** confirms the diagnosis in ca. 33% of patients.

Table 19.2 Measurement of laboratory parameters in acute pancreatitis

Initial assessment	Follow-up test
<ul><li>Blood count</li><li>CRP</li><li>Arterial blood gas analysis</li><li>Sodium, potassium, calcium</li><li>Creatinine</li><li>Lipase</li><li>ALT</li><li>Albumin</li><li>Triglycerides</li><li>LDH</li><li>Glucose</li></ul>	<ul><li>Blood count</li><li>CRP</li><li>Arterial blood gas analysis</li><li>Sodium, potassium, calcium</li><li>Creatinine</li></ul>

ALT: alanine aminotransferase; CRP: C-reactive protein; LDH: lactate dehydrogenase.

- **Ultrasonographic** evidence of biliary tract calculi and raised cholestasis parameters suggest a biliary cause of the pancreatitis.
- According to the current guidelines of the different societies for digestive and metabolic diseases, a **contrast CT scan** is not usually necessary to diagnose acute pancreatitis.
- **ERCP** is indicated in obstructive jaundice and persistent cholestasis.

Treatment Approach

■ Indications

- Treatment is strictly **conservative** and includes standardized basic therapy along with close patient monitoring (**Fig. 19.3**).
- All possibilities for intensive medical monitoring and treatment must be exhausted.
- When the cause is **biliary**, the optimal timing of cholecystectomy is controversial.
- With the **edematous** form, laparoscopic cholecystectomy can usually be performed following ERCP.
- In the **necrotizing** form, the inflammation should first subside completely and elective cholecystectomy should be performed after 3–6 weeks at the earliest.
- Patients with **septic complications** due to infected necrosis require surgical therapy. The most important deciding factor is progressive multiorgan failure despite maximum intensive therapy or aspiration evidence of infected necrosis in the case of sepsis.

- Confirmed infection of necrotic areas: interventional radiology procedure or surgery

- Marked necrosis (> 30%) or suspected superinfection: diagnostic fine-needle aspiration

19

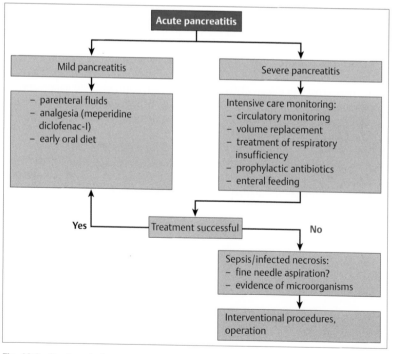

Fig. 19.3   Treatment of acute pancreatitis.

■ Conservative Treatment

- **Parenteral nutrition:** Fat emulsions should be avoided if there is marked hypertriglyceridemia. **Caution:** uncontrolled blood glucose is not infrequent.
- **Fluids and electrolytes:** At the start of the disease, a considerable intravascular fluid deficit can occur (up to 8 L/day), which is due to major fluid sequestration in the retroperitoneum.
- **Analgesia:** Morphine agonists should be avoided as they cause an increase in pressure at the sphincter of Oddi.
- Septic complications can be significantly reduced by early antibiotic therapy.

■ Surgical Treatment

- The aim of surgery is interventional decompression (abscess) or operative removal of all intra- and peripancreatic necrotic tissue and pancreatogenic secretions.
- At operation, after irrigation of the abdominal cavity and omental bursa, large-lumen silicone drains should be placed, especially along the typical retroperitoneal pathways of necrosis with continuous postoperative lavage, scheduled relaparotomy (etappenlavage), or further revision with an open abdomen ("laparostomy").
- During debridement, as much vital pancreatic parenchyma as possible should be preserved to prevent later organ insufficiency. In recent years, there has been a change with regard to the indication for necrosectomy to operations performed more and more rarely and later. This has been associated with a marked reduction in mortality from 39% to 12%.

■ Complications

- Infected pancreatic necrosis increases mortality

- Typical late complications of acute pancreatitis are **pancreatic abscess** or **pancreatic necrosis** and the development of **pseudocysts**.
- Infected pancreatic necrosis increases the mortality of acute pancreatitis to ca. 40%, so a central aim of treatment is to prevent infection of necrotic tissue.
- **Acute necrotizing pancreatitis** as a severe early form of acute pancreatitis is characterized by massive systemic absorption of vasoactive and toxic substances that lead to metabolic, renal, cardiocirculatory and pulmonary reactions (imminent multiorgan failure).
- Bacterial colonization of the necrotic tissue by enterogenic microorganisms often occurs with subsequent **sepsis.** Relevant investigations are contrast-enhanced CT scanning (to assess the extent and boundaries of the necrotic areas) and ultrasound-guided aspiration of the necrotic tissue (bacteriology).
- C-reactive protein measurement is regarded as the best parameter for monitoring the development of necrosis.

■ Chronic Pancreatitis

Epidemiology

- The prevalence is ca. 27 cases per 100 000 population.

Etiology

- The etiology of chronic pancreatitis corresponds to the acute form. Chronic **alcohol abuse** is the predominating factor (70%).
- The **pathogenesis** of chronic pancreatitis is relatively uniform despite the different causes.
  - ► The starting point for the pathological changes in organ structure found later is intraluminal precipitation of proteins in the acini and duct system.
  - ► Calcium deposition gives rise to calculi and parenchymal calcification. In addition, proliferation of the pericanalicular connective tissue with invasion of the lumen leads to stenosis and occlusion of the duct system, which can be detected as irregularities in the caliber of the large and small pancreatic ducts.
  - ► Incomplete duct obstruction can result in cystic dilatation of the duct system. The elevated pressures as a result of the impaired drainage of secretion can cause acute exacerbations, which lead to permanent loss of exocrine pancreatic tissue due to sclerosis of the parenchyma.
  - ► This can be followed later by destruction of the islet system.

19

Diagnostic Approach

- **Clinical investigation:** current diagnostic methods employed to assess the functional exocrine and endocrine organ reserve include: stool elastase, pancreolauryl test, stool weight per day, daily blood glucose profile, oral glucose tolerance test, measurement of HbA_{1c}
- **Radiography:** Calcification in the pancreas compartment can often be identified even on plain abdominal x-ray photos. A chest x-ray is done to rule out pleuropulmonary complications (pleural effusion).
- **Ultrasonography** forms the basis of diagnostic imaging and provides information about the size and shape of the pancreas, pancreatic duct calculi, cystic changes, dilatation of the duct system, and pancreatogenic ascites.
- **Contrast-enhanced CT** is now regarded as the standard diagnostic imaging procedure. It helps to provide a more accurate assessment of the tail of the pancreas and pre-existing pathomorphological changes when surgery is being planned.
- **ERCP** is used to detect occlusions and stenosis of the pancreatic duct system.

Treatment Approach

■ Indications (Fig. 19.4)

Indications for Surgery
- Pain syndrome that can no longer be controlled by conservative means
- Suspected malignancy
- Complications of chronic pancreatitis (e.g., adverse effects on neighboring organs, fistulas, pseudocysts)

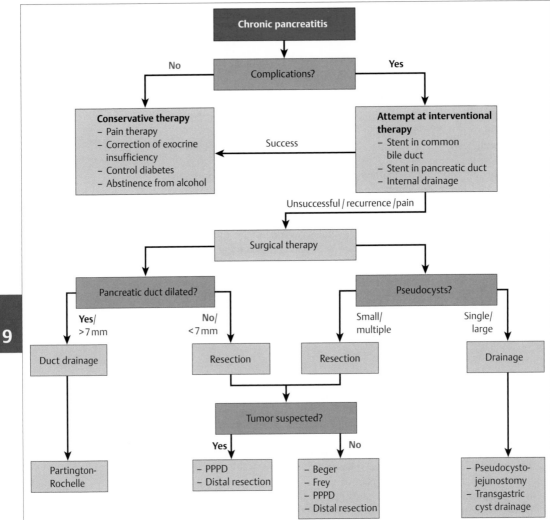

Fig. 19.4 Treatment algorithm in chronic pancreatitis (modified from Grützmann and Saeger 2008). PPPD: pylorus-preserving pancreatoduodenectomy.

■ Conservative Treatment

- Exocrine pancreatic insufficiency alone is not an indication for operative management.

- The initial stage of chronic pancreatitis is treated medically. The main features of treatment are:
  - ► Elimination of noxious agents
  - ► High-protein and low-fat diet
  - ► Adequate replacement of pancreatic enzymes

■ Surgical Treatment

Aims of Surgery
- Long-term reduction in pain, freedom from pain
- Improved quality of life, less hospitalization, resocialization

- Elimination and avoidance of complications
- Preservation of residual endocrine and exocrine pancreatic function

Drainage Procedures

- A drainage operation (decompression) should counteract or completely eliminate the pain-inducing congestion that results from the calcification.
- The Partington–Rochelle **side-to-side pancreaticojejunostomy** is a typical procedure (**Fig. 19.5**), in which the opened pancreatic duct is anastomosed with a Roux loop over its entire length. A precondition for effective drainage is opening of the dilated pancreatic duct over a distance of 7–10 cm. Multiple areas of stenosis with dilatation between them ("chain of lakes") are more frequent. Inadequate drainage of side ducts leads to persistence of the primary inflammatory event with possible later scarring and occlusion of the anastomosis. Smaller pancreatic cancers producing stenosis are not discovered with these operation methods.

Resection Procedures

- In the case of chronic inflammatory processes in the head of the pancreas, apart from classical **resection of the head of the pancreas** (Whipple procedure) or **pancreatectomy, duodenum-preserving resection of the head of the pancreas** (Beger procedure) can also be performed. The indications are stenosis of the duodenum, pancreatic duct or common bile duct with cholestasis, chronic pain syndrome, and narrowing of the retroperitoneal blood vessels (portal vein). Subtotal resection of the head of the pancreas is performed between the duodenal border of the portal vein and the intrapancreatic segment of the common bile duct. The head of the pancreas is then reconstructed with an interposition jejunal graft (**Fig. 19.6**).
- In **distal resection**, depending on the extent of the inflammatory changes, the tail and body of the pancreas and, if appropriate, parts of the head are resected with or without the spleen.
- **Proximal resections** include partial or total pancreatoduodenectomy. The disadvantage of these resections is the reduction in the still functioning organ substance, which leads to an increased incidence of exocrine and endocrine pancreatic insufficiency.
- Apart from the classical Whipple resection, the other operation methods are contraindicated when a malignant tumor in the head of the pancreas is suspected.

- Only Whipple resection if a malignant tumor in the head of the pancreas is suspected.

19

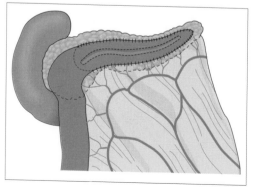

Fig. 19.5 Partington–Rochelle side-to-side pancreaticojejunostomy.

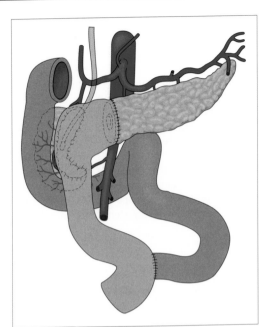

Fig. 19.6 Beger operation. Drainage of the enucleated head of the pancreas after duodenum-preserving pancreatic head resection with mobilized jejunum using Roux-en-Y technique.

Combination of Resection Procedures and Extended Drainage Operation

- Combined procedures, such as combination of side-to-side pancreaticojejunostomy with limited local resection of the head of the pancreas (Frey operation), are used more often when the pancreatic duct contains both dilatation and stenosis and there is an inflammatory mass in the head of the pancreas (**Fig. 19.7**).

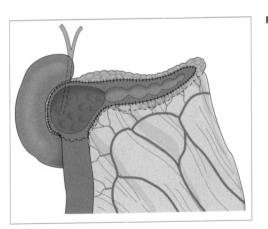

Fig. 19.7 Frey operation

■ Pancreatic Pseudocysts

Definition

- In contrast to genuine pancreatic cysts (dysontogenetic cysts, retention cysts, cystadenomas, and cystadenocarcinomas), the wall of a pseudocyst is not lined with epithelium. The boundary with the surrounding parenchyma consists only of a fibrous membrane.
- Pancreatic pseudocysts can be post-traumatic or can occur as a result of acute and chronic pancreatitis.

Symptoms

- Small cysts usually remain clinically silent and are identified only as an incidental finding on ultrasound or CT scans.
- Larger cysts are apparent clinically as a palpable abdominal mass. Besides pain, indirect symptoms can occur, which are caused by compression of neighboring structures, for example, stomach, duodenum, or common bile duct.
- Complications such as hemorrhage due to erosion (from the splenic artery, gastroduodenal artery, gastroepiploic artery), abscess formation, or cyst rupture are rare.

- Small cysts are usually an incidental finding.
- Larger cysts are palpable.

Diagnostic Approach

- Clinical examination: possible palpable upper abdominal mass
- Ultrasonography, endosonography
- CT
- ERCP, GI endoscopy

19

Treatment Approach

■ Indications

- Operation is indicated when **complications** are imminent (relative indication for surgery), for instance, when there is a risk of rupture as a result of a rapid increase in the size of the pseudocyst, and when the cyst is > 6 cm, shows no tendency to regress after more than 6 weeks, and causes clinical symptoms. Malignancy should be ruled out.

- Operation for imminent complications and clinical symptoms

■ Surgical Treatment

- Smaller symptomatic pseudocysts are resected.
- So-called internal drainage is possible technically only when the cyst wall is sufficiently strong (usually after 6–8 weeks) to provide a suitable site for suture of the planned anastomosis. Depending on the location of the pseudocyst, internal drainage can be through
  - ► a cystogastrostomy,
  - ► a cystojejunostomy using a Roux-en-Y loop, or
  - ► a cystoduodenostomy.
- In each case, the lowest point of the cyst must be used for anastomosis to guarantee complete evacuation of the cyst contents.

Minimally Invasive Procedures
- Ultrasound-guided cyst aspiration
- Percutaneous catheter drainage (if necessary medically assisted by somato-statin)
- Endoscopic cystoenterostomy with placement of an internal drainage catheter (usually into the stomach)

■ Carcinoma of the Pancreas

Epidemiology

- Cancer of the pancreas accounts for ca. 10% of all gastrointestinal neoplasms and is currently the fourth most common type of malignancy causing death, with a survival rate of less than 5%.
- Incidence 10 per 100 000 population
- Men and women equally often

Etiology

- The etiology remains unclear and is probably multifactorial (nicotine, alcohol, hereditary).

Classification (Table 19.3)

Table 19.3   TNM classification of exocrine pancreatic carcinoma

T—primary tumor	
Tis	Carcinoma in situ (Tis also includes the "PanIN-III" classification)
T1	Limited to pancreas ≤ 2 cm
T2	Limited to pancreas ≥ 2 cm
T3	Tumor extends beyond the pancreas but without involving the celiac trunk or superior mesenteric artery
T4	Infiltration of the celiac trunk or superior mesenteric artery
N—regional lymph nodes	
N0	No regional lymph node metastases
N1	Regional lymph node metastases
M—distant metastases	
M0	No distant metastases
M1	Distant metastases

- Depending on the site of origin, pancreatic carcinoma is classified into:
  - **Ductal adenocarcinoma** of the exocrine pancreatic parenchyma (rarely acinar carcinoma)
  - **Periampullary carcinoma** (significantly better prognosis)
  - **Islet cell carcinoma**
- Depending on the location, ductal adenocarcinomas are divided into cancers of the head (ca. 70%), body (ca. 10%) and tail (ca. 20%) of the pancreas.
- Periampullary carcinomas arise from the duodenal C, the common bile duct, the papilla of Vater, or the adjacent duodenal mucosa. It is often not possible to determine the exact site of origin.

Symptoms

- Apart from nonspecific evidence of malignant disease (anorexia, weight loss, fall in energy), upper abdominal pain and back pain (due to congestion of secretions or infiltration of the solar plexus) can occur.
- Painless jaundice with a palpable nontender gallbladder (Courvoisier sign) is regarded as the classical clinical symptom.

Diagnostic Approach

- The fact that pancreatic cancer becomes symptomatic only late in its course continues to be a problem.
- The primary screening method is **upper abdominal ultrasonography**, which can identify ca. 70% of pancreatic tumors. However, tumors with a diameter of less than 2 cm and malignancies located in the tail of the pancreas are often not recognized on ultrasonography. If this is suspected, a **contrast-enhanced CT** (ideally three-phase CT) is indicated to assess the relationship to vessels; it is also better at demonstrating tumor growth extending beyond the pancreas as well as lymphomas.
- **ERCP** is characterized by high sensitivity and specificity.
- When differentiation between neoplastic and inflammatory changes is uncertain, **cytological examination** of tumor aspirate obtained endosonographically can be helpful.
- The marker Ca 19–9, which is elevated in 70%–80% of advanced cases, is regarded as a specific **tumor marker** for pancreatic cancer. However, it is unsuitable as a screening parameter as elevated levels are also observed with pancreatitis, cholestasis, and other tumors of the gastrointestinal tract.
- Percutaneous **fine-needle aspiration** is obsolete today as laparoscopy or explorative laparotomy is performed in case of doubt.

> Pancreatic cancers often become symptomatic only late in the course of the disease.

19

Treatment Approach

■ Indications

Surgical Treatment

- Operation is regarded as the only potentially curative treatment for pancreatic cancer. The exclusion criteria are peritoneal carcinomatosis, liver metastases, and other distant metastases. Local vascular invasion is not a strict contraindication as it may be possible to treat it with resection and vascular reconstruction.
- Tumors in the head of the pancreas and periampullary carcinomas are treated by **partial pancreatoduodenectomy** (Whipple operation or pylorus-preserving resection of the head of the pancreas).
- The standard procedure for cancers of the body and tail is **distal** pancreatectomy with **splenectomy**. With both procedures, improved late results have been obtained with systematic lymphadenectomy but not by extended intra- and retroperitoneal lymphadenectomy.
- Local **papilla excision** can be considered for small cancers of the papilla and in patients who are too high-risk for partial pancreatoduodenectomy.
- **Total pancreatectomy** has not yielded better survival rates but is burdened with the often considerable problems of postoperative exocrine and endocrine pancreatic insufficiency.

> Surgery is the only potentially curative method of treatment

Adjuvant Therapy
- Radiotherapy and chemotherapy have not led to any improvement in the long-term prognosis of pancreatic cancer.

■ Surgical Treatment

Whipple Partial Pancreatoduodenectomy

- In this procedure, the following structures are removed in an en-bloc resection (**Fig. 19.8**):
  - ► The head and parts of the neck and body of the pancreas, depending on tumor location
  - ► The duodenum together with a short segment of proximal jejunum
  - ► Peripancreatic lymph nodes and the lymph nodes of the hepatoduodenal ligament
  - ► The gallbladder together with the bile ducts
  - ► The distal half of the stomach together with the right-hand side of the greater omentum
- The operative procedure is divided into two stages: resection and reconstruction.
- The best access is transverse upper abdominal laparotomy.

Operative Technique

- The local extent of tumor must first be assessed with regard to resectability. The sub- and retropancreatic course of the superior mesenteric vein must be exposed and the portal vein or confluence must be separable from the pancreas.
- This is followed by examination of lymph node status, distinguishing compartment 1 (peripancreatic lymph nodes) from compartment 2 (collecting lymph nodes) (see **Fig. 19.2**). If lymph nodes along the celiac trunk or paraaortic lymph nodes are involved, resection is probably of doubtful benefit.

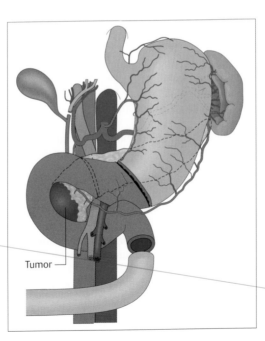

Fig. 19.8 Extent of the resection in partial pancreatoduodenectomy without pylorus preservation. The mesenteric vessels are spared.

Tumor

Liver metastases and peritoneal carcinomatosis are contraindications to pancreatic resection.

- After examining for resectability, resection begins with cholecystectomy and skeletonization of the hepatoduodenal ligament. Whether distal gastrectomy or postpyloric division of the duodenum is performed depends on the local situation.
- The reconstructive phase of the operation begins with pancreaticojejunostomy or pancreaticogastrostomy.
- This is followed by end-to-side hepaticojejunostomy, then gastrojejunostomy with or without Braun anastomosis depending on the reconstruction (**Fig. 19.9**).

Distal Pancreatectomy with Splenectomy

Operative Technique

- This operation is performed from left to right and begins with splitting of the gastrocolic ligament.
- After assessing resectability, the gastrosplenic ligament is divided and the tail of the pancreas is mobilized together with the spleen.
- Ligature of the splenic vessels and division of the pancreas is performed at a sufficient distance from the tumor.
- The remainder of the pancreas is either closed fish-mouth fashion with sutures or anastomosed to a Roux-en-Y small bowel loop.

19

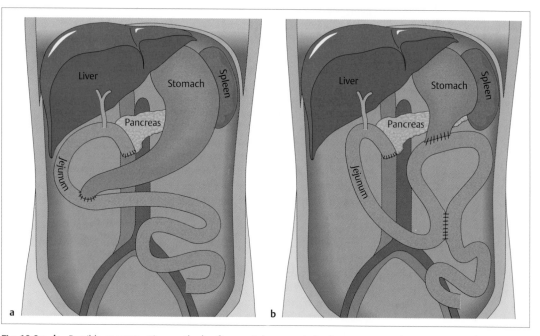

Fig. 19.9 a, b   Possible reconstruction methods after partial pancreatoduodenectomy: **a** pylorus-preserving, **b** with distal gastrectomy as pancreatojejunostomy (pancreaticogastrostomy is an alternative possibility).

■ **Palliative Measures**

- Palliative operations aim to eliminate biliary and gastrointestinal obstruction. Creation of a **gastroenterostomy** (when the duodenum is blocked) and/or a **biliary-enteric anastomosis** (when there is a non-stentable common bile duct stenosis) is indicated.
- Percutaneous transhepatic catheter drainage of the bile ducts is performed only in exceptional cases for preoperative decompression of obstructive jaundice.

Prognosis

- Poor prognosis because of late diagnosis
- The prognosis of pancreatic carcinoma is poor. The average survival is 3–6 months. The main reason is the late diagnosis of the tumor with the result that 70%–80% of the cancers are no longer operable with curative intent when they are diagnosed.
- Tumor recurrence can be anticipated in more than 95% of patients even after resection.
- The best results of operative treatment are achieved with cancer of the papilla (20%–30% 5-year cure rate).

■ Endocrine Pancreatic Tumors

- Pancreatic neuroendocrine tumors must be regarded as potentially malignant.
- **Incidence:** pancreatic neuroendocrine tumors are rare (4–12 new cases per million population).
- The **etiology** is unknown.
- **Classification:** A biological distinction is made between benign pancreatic neuroendocrine tumors, well differentiated neuroendocrine cancers, and poorly differentiated neuroendocrine cancers (2%–3%). Benign neoplasms, which arise from the endocrine islets of the pancreas, produce peptide hormones and biogenic amines. These rare tumors occur not only in the pancreas but also in other locations in the digestive tract and in other organs such as ovary, spleen, and lung.
- The most well-known pancreatic tumors are:
  - ► **Insulinoma:** lead symptom: hypoglycemia
  - ► **Gastrinoma:** lead symptoms: recurrent multiple, atypically located ulcers, diarrhea, Zollinger–Ellison syndrome
  - ► **Vipoma:** lead symptoms: watery diarrhea, hypokalemia, metabolic acidosis as a result of secretion of vasoactive intestinal polypeptide; Verner–Morrison syndrome (see Chapter 22)
- **Pancreatic neuroendocrine tumor frequency distribution:**
  - ► Hormonally active, well differentiated 20%–60%
    - – Insulinoma 25%–40%
    - – Gastrinoma 15%–20% (vipoma, glucagonoma 5%–15%, somatostatinoma)
  - ► Hormonally inactive, well differentiated 40%–80%
  - ► Poorly differentiated < 5%
- **Symptoms:** hormonally inactive tumors (40%–60% of the total) are discovered as a space-occupying lesion or because of lymphatic and hepatic metastases. The majority of hormonally active pancreatic neuroendocrine tumors become apparent as a result of the overproduction of insulin, glucagon, and other hormones.

Diagnostic Approach

- Ultrasonography (contrast-enhanced ultrasonography, endosonography)
- CT
- Positron emission tomography (PET)-CT
- MRI
- Measurement of the blood levels of the produced substances, chromogranin A
- Since pancreatic neuroendocrine tumors are usually small and the pancreas is often altered in its structure, imaging yields a result in fewer than 50% of cases.

- Diagnostic imaging yields a result in fewer than 50% of cases.

Treatment Approach

- It is often not possible to localize the tumors because of their small size.
- When localization is successful, for example, by means of intraoperative ultrasonography, **enucleation** or one of the typical **resection procedures** is performed.
- While radiotherapy has no role, remissions can be achieved with **chemotherapy.**
- **Symptomatic** forms of treatment are also employed, for instance, inhibition of hormone production by somatostatin analogues.

Prognosis

- Overall the prognosis of endocrine pancreatic tumors is much better than that of exocrine tumors (ca. 60% 5-year survival rate).

19

■ Pancreatic Trauma

Etiology

- Injuries of the pancreas usually occur as part of blunt upper abdominal trauma. The pancreas is compressed against the spine, usually owing to violent impact with the steering of a car or motorcycle or bicycle handle bars, and suffers contusions or tears.
- The possibility of involvement of neighboring organs (duodenum, bile ducts, spleen) must always be borne in mind.

Diagnostic Approach

- Because of the inaccessible location of the organ, diagnosis of pancreatic injury is often made late or not at all. Bleeding or pancreatitis can be the result.
- **Ultrasonography** and **angio-CT** along with raised levels of **pancreatic enzymes** in the serum and urine provide evidence of pancreatic injuries; **ERCP** can also be considered.

- **Indication:** terminal renal failure due to
  - ► Chronic glomerulonephritis
  - ► Diabetic nephropathy
  - ► Interstitial nephritis
- **Procedure:** Heterotopic KTx to the iliac fossa is performed. The recipient's iliac vessels are used for vascular anastomosis. The ureter of the donor organ is implanted in the bladder mucosa with an antireflux technique, and if necessary drained externally in addition.
- **Prognosis:** The 10-year transplant survival is 52.5%–77.5% after living kidney donation and 41.2%–44.5% after postmortem KTx.

■ Liver Transplantation

- Most frequent indications: posthepatitis cirrhosis and postalcohol cirrhosis

- The first successful liver transplant (LTx) was performed in Denver by Starzl in 1963. Survival of over 31 years after LTx is now reported.
- **Donor organs:** postmortem donors (over 85%) and living donors
- **Allocation:** According to five medical urgency categories (**MUC; Table 20.1**). The severity of the disease is assessed according to the **CPT** (Child Pugh Turcotte) score.
- **Indications:** acute liver failure, chronic liver disease, and malignant intrinsic liver tumors without extrahepatic manifestations (**Table 20.2**)
- Acute **liver failure** due to
  - ► Fulminant hepatitis (HBV or HCV)
  - ► Acetaminophen (paracetamol) intoxication
  - ► Amanita poisoning
- Advanced **liver disease** due to
  - ► HBV and HCV infection
  - ► Alcoholic hepatitis
  - ► Autoimmune hepatitis
  - ► Primary sclerosing cholangitis (PSC)
  - ► Primary biliary cirrhosis

- Milan criterias. HCC < 5 cm or up to three HCC nodules each < 3 cm

- Intrinsic liver **tumors:**
  - ► Hepatocellular carcinoma (HCC). The Milan criteria (HCC < 5 cm or up to three HCC lesions each < 3 cm) should be observed.
  - ► Metastases from a neuroendocrine tumor
  - ► Bile duct carcinoma (with restrictions)
- **Procedure:** Size compatibility is important in LTx. Reductions in the size of the donor liver are necessary in children or slim adults. The **split LTx** procedure has also been used since the 1980s, for instance, to transplant one-half

20

Table 20.1   Urgency levels in the Eurotransplant (ET) area

Registration status (MUC)	Description
HU (MUC 1)	Registration only through ET office after examining criteria
T2 (MUC 2)	Chronic liver dysfunction with acute deterioration
T3 (MUC 3)	Chronic liver dysfunction with complications
T4 (MUC 4)	Chronic liver dysfunction without complications
NT (MUC 5)	Provisionally not transplantable

MUC: medical urgency codes.
Source: From www.eurotransplant.nl

Table 20.2 Indications for liver transplantation

Indication
Acute or subacute hepatitis
Acute liver failure
Secondary biliary cirrhosis
Primary biliary cirrhosis
Sclerosing cholangitis
Bile duct atresia
Alcoholic cirrhosis
Autoimmune cirrhosis
Posthepatitis cirrhosis
Hepatocellular carcinoma
Biliary tract carcinoma
Metabolic disease
Budd–Chiari syndrome
Polycystic liver disease
Other liver disease

This table lists the underlying diseases (more than one possible) of new registrations without repeat registrations.
Source: From: www.dso.de

of the liver into a child and the other half into an adult. The minimum required liver mass should be over 0.8% of the recipient's body weight.

- In **living-donor liver donation**, the organ is obtained from the donor in the form of a hemihepatectomy. The liver lobe is transplanted using a piggy-back technique, preserving the recipient's vena cava (**Fig. 20.2**). This technique can be employed especially in right LTx, where numerous adhesions can render dissection extremely difficult.
- As a bridging method until LTx, when a donor organ is not available, the extracorporeal liver replacement system known as the molecular absorbents recirculating system (MARS) can be used. A portosystemic shunt or a transjugular intrahepatic portosystemic stent (TIPSS) is used to treat the portal hypertension and its symptoms and complications.
- **Prognosis:** The 1-year and 5-year transplant survival rates after LTx are > 90% and 86%, respectively.

■ Pancreas Transplantation

- The first successful pancreas transplant (PTx) was performed in 1967 by Kelly and Lillehei. Survival of over 18 years after PTx is now reported. The pancreas is usually transplanted simultaneously with a kidney (SKPTx).
- **Indications:**
  - ► Patients after KTx with type 1 diabetes mellitus (as PTx)
  - ► Patients with unstable type 1 diabetes mellitus, or with type 1 diabetes mellitus when more than two late complications of diabetes are present (as PTx)
  - ► Younger patients with unstable type I diabetes mellitus, as pre-emptive SKPTx, before irreversible late complications of diabetes, such as nephropathy or retinopathy, have occurred

- PTx is often performed simultaneously with KTx.

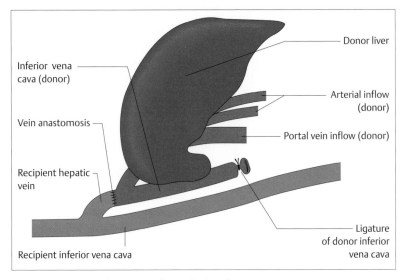

Fig. 20.2   Liver transplantation and piggy-back technique.

- **Procedure:** The pancreas is transplanted as an entire organ with attached blindly closed duodenum either heterotopically into the iliac fossa or in its physiological position. As with heterotopic kidney transplantation, the vascular anastomosis is to the iliac vessels. Exocrine drainage is through a duodenocystostomy, or into the jejunum through a side-to-side anastomosis when it is in paratopic location (**Fig. 20.3**).
- An **alternative** is transplantation of isolated pancreatic islet cells. Up to now, however, islet cell transplantation has usually been performed only at the same time as or after kidney transplantation. The past 10 years have shown that independence from insulin treatment can be achieved in principle in humans, even though this has hitherto been successful long-term in only a few cases.
- **Prognosis:** The 1-year and 10-year patient survival rates after PTx are > 95% and 80%, respectively.

■ Small Bowel Transplantation

- Indicated in short bowel syndrome when TPN becomes impossible due to catheter problems.

- The first successful small bowel transplant (SbTx) was performed in 1967 by Lillehei. Survival of over 10 years after SbTx is now reported. SbTx was developed successfully only after potent immunosuppressive agents were developed. Marked transplant rejection prevented long-term successful outcomes previously.
- **Indications:**
  - ▶ Patients with short bowel syndrome in whom total parenteral nutrition (TPN) is no longer feasible
  - ▶ As combined SbTx and LTx in patients with complications of TPN such as fatty liver, cholestatic liver cirrhosis, and malnutrition
- **Procedure:** The small bowel is transplanted orthotopically. An ileostomy is fashioned in the distal transplant so that endoscopic biopsies can be taken regularly in the postoperative observation period to assess rejection. The donor superior mesenteric artery is anastomosed to the abdominal aorta

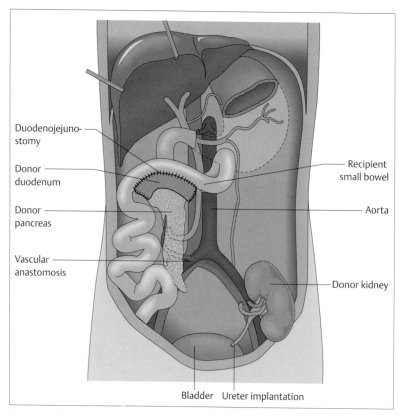

Duodenojejuno-
stomy

Donor
duodenum

Donor
pancreas

Vascular
anastomosis

Recipient
small bowel

Aorta

Donor kidney

Bladder   Ureter implantation

Fig. 20.3   Simultaneous kidney and pancreas transplantation (SKPTx) with anastomoses.

20

and the superior mesenteric vein to the portal vein or infrahepatic vena cava
(**Fig. 20.4**).

* Immediate postoperative enteral nutrition is important for regeneration of the
  intestinal villi and for correct intraluminal bacterial colonization of the transplant to avoid infections. Other problems are a considerable postoperative
  volume requirement and subsequent fluid loss and loss of bicarbonate through
  the ileostomy. Metabolic acidosis often develops and must be controlled.

* **Prognosis:** The 1-year patient survival rates after SbTx are about 60%–70%.

■ Multivisceral Transplantation

* Multivisceral transplantation (MTx) is performed rarely and nearly exclusively in large transplantation centers.

* On the one hand, combined liver and small bowel transplantation or multivisceral transplantation is difficult technically and, on the other hand, postoperative success is determined critically by postoperative immunosuppression, as with SbTx.

• MTx is performed rarely.

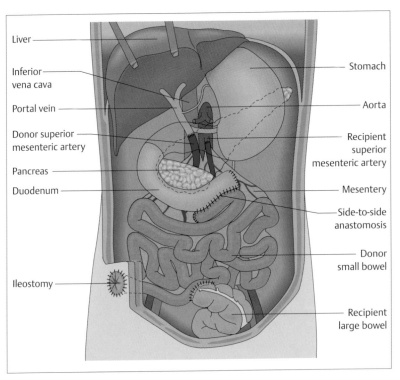

Fig. 20.4   Small bowel transplantation (SbTx) with anastomoses.

20

Immunosuppression

- Regular drug monitoring

- Regular drug monitoring is essential after transplantation.
- In the course of the past 20 years, immunosuppressive agents underwent marked development. The following are employed currently:
  - ► Nonspecific immunosuppressive drugs (prednisolone)
  - ► Calcineurin inhibitors (ciclosporin, tacrolimus)
  - ► Mammalian target of rapamycin inhibitors (mTOR inhibitors, e.g., rapamycin, everolimus)
  - ► Inositol monophosphate dehydrogenase inhibitors (mycophenolate mofetil = MMF)
  - ► Monoclonal IL-2 receptor antibodies (daclizumab, basiliximab)
  - ► Monoclonal and polyclonal T-cell antibodies (OKT 3, ATG)
  - ► Anti-proliferative drugs (azathioprine)
- A distinction is made between initial immunosuppression (induction) and low-dose long-term immunosuppression (maintenance therapy). The long-term goal is combined treatment with the lowest possible dose of the individual drugs and thus the fewest possible side effects. Successful long-term monotherapy with low-dose immunosuppressive agents is also reported.

Complications after Transplantation

- Complications due to operative technique, rejection reactions, and drug side-effects

- Possible complications:
  - ► Nonfunction or dysfunction of transplanted organs
  - ► Rejection reactions (hyperacute, acute, chronic)

- Anastomosis complications (stenosis, leakage)
- Recurrence of the underlying disease (especially hepatitis and malignancies)
- Bacterial and mycotic infections
- Cytomegalovirus (CMV) infection (especially in CMV-negative recipients)
- Skin malignancies and lymphoproliferative diseases
- Neurological and psychiatric behavioral disorders (medication-induced)
- Cardiovascular disease
- Diabetes mellitus (steroid-induced)
- Osteopenia (steroid-induced)

- **Caution:** Masking of acute abdominal inflammation—such as appendicitis, sigmoid diverticulitis, and cholecystitis—with immunosuppression. In particular, clinical symptoms and signs and laboratory parameters do not reflect the actual extent of inflammation.
- When operative procedures are performed on immunosuppressed patients, consistent drug monitoring is advisable along with perioperative steroid treatment. In this case, too, careful drug monitoring is critical for successful treatment.

- Immunosuppression can mask abdominal inflammation.

Further Reading

Deutsche Stiftung Organtransplantation (DSO). Im Internet: http://www.dso.de
Eurotransplant International Foundation. Im Internet: http://www.eurotransplant.nl
Starzl TE. The birth of clinical organ transplantation. Am Coll Surg 2001; 192: 431–446
Taylor AL et al. Immunosuppressive agents in solid organ transplantation: mechanisms of action and therapeutic efficacy. Critical Reviews in Oncology-Hematology 2005; 56: 23–46
Wolff M et al. Liver transplantation in Germany. Zentralbl Chir 2003; 128: 831–841

20

21 Peritonitis

B. Thiel

Anatomy of the Peritoneum

- Parietal layer: anterior and posterior abdominal wall with diaphragm
- Visceral layer: intraperitoneal abdominal and pelvic organs
- Total surface area of the peritoneum: 2 m^2

Histology

- Thin layer of loose connective tissue rich in lymphatic and blood vessels
- Covered with a single layer of squamous epithelium, known as mesothelium because of its mesodermal origin
- There are small openings between the mesothelial cells (8–12 mm diameter), which connect the abdominal cavity with lymph capillaries so that particles and cells (e.g., blood) can be absorbed.

Nerves

- **Parietal peritoneum:**
  - ► Numerous nerve endings, especially on the anterior and lateral abdominal wall
  - ► The joint nerve supply of the parietal peritoneum with the overlying abdominal wall explains the reflex muscle guarding that occurs with peritoneal irritation.
  - ► Irritation leads to persistent sharp pains.
- **Visceral peritoneum:**
  - ► Scant sensory afferents following the course of the mesenteric arteries
  - ► The nerves produce dull, poorly localized, burning, boring, wavelike pain due to traction on the mesenteries, bowel distention, muscle spasm or ischemia, with concomitant autonomic symptoms.

Vascular Supply

- **Arteries:** branches of the arteries that supply the abdominal wall, diaphragm, pelvis, and mesentery
- **Veins:** segmental or longitudinal drainage of the parietal layer to the territory of the upper and lower vena cava. The visceral layer drains through the territory of the portal vein.
- **Lymphatic drainage:** parallel to the arteries; the main flow is through the thoracic duct.

Definition

- Sepsis is a complex immunological reaction to a localized infection that extends through several phases.
- **Abdominal sepsis** represents a special form. It is defined as an intra-abdominal infection with a concomitant extraperitoneal reaction. Peritonitis is the correlate of abdominal inflammation.

Epidemiology

- The prevalence of severe sepsis and septic shock in intensive care units is about 10%.
- 90-day mortality: 54%
- With ca. 60 000 deaths annually. Septic diseases are in third place in mortality statistics.
- The incidence of postoperative peritonitis is 1% after laparotomy.

Etiology

- Contamination of the abdominal cavity with bacteria sets a series of complex immune mechanisms in motion:
  - ▸ Transport of the bacteria away by lymph fluid
  - ▸ Phagocytosis of the pathogens, sequestration of bacteria
  - ▸ Encapsulation of the bacteria in a fibrinous exudate
  - ▸ Early inflammatory immune response through activation of peritoneal macrophages, leukocytes, and mesothelial cells
  - ▸ Release of inflammatory mediators such as cytokines, growth factors, eicosanoids (cellular defense mechanisms)
  - ▸ Activation of the complement system, kallikrein–kinin system, the coagulation cascade, the renin–angiotensin system, and fibrinolysis (humoral defense mechanisms)
- If the local peritoneal reaction does not suffice to control the contamination and if an excessive immune reaction occurs with an imbalance between pro- and anti-inflammatory cytokines, a systemic inflammatory reaction with release of inflammatory mediators into the blood results. This leads to an increase in permeability, exudation and fluid losses, which can lead via dehydration and shock to multiorgan failure and death.

Classification (Table 21.1)

21

Table 21.1   Classification of peritonitis according to further criteria

Phenomenology	Extent	Severity
• Biliary • Fibrinous • Purulent • Fecal	• Local • Diffuse	• Without multiorgan failure • With multiorgan failure

Primary Peritonitis

- Primary peritonitis is rare (1%–2% of peritonitis patients).
- Bacterial invasion does not arise from an intraperitoneal hollow organ but is hematogenous and lymphatogenous in the framework of serious underlying diseases, and is increasingly iatrogenic and intraluminal (peritoneal dialysis, intraperitoneal chemotherapy, bacterial invasion through the female genitalia). It is usually a monoinfection.
- Adults with liver cirrhosis may be affected by spontaneous bacterial peritonitis.
- Tuberculous peritonitis

• Primary peritonitis is rare

- **Bacterial spectrum:**
  - ► Liver cirrhosis: *Escherichia coli* and other enterobacteria
  - ► Children: hematogenous spread, pneumococci, β-hemolytic streptococci
  - ► Women: ascending infection from the genital tract, β-hemolytic strepto-cocci, gonococci, chlamydia

Secondary Peritonitis (Fig. 21.1)

- The most common form of peritonitis is secondary peritonitis.

- Secondary peritonitis is the most common form.
- Usually due to **spread of pathogens** from an intra-abdominal hollow organ or from the exterior. Caused by organ perforation (gastric or duodenal ulcer, appendicitis, sigmoid diverticulitis, ischemic bowel wall necrosis, or chole-cystitis), iatrogenic (overlooked injuries of the biliary tract or bowel during laparoscopy), infection of intra-abdominal organs (intraoperative contami-nation) or trauma.
- Postoperative peritonitis (suture leakage, anastomosis leakage, organ injury, intraoperative contamination)
- Diffuse or local peritonitis due to an abscess
- **Bacterial spectrum:** mixed flora
- Mortality of postoperative peritonitis is higher at 60% than that of peritonitis due to perforation, which is 14%.

Tertiary Peritonitis

- Persistent peritonitis in patients on immunosuppression despite source con-trol, in the form of a self-maintaining inflammatory reaction, although the source of infection has been treated

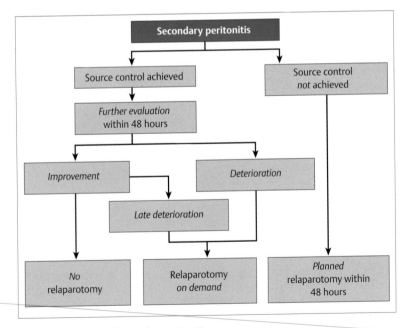

Fig. 21.1   Treatment of secondary peritonitis.

Symptoms

Lead Symptoms

- **Pain:**
  - ► Visceral layer:
    - – Autonomic sympathetic and parasympathetic fibers
    - – Not lateralized
    - – Poorly localizable
    - – Cramping or colicky
    - – Autonomic symptoms
    - – Changing location
  - ► Parietal layer:
    - – Segmental somatic nerves of spinal origin on either side
    - – Lateralized
    - – Patient can point to the site of pain
    - – Burning, sharp
    - – Can be localized to the affected organ
- **Disturbed peristalsis:**
  - ► Acute change in bowel habit, diarrhea, constipation, inability to pass feces or gas
  - ► The pain symptoms cause paralysis of bowel peristalsis through viscerospinal reflexes.
  - ► Marked meteorism with a distended abdomen
- **Guarding:**
  - ► Local resistance
  - ► Increased abdominal wall tension due to reflex increase in muscle tone
  - ► Boardlike abdomen
  - ► Must be distinguished from meteoristically distended but soft and non-tender abdomen, ascites

Lead symptoms:
- Pain
- Bowel motility disorder
- Guarding

Concomitant Symptoms

- Nausea, tachycardia, tachypnea, hypotension, pallor, sweating, vomiting, fever

Special Evidence of Postoperative Peritonitis

- Deterioration of general condition
- Postoperative recovery delayed
- Abnormal abdominal examination
- Change in drain secretion

21

Diagnostic Approach

- The clinical picture of peritonitis is often represented by the term "acute abdomen." The need for immediate operative treatment becomes apparent. The diagnostic investigations presented here must be performed promptly and accord closely with the clinical picture. If the patient's condition worsens, diagnostic investigations should not be concluded but action is required.
- The terms diffuse peritonitis and acute abdomen include a very broad range of conditions but do not enable assessment of the prognosis or provide a basis for deciding on suitable treatment. Different prognostic indices for assessing the severity of peritonitis have therefore been evaluated.

- The Mannheim Peritonitis Index is a widely used peritonitis score:
- MPI < 20 points, mortality close to 0
- MPI > 29 points, mortality > 50%

Scoring Systems

- The following scoring systems can be used:
  - ► MPI (Mannheim Peritonitis Index)
  - ► APACHE-II (Acute Physiology And Chronic Health Evaluation)
  - ► SOFA (Sepsis-related Organ Failure Assessment)
  - ► SIRS score (Systemic Inflammatory Reaction Syndrome)
  - ► TISS-28 (Therapeutic Intervention Scoring System)
- The **Mannheim Peritonitis Index** is used most widely clinically; this presents the risk of death on the basis of surgical details. This index can be obtained without complex diagnostic investigations and laboratory parameters. It is calculated as shown in **Table 21.2**, and the maximum score is 47. Other indices for assessing intra-abdominal infections and sepsis usually have an intensive care medicine orientation and require precise documentation of laboratory and other parameters.
- The **APACHE-II score** is also widespread but is used more to assess the course of septic intensive care patients. Twelve parameters must be recorded and calculated (temperature, mean arterial blood pressure, heart rate, respiratory rate, oxygenation, arterial pH, serum sodium, potassium, creatinine, hematocrit, leukocytes, Glasgow Coma Scale). These cannot be evaluated very quickly in an acute situation.

■ Clinical Examination

- Peritonitis is a clinical diagnosis.

- **History:** targeted, ulcer history, medication use, underlying diseases, onset of pain, localization, course, previous surgery
- **Inspection:** reduced general condition, anxiety, agitation, protective posture with legs drawn up, shallow breathing, dehydration, pain on jolting
- **Palpation:** meteorism, rebound tenderness, tenderness, resistance, guarding, boardlike abdomen
- **Auscultation:** absence of bowel sounds, "silent abdomen"
- **Temperature:** hypothermia with severe sepsis
- **Rectal examination:** abscess in pouch of Douglas, pain on moving cervix, rectal abscesses with low anastomosis

Table 21.2   Calculation of the Mannheim Peritonitis Index

Prognostic factor		Score (points)
Age over 50 years		5
Female		5
Organ failure		7
Malignancy		4
Preoperative duration of peritonitis > 24 h		4
Source not arising from the colon		4
Diffuse spread		6
Exudate	Clear	0
	Cloudy	6
	Feculent or putrid	12

■ Laboratory Tests

Procalcitonin (Table 21.3)
- Since unraised or slightly raised procalcitonin (PCT) levels are found with viral infections, chronic inflammation, and acute nonbacterial inflammation, measurement of the PCT can be used for differentiating the following conditions:
  - ▸ Infectious/noninfectious diseases
  - ▸ Bacterial/viral infections
  - ▸ Acute bacterial infections / chronic inflammatory reactions
  - ▸ Bacterial/viral meningitis
  - ▸ Fever of unknown origin in neutropenic patients
- The PCT level is used subsequently to assess therapy.

• PCT level has now become an important measure of sepsis

Interleukin-6
- Interleukin (IL)-6 induces acute phase protein synthesis in the liver.
- Advantage: increases up to 48 hours earlier than C-reactive protein (CRP), rapid dynamics; regarded as an early marker of inflammation, magnitude of initial IL-6 level is also regarded as a survival marker in patients with sepsis.

Lipopolysaccharide Binding Protein (LBP)
- LBP is an acute phase protein that binds lipopolysaccharides (endotoxins) of the bacterial cell wall during infections; according to the most recent studies, it is also elevated in fungal infections.
- The magnitude of the LBP level correlates with the removal of lipopolysaccharides (from bacterial cell walls) and thus with the extent of infection. LBP is a better initial marker of infection in babies (younger than 48 hours) than IL-6 or PCT and it is equivalent to PCT measurement in babies over 48 hours old.

Other Laboratory Parameters
- Blood count, CRP, creatinine, urea, electrolytes, lipase, prothrombin time (PT), partial thromboplastin time (PTT), international normalized ratio (INR), lactate, lactate dehydrogenase (LDH), liver function tests, creatine kinase (CK), blood grouping, blood crossmatch

21

■ Diagnostic Imaging

- **Ultrasonography:** little time lost, free fluid, search for septic focus, organ changes (tumor, appendicitis, cholecystitis)
- **Radiography of abdomen** in two planes (erect and left lateral decubitus): free air, fluid level (paralysis), aerobilia, obstruction, meteorism (Ogilvie syndrome)
- **Contrast-enhanced imaging:** blockage or leakage of contrast agent (water-soluble) in retrogradely filled colon (diverticulitis, tumor, perforation); gastrointestinal series with oral contrast is not useful when peritonitis is marked.
- **CT:** intravenous contrast, transrectal contrast, not useful orally if peritonitis present preoperatively, used today more than conventional contrast imaging, rapid and comprehensive investigation of the abdomen (differentiation of etiology, pancreatitis, perforation, tumor, etc.), severity of the disease (necrotic areas, multiple abscesses, perfusion disorders centrally or peripherally, extent of bowel damage)
- **Chest x-ray:** preoperative preparation, differential diagnosis

• If clinical condition deteriorates, discontinue investigations and institute immediate surgical treatment

Table 21.3   Probability of sepsis depending on serum procalcitonin (PCT)

Serum PCT	Sepsis
< 0.5 ng/mL	unlikely
> 0.5 ng/mL, < 2 ng/mL	possible
> 2 ng/mL	very likely

- **Endoscopy:** rare, as usually takes too long to set up while clinical signs are increasing
- **Laparoscopy:** usually for localized peritonitis (appendicitis, ovarian process)
- **ECG:** to rule out cardiac causes

Intervention during Diagnostic Investigations
- Because of the peritoneum's defense mechanisms, inflammation can remain locally limited. In addition, if the patient is unstable clinically, a locally limited condition, for example a diverticular abscess, can be drained by inserting a CT-guided drain when a CT scan is performed as investigation. This measure may provide a somewhat greater therapeutic window and can stabilize the patient. However, this does not replace treatment of the septic focus.

Treatment Approach

■ Conservative Treatment

Primary Peritonitis

- Primary peritonitis is treated medically.

- Surgical eradication of a septic focus is not possible.
- Pneumococci or β-hemolytic streptococci: **penicillin G**
- Liver cirrhosis: a third-generation **cephalosporin** (ceftriaxone, cefepim) combined with **metronidazole**
- Supportive measures
- Recurrent spontaneous primary peritonitis: possibly recurrence prophylaxis, for example, with norfloxacin 400 mg/d; this reduces the frequency of recurrence by up to 66%. Long-term prophylaxis should be given only when recurrences are frequent or prior to liver transplantation. Short-term antibiotic prophylaxis is indicated with endoscopies or other invasive investigations.

Secondary Peritonitis (Fig. 21.1)

- Start empirical antibiotic therapy as soon as possible.

- Antibiotic therapy is an important component of the treatment of peritonitis. If an intra-abdominal infection is suspected, a blood culture should be taken prior to antibiotic therapy; however, the therapy should be started as soon as possible after the diagnosis is made. Empirical therapy is begun. The selected antibiotic regimen should be adjusted after the results of microbiological tests are obtained. During the therapy, the antibiotic regime should be re-evaluated after 48–72 hours using clinical and microbiological criteria.
- The duration of treatment is guided by the clinical course but should generally not exceed 7–10 days. The dictum that antibiotic therapy should continue until 2 days after a drop in fever and leukocytes, is no longer current.

21

Antibiotic Selection Criteria
- Duration of disease
- Origin of the cause, location
- Resistant bacterial spectrum in own hospital
- Patient's risk profile
- Locally limited or recent perforation:
  - ▸ For example, appendicitis, stomach perforation, or acute cholecystitis
  - ▸ Lower bacterial counts and clear or slightly cloudy secretion
  - ▸ Mixed aerobic/anerobic infections tend to be rarer when the perforation originates in the stomach or duodenum.
- Diffuse, moderately severe peritonitis:
  - ▸ For example, perforation of the biliary tract or jejunum
  - ▸ With moderate bacterial counts
  - ▸ Mixed aerobic/anerobic infections in 50% of cases
- Diffuse severe peritonitis:
  - ▸ Perforation of the distal small bowel and colon
  - ▸ High bacterial counts
  - ▸ Mixed aerobic/anerobic infections almost without exception from, for example, *E. coli*, klebsiellas, enterobacter, enterococci, streptococci, *Pseudomonas aeruginosa*, *Bacteroides* spp., *Clostridium* spp. and *Candida* spp.
  - ▸ Turbid, feculent exudate
  - ▸ Risk factors: duration of peritonitis > 2–4 hours, carcinoma, organ failure, not completely treatable

Antibiotic Therapy
- **Locally limited** peritonitis, as briefly as possible with, for example:
  - ▸ Aminopenicillin with β-lactamase inhibitors (BLIs)
  - ▸ Acylaminopenicillin with BLIs
  - ▸ Carbapenems
  - ▸ Cephalosporins as monotherapy or in combination with metronidazole
- **Moderately severe** peritonitis 3–5 days, and longer for severe disease, with, for example:
  - ▸ Acylaminopenicillin with BLIs
  - ▸ Carbapenems
  - ▸ Third-generation cephalosporins in combination with metronidazole

21

■ Surgical Treatment

- In secondary peritonitis, early surgical intervention is crucial for the prognosis and course of the peritonitis and existing sepsis. Surgical therapy consists of
  - ▸ Early operative intervention with eradication of the **septic focus** (elimination of the cause)
  - ▸ Mechanical **cleansing of the abdominal cavity** (reduction of bacteria and endotoxin, abdominal lavage)
  - ▸ Postinterventional **drainage** of the infectious focus (laparostomy if appropriate)

• Early surgical intervention crucial for prognosis and course of the peritonitis

Eradication of the Septic Focus

- Emergency operation; start of treatment must not be delayed by diagnostic investigations
- Vertical laparotomy for complete exploration, transverse upper abdominal laparotomy also with necrotizing pancreatitis

• Anatomical restoration
• Control of the source of infection

- Bacterial swab, gross cleansing, complete exploration
- The further procedure depends on the extent and location of the findings, and whether and how eradication of the focus is achieved (**Table 21.4**).
- Through these measures, definitive anatomical restoration is achieved or continuing contamination is prevented. This enables surgical control of the source of infection. In addition, infected soft tissue should be debrided and foreign bodies should be removed, but excessively radical resection of the surrounding tissue does not confer the hoped-for improvement in prognosis.

Cleansing of the Abdominal Cavity

- Cleansing of residues
- Reduce number of bacteria.

- The aim is to cleanse the abdomen of residues of peritonitis, such as fibrin deposits, and to reduce the number of bacteria and amount of endotoxin.

Procedure
- Peritoneal lavage with several liters of Ringer solution at body temperature, including all compartments
- Careful division of adhesions
- The irrigation volume is controversial: on the one hand, dilution of the bacterial count and endotoxin is desirable but, on the other hand, excessive irrigation volumes can worsen the patient's clinical condition.
- The fibrin deposits should be removed as far as possible but radical removal causing serosal defects and bleeding must be avoided.
- Decompression of the paralytic bowel by careful massaging may be necessary before the abdomen is closed but should be avoided when the bowel wall is severely damaged and edematous.
- Drain insertion is controversial. A distinction must be made between irrigation drains, which are relatively rigid tubes that allow continuous irrigation of a focus of infection and pure outflow drains, such as Easy-Flow drains, which are placed to control the infection of the abdominal cavity.

Table 21.4   Measures for controlling the source of infection

Location	Surgical procedure, source control
Gastric ulcer, duodenal ulcer	Excision/oversewing
Hepatobiliary source	Cholecystectomy, diversion through T-tube, extrahepatic drainage
Duodenal stump leakage	Extraperitonealization, drainage
Pancreatitis	Compartment formation, necrosectomy, drainage
Small bowel	Short segment resection of the perforation or gangrene
Cecal pole to splenic flexure	Resection with primary anastomosis usually suffices
Lower gastrointestinal tract	Discontinuity resection, resection with anastomosis
• with mild peritonitis	• resection and primary anastomosis, with proximal loop ileostomy
• with severe peritonitis	• Hartmann procedure (resection with terminal colostomy, restoration of continuity in 3–6 months)

Extended Treatment Concepts

The measures described above are intended to avoid relaparotomy, which is associated with complications and increased mortality. With more prolonged purulent peritonitis or when the source cannot be securely controlled, this must be followed by a phase of further revision and lavage. There are several ways of doing this.

- The criteria for selecting the appropriate procedure are difficult to objectify and depend on the surgeon's experience.
  - ► With local processes, a single-stage procedure with source control is employed, with postoperative continuous closed irrigation if necessary.
  - ► If an ischemic process is present, a staged procedure with planned revision can be performed to allow re-evaluation of the uncertain intra-abdominal situation.
  - ► Simpler cases of peritonitis with a better prognosis should be treated with a single-stage standard procedure (with relaparotomy on demand). Severe forms (MPI > 26) should be treated more aggressively with decompression, scheduled peritoneal lavage, and temporary abdominal closure.

Continuous Peritoneal Lavage

- **Closed** postoperative peritoneal lavage:
  - ► Insertion of several irrigation drains after source control
  - ► Closure of the abdomen
  - ► Irrigation volumes ca. 1 L per hour with hyperosmolar solution, for 2–5 days until the irrigation fluid is clear
  - ► **Advantages:** continuous cleansing of the abdomen from bacteria, endotoxins, mediators, secretions, blood and detritus, avoidance of further laparotomies and anesthesia, enteric feeding can be increased while irrigation is running
  - ► **Disadvantages:** high enteral protein loss, development of irrigation tracks, temporary development of high intra-abdominal pressures, inability to check on the progress of complications
- **Open** postoperative peritoneal lavage:
  - ► Insertion of irrigation drains anteriorly and far posteriorly for inflow
  - ► No abdominal closure
  - ► Outflow is through the laparostomy
  - ► **Advantages:** lower abdominal pressure, inspection of the site is possible, less irrigation track development
  - ► **Disadvantages:** water retention, potassium loss, enormous staff demand, outflow/leakage of the irrigation fluid, dehiscence of the wound edges, difficult secondary approximation of the wound edges
- Because of the disadvantages, especially the enormous staff requirement, the two procedures are employed rarely, for example, when there is extensive necrotizing pancreatitis with abdominal hypertension (compartment development).

Programmed Relaparotomy

- **Indications:** definite source control not possible surgically, secondary diffuse fecal peritonitis, risk of abdominal compartment development (with edematous inflammation of the bowel), increasing loss of abdominal wall due to necrosis and infection (apply vacuum dressings, e.g., VAC)
- At the first source-control procedure, the surgeon establishes whether a further intervention must take place, especially when the source cannot be

21

eradicated or the peritonitis is severe (possibly ischemic bowel, extensive progressive necrosis).

- The interval between relaparotomies is initially 24 hours, later up to 48 hours depending on the situation.
- Insertion of drains, which are liable to complications, can be omitted.
- Repeat lavage with up to 20 L.
- Fibrin deposits are removed carefully and adhesions between bowel loops are divided.
- **Advantages:** regular inspection of the source site, inspection of anastomoses, removal of secondary fibrin deposits and fluid collections
- **Disadvantages:** wound margin necrosis and wound dehiscence due to repeated wound closure, consequences of repeated manipulation in the inflamed abdomen (bowel injury, fistula formation, bleeding), general risks of reoperation, increased mortality with increasing number of laparotomies
- **Temporary abdominal closure options:** To diminish wound healing problems with repeated laparotomies, the abdominal cavity is often left open as a laparostomy and a temporary closure is sutured in place or special dressings are applied.
  - ► **Adhesive plastic drape:** An adhesive plastic drape is applied. The drape does not adhere to the bowel and the wound margins can be drawn together so that an abdominal compartment can be avoided. The situation in the abdomen can be assessed and the abdominal closure can be changed easily and quickly at relaparotomy. Suitable when treatment is over a short period.
  - ► **Plastic zippers, slide fasteners:** These procedures involve suturing zippers or, ideally, slide fasteners to the wound fascial margins so that a suture does not always have to be opened and resutured at the daily relaparotomy. Alterations in the wound margins are reduced and there is less necrosis of the wound margins. Narrower sliding closures are sutured every 3 days so that the fascial margins are gradually approximated.
  - ► **Vacuum dressings with special intestinal dressing (e.g., VAC therapy):** This temporary abdominal closure achieves good control of secretion from the laparostomy. This is an enormous advantage from the nursing aspect and at the same time, bacteria, endotoxins, and fluids are removed from the abdomen.

    If the fascia is open and the greater omentum has been consumed by the infection and necrosis, a special drape is placed on the bowel loops to protect them.

    A special sponge is placed over this, which acts as a medium to aspirate the secretion for suction through a vacuum. The sponge is tailored to the size of the laparostomy. This is covered by a sealing film. The film is perforated in one place where a tubing system connected to a vacuum pump is attached. This produces steady suction on the laparostomy without vacuum peaks. Depending on the condition of the bowel loops and the patient's situation, the pump is set to continuous or intermittent variable vacuum.

    Because of the vacuum, secretions are removed continuously from the abdominal cavity and the wound margins come closer together. Granulation in the wound is also stimulated. If the fascial margins are too far apart to allow wound and fascial closure, the rapid granulation enables cutaneous wound closure when the wound is clean. Definitive surgical closure can then take place under better conditions when the patient is stable.

21

- ▶ **Palisade dressings (wound dressings made of tube drains):** If there is very diffuse fecal peritonitis and if the source cannot be brought under control, early and frequent reintervention is scheduled. At the beginning of such an aggressive therapy regimen, an adhesive drape or vacuum dressing is not effective. To protect the abdomen and nevertheless drain secretions, palisade dressings can be used. Tube drains to the width of the open abdomen are sutured together in parallel, placed in the wound, and covered with abdominal sponges. Once gross cleansing has been concluded, other methods (e.g., VAC therapy) can follow. Palisade dressing requires a lot of nursing time, so it is no longer used frequently.
- ▶ **Sterile plastic bag:** If the abdomen has to be left completely open to avoid a compartment syndrome, the bowel loops can be enclosed in a sterile bag. During open postoperative continuous peritoneal lavage, the abdomen is covered by a sterile plastic bag. Newer closure options will supersede this method.
- The **advantage** of temporary abdominal closure is problem-free control of possible complications and the possibility of gradual approximation of the wound margins. The disadvantages are the lack of objective criteria for the time of closure. The accepted criteria are the reduction of fibrin deposits and the secretion becoming clearer.

Relaparotomy on Demand

- Source control at the first operation must be possible, and the operation is performed only once.
- After source control, the peritoneum plays a crucial part in fighting the peritonitis.
- The decision on whether a single-stage or repeated treatment method should be used depends on the surgeon's experience.
- Close monitoring of the patient's clinical course and laboratory parameters
- Early monitoring of the situation with ultrasonography or CT
- Insertion of drains to control secretions
- Repeat laparotomy in < 48 hours if the patient deteriorates
- **Advantages:** avoidance of serious operative complications such as bowel injury, fistula formation and bleeding. Intensive care parameters such as protein and electrolyte loss of control or abdominal wall dehiscences are rarer.
- **Disadvantages:** There are no objective parameters for determining the need for relaparotomy on demand, and whether to perform relaparotomy depends on the surgeon's experience. The decision for relaparotomy may be delayed by prolonged diagnostic investigations or changing personnel and the patient's condition can suddenly deteriorate. Operative complications only become apparent later.

■ Supportive Therapy

- Apart from treating the cause (eradication of septic focus, antibiotic therapy), the treatment of peritonitis often means treatment of sepsis and requires further measures. The first priority is consistent hemodynamic therapy to achieve an adequate cellular oxygen supply.

21

Volume Replacement
- Giving crystalloids and colloids increases cardiac output and the systemic oxygen supply in septic shock. Volume therapy may suffice to stabilize the hemodynamic situation. Administration of human albumin in septic shock is no longer recommended.

Transfusion of Erythrocyte Concentrate
- Once the diminished tissue perfusion has been corrected, if the hemoglobin level is < 7 g/dL it may be necessary to increase it, especially in patients with septic shock and ischemic heart disease.

Vasopressors
- Dobutamine: if volume administration alone does not suffice, to increase myocardial contractility in sepsis.
- Norepinephrine: if the mean pressure cannot be maintained at an adequate level. Can be used even earlier in unstable patients.

Ventilation
- The decision on whether ventilation is indicated should be made early, especially in patients with severe sepsis and ALI/ARDS (acute lung injury / acute respiratory distress syndrome) and should have positive end-expiratory pressures.
- The ventilation of patients with ALI/ARDS should be managed according to ARDSNet guidelines:
  - Reduce tidal volume to 6 mL/kg body weight.
  - Keep plateau pressure below 30 cm H_2O.
  - Tidal volume should be reduced to 4 mL/kg desirable weight to keep the plateau pressure below 30 cm H_2O.
  - Maintain SaO_2 or SpO_2 between 90% and 95%.

Nutrition
- Enteral feeding should be attempted as soon as possible.

■ Adjunctive Treatment

- Low-dose **hydrocortisone** at a dosage of 200–300 mg/d
- **Recombinant activated protein C** (Drotrecogin alfa) 24 mg/kg per hour for patients with severe sepsis (Apache score > 25) and failure of two organ systems
  - Inhibits coagulation factors Va and VIIIa and reduces thrombin production
  - Has a fibrinolytic action
  - Reduces production of proinflammatory cytokines
  - Increased bleeding tendency so postoperative use only after 12 hours
  - Patients with less severe sepsis show increased mortality.
- **Intensified insulin therapy** (80–110 mg/dL) for patients with severe sepsis
- Not found to be effective: antithrombin, ibuprofen, prostaglandins, pentoxifylline, *N*-acetylcysteine, plasmapheresis, and hemofiltration in the absence of acute renal failure (**Table 21.5**)

Table 21.5 Diagnostic criteria for sepsis, severe sepsis, and septic shock according to the ACCP/SCCM consensus conference criteria

Criterion	Clinical features
I. Evidence of an infection	• Diagnosis of infection by microbiological confirmation or clinical criteria
II. Systemic inflammatory response syndrome (at least two clinical signs)	• Fever ($\geq 38°C$) or hypothermia ($\leq 36°C$), confirmed by rectal or intravascular or intravesical measurement • Tachycardia: heart rate ≥ 90/min • Tachypnea (rate ≥ 20/min) or hyperventilation ($PaCO_2 \leq 4.3$ kPa / ≤ 33 mmHg) • Leukocytosis ($\geq 12\,000$/mm³) or leukopenia (≤ 4000/mm³) or > 10% immature neutrophils on differential blood count
III. Acute organ dysfunction (at least one clinical sign)	• Acute encephalopathy: impaired level of consciousness, disorientation, agitation, delirium • Relative or absolute thrombocytopenia: drop in platelet count by more than 30% within 24 hour or platelet count $\leq 100\,000$/mm³ (thrombocytopenia due to acute bleeding or immunological causes must be ruled out) • Arterial hypoxemia: $PaO_2 \leq 10$ kPa (≤ 75 mmHg) on room air or a PaO_2/FiO_2 ratio of ≤ 33 kPa (< 250 mmHg) on oxygen (overt cardiac or pulmonary disease as the cause of the hypoxemia must be ruled out) • Renal dysfunction: diuresis of ≤ 0.4 mL/kg/h for at least 2 hours despite adequate volume replacement and/or a rise in serum creatinine to over twice the local normal reference range • Metabolic acidosis: base excess ≤ -5 mol/L or lactate concentration more than 1.5 times the local normal reference range

Sepsis: criteria I and II
Severe sepsis: criteria I–III
Septic shock: criteria I and II and systolic arterial pressure ≤ 90 mmHg or mean arterial pressure ≤ 65 mmHg for at least 1 hour or need for vasopressor use to maintain systolic arterial pressure ≥ 90 mmHg or mean arterial pressure ≥ 65 mmHg. The hypotension is present despite adequate volume administration and cannot be explained by other causes.

21

Further Reading

Knaebel H-P et al. Aktueller Stand der Diagnostik und Therapie der Peritonitis. Zentralbl Chir 2007; 132: 419–426

Reinhart K, Brunkhorst FM et al. Diagnose und Therapie der Sepsis. Leitlinien der Deutschen Sepsis-Gesellschaft e.V. und der Deutschen Interdisziplinären Vereinigung für Intensiv- und Notfallmedizin. AWMF-RegNr. 079/001

Westerholt A, Maier S, Heidecke C-D. Peritonitis, Sepsis, septischer Schock. Allgemeine und Viszeralchirurgie up2date 2007; 4: 237–252

22 Neuroendocrine Tumors and Gastrointestinal Stromal Tumors

J.M. Mayer

■ Neuroendocrine Tumors

Definition

- Derived from neuroendo-crine cells of endodermal origin
- Produce peptide hor-mones and neurotransmit-ters

- Derived from neuroendocrine cells
- Scattered in small groups or diffusely in the epithelia of the gastropancreatic system
- Produce peptide hormones and neurotransmitters
- Rarely manifested in the bronchial system or thymus
- Pearse coined the term APUD system (amine precursor uptake and decar-boxylation), which he used to describe functional characteristics of the neu-roendocrine cells similar to neurons, and therefore assumed that they were of neuroectodermal origin.
- Neuroendocrine cells arise during evolution from the endoderm and not, as previously assumed, from the neural ridge.
- The term carcinoid goes back to Oberndorfer, who wanted to stress the relatively benign character of these tumors compared with carcinoma.
- In clinical parlance, the term carcinoid is often restricted to a serotonin-producing tumor with the corresponding carcinoid syndrome.

Epidemiology

- Rare entity
- Malignancies of the ap-pendix, small bowel, and pancreas often with neu-roendocrine differentiation

- Incidence: ca. 1–2 cases per 100 000 population per year
- Neuroendocrine carcinomas account for 77% of all appendix malignancies, 34% of all small bowel malignancies, 20% of all pancreatic malignancies, and 1% of all gastric and colon malignancies.

Etiology

- The tumors are caused by genetic changes in different tumor suppressor genes.
- They occur sporadically or as part of hereditary MEN I syndrome.

■ Multiple Endocrine Neoplasia Type I (MEN I) (Werner Syndrome) (Table 22.1)

- MEN I syndrome in up to 30% of all patients with NETs
- Neuroendocrine pancreat-ic tumors, primary hyper-parathyroidism, hypophy-seal tumors

- **Epidemiology:** MEN I syndrome is present in up to 30% of all patients with neuroendocrine tumors (NETs).
- **Precondition:** Germ line mutation of the MEN I tumor suppressor gene
- **Pathogenesis:** Tumor develops owing to loss of the second wild-type MEN I allele at somatic level (usually through loss of heterozygosity).
- **Symptoms:**
  - ► Early tumor manifestation (adolescents, young adults)
  - ► Synchronous and metachronous second tumors

Table 22.1 Indications for MEN I genetic analysis in patients with neuroendocrine tumors (NETs)

Is hereditary MEN I syndrome present?	Is positive gene carrier status present?

• Patient with confirmed typical MEN I NET plus an additional criterion:
  ► multifocal tumor
  ► typical second neoplasm
  ► age <40 years
  ► positive family history
  ► recurrent second tumor
	• In the context of family investigation in all first-degree relatives of MEN I patients
	• First-degree relatives of MEN I mutation carriers

  ► Primary hyperparathyroidism (90%)
  ► Neuroendocrine pancreatic tumors (50%), for example gastrinoma, insulinoma
  ► Pituitary tumors (40%)
• **Follow-up:** Regular investigation for second tumors (measurement of serum calcium, gastrin, insulin, prolactin, CT of abdomen)

Classification (Tables 22.2, 22.3)

Table 22.2 WHO classification of neuroendocrine tumors of the digestive tract (2000)

Grade	WHO classification	Synonym
1	Highly differentiated neuroendocrine tumor	Carcinoid
2	Highly differentiated neuroendocrine carcinoma	Malignant carcinoid
3	Poorly differentiated neuroendocrine carcinoma	Small cell carcinoma

Table 22.3 Classification according to embryogenesis

	Organs	Special features
Foregut	Bronchus, esophagus, stomach, duodenum, pancreas	Multihormonal potency (especially 5-hydroxytryptophan
Midgut	Jejunum, ileum, appendix, proximal colon	Carcinoid syndrome (serotonin) frequently
Hindgut	Distal colon, rectum	Usually functionally inactive

Source: From Williams ED, Sandler M. The classification of carcinoid tumors. Lancet 1963;1:238–239.

Symptoms

• Characteristic symptoms due to the hormonal activity of the tumors
• Particularly with tumors located in the foregut and midgut
• Not all secreted substances cause clinical symptoms
• Most frequently, colic and diarrhea (50%–70%), flushing (20%–30%), and cardiac tachyarrhythmias (10%)
• Because of the liver's first-pass effect, the hormones become symptomatic only when liver metastases are present, for example, in carcinoid syndrome.

• Hormone-induced symptoms only with liver metastases: colic, diarrhea, flushing, tachycardia

22

- Hormonally inactive tumors usually become symptomatic only at an advanced stage with nonspecific symptoms such as obstruction or obstructive jaundice, intussusception, adhesion, or bleeding.

Diagnostic Approach

■ Laboratory Tests

- **Usually functionally inactive**
- The majority of NETs are functionally inactive and do not cause a hypersecretion syndrome (typical peptide hormones and neurotransmitters are nevertheless usually detectable in the specimen on immunohistochemistry).

Chromogranin A

- **Highly sensitive marker**
- Component of the secretory granules of neuroendocrine tumors, together with other peptide hormones
- Nearly always detectable with metastatic tumors

5-Hydroxyindole Acetic Acid (5-HIAA)

- Main degradation product of serotonin (detected in 24-hour urine)
- Regularly elevated levels in carcinoid syndrome and thus a sensitive and specific marker, especially for NETs of the midgut

Neuron-Specific Enolase and Synaptophysin

- Expressed in the cytoplasm independent of specific hormone secretion
- Highly specific markers for NETs

Peptide Hormones

- Expressed by both neuroendocrine cells and NETs
- More than 12 different peptide hormones known currently, but only a few are expressed by NETs (e.g., gastrin, insulin, glucagon, somatostatin, vasoactive intestinal peptide)

■ Diagnostic Imaging

Computed Tomography, Magnetic Resonance Imaging, and Positron Emission Tomography

- **High-resolution diagnostic imaging**
- Cross-sectional imaging methods such as CT, MRI and PET are used for localization and to look for metastases.
- Because of the multislice technique, similar sensitivity and specificity can now be obtained with CT as with endosonography.

Scintigraphy

- **Somatostatin receptor scintigraphy, only if receptor-positive**
- Somatostatin receptor scintigraphy can discover both the primary tumors and metastases in the event of receptor positivity.
- Basis: overexpression of somatostatin receptors in NETs.
- Tumors > ca. 1 cm diameter are detectable.
- Sensitivity is between 70% and 90% and specificity is up to 90%.
- Hindgut tumors and poorly differentiated neuroendocrine carcinomas are often receptor-negative and therefore elude scintigraphy.

■ Invasive Investigations

Endoscopy
- For diagnostic localization in the esophagus, stomach, duodenum, pancreas, small bowel, colon, and rectum
- To obtain material for histology:
  - ► Uniform cell picture, neurosecretory granules
  - ► Only clear criteria of malignancy: infiltration of neighboring organs or established metastasis
  - ► Characterization of the degree of malignancy from a biopsy is therefore difficult.
  - ► The degree of malignancy is assessed by other parameters such as tumor size and location, rate of mitosis, proliferation index (K_i-67), and immunohistochemical stains (peptide hormones, chromogranin A, synaptophysin, neuron-specific enolase).
- Endosonographic determination of the depth of infiltration and of enlarged locoregional lymph nodes

- Endoscopy with endosonography
- Histological assessment of malignancy is difficult

Treatment Approach

■ Conservative Treatment

Symptomatic Treatment
- Long-acting **somatostatin analogues** (octreotide, lanreotide) and interferon-α to control the hypersecretion syndromes appear to possess an anti-proliferative effect in addition.

- Somatostatin analogues to control the hypersecretion syndromes

Chemotherapy
- Response rate to chemotherapy of well-differentiated neuroendocrine tumors is low at < 30%.
- Effective substances: doxorubicin, fluoropyrimidine, streptozotocin, alkylating agents
- Rapidly growing anaplastic carcinomas: combined therapy with cisplatin and etoposide

Radiotherapy
- Peptide receptor-mediated radiotherapy as a further conservative treatment possibility
- Administration of a somatostatin analogue labeled with a source of β-radiation (e.g., ^{90}yttrium), which is taken up by the tumor tissue rapidly and selectively. The following are suitable for such therapy:
  - ► Patients with hepatic/extrahepatic metastases and slowly growing tumors that have been shown to respond poorly to chemotherapy, and in whom the surgical possibilities for tumor resection have been exhausted
  - ► Patients with hepatic metastases who exhibit disease progression on octreotide therapy or combined biotherapy
  - ► Patients with marked clinical symptoms (diarrhea, flushing, weight loss) who continue to be symptomatic despite high-dose octreotide therapy

- Peptide receptor-mediated radiotherapy as palliative therapy

22

Radiotherapy
- Percutaneous radiotherapy is possible after failure of all the aforementioned treatment methods.
- High-precision radiation using stereotactic methods: high local effect, low morbidity of the surrounding healthy tissue, and sometimes high response rates

■ Surgical Treatment

- RO resection is the only curative approach

- Complete endoscopic removal of small tumors
- Surgical RO resection is the only curative approach
- RO resection of metastases with curative intent is rational
- With inoperable tumors and advanced metastasis, tumor debulking to prolong life or for palliation of tumor-associated hormone effects
- Chemoembolization, thermoablation, or alcohol injection of inoperable liver metastases

Prognosis

- The biological behavior and thus the prognosis of the different endocrine tumors are highly variable.
- The degree of differentiation, location, and presence of metastases are the most important prognostic parameters.

Stomach (Table 22.4)

Etiology

- NETs develop from the histamine-producing enterochromaffinlike (ECL) cells of the stomach.
- The main cause of tumor development in types I and II is hypergastrinemia caused by type A gastritis or gastrinoma.
- Tumor develops via the hyperplasia–dysplasia–neoplasia sequence.
- The pathogenesis of type III and IV is as yet unclear.

Symptoms

- Small tumors are usually asymptomatic.
- Large lesions become apparent depending on their location.
- Metastases occur only with tumor size over 2 cm.
- Flushing symptoms are possible with liver metastases.

Prognosis

- Types I and II have a good prognosis; annual endoscopic follow-up recommended following removal.
- Type III: average survival is 2–4 years.
- Type IV corresponds to a small cell carcinoma with very poor prognosis; ca. 75% of patients die in the first year after the diagnosis is made.

Duodenum and pancreas—Insulinoma (Table 22.5)

Epidemiology

- Most common NET of the pancreas

- Incidence: 0.5 per 1000 000 population per year
- Usually occurs between the ages of 30 and 60 years
- The most common NET of the pancreas, accounting for 40%–70%

Table 22.4 Neuroendocrine tumors of the stomach

Type	Incidence Age distribution M : F	Associated with	Additional findings	Functional	Tumor localization/characteristics	Differentiation	Metastases	Treatment
I	70–80% 50–60 y F > M	Type A gastritis, pernicious anemia	Hypergastrinemia, ECL cell hyperplasia	Inactive	Body/fundus usually < 1 cm Multiple, mucosa/submucosa	Highly differentiated, benign/low malignancy	Up to 8%	Endoscopic removal, excision if appropriate
II	3% ca. 45 y M = F	MEN I	Hypergastrinemia, ECL cell hyperplasia	Inactive	Body/fundus > 1–2 cm Multiple, mucosa/submucosa	Highly differentiated, benign/low malignancy	Up to 8%	Endoscopic removal, excision or resection if appropriate
III	15% ca. 50 y M > F	Sporadic		Inactive	Ubiquitous ca. 30% > 2 cm Solitary	Highly differentiated, low malignancy	Up to 8%	Subtotal gastrectomy, gastrectomy with lymphadenectomy if appropriate
IV	< 2% > 60 y M > F	–		Inactive	Usually > 5 cm	Poorly differentiated, highly malignant	Up to 8%	Extent of resection corresponds to adenocarcinoma of the stomach

ECL: enterochromaffinlike.

22

Etiology

- Usually very small tumors with autonomic insulin and proinsulin secretion, located almost exclusively in the pancreas
- 5%–10% of the tumors occur as part of MEN I syndrome and are then usually multiple.

Symptoms

- Whipple triad: hypoglyce-mic symptoms, fasting blood glucose < 40 mg/dL, improvement after admin-istration of glucose

- The Whipple triad is typical
  - ► Hypoglycemic symptoms
  - ► Fasting blood glucose < 40 mg/dL
  - ► Instant improvement after administration of glucose
- Neuroglycopenic symptoms such as poor concentration, dizziness, tremor, loss of consciousness, or seizure are common.
- Tendency to obesity due to increased food intake

Diagnostic Approach

- Fasting test: low blood glucose level, high insulin level
- Intraoperative ultrasonog-raphy very sensitive with the often-small tumors

- Fasting test: regular measurement of blood glucose, insulin, and C-peptide (to rule out factitious hypoglycemia). Blood glucose levels below 40 mg/dL with simultaneously elevated insulin and C-peptide levels over 7 µg/mL are proof.
- Preoperative localization investigations are difficult because the lesions are usually small.
- Endosonography is the most sensitive method.
- Somatostatin receptor scintigraphy is successful in only 60% of cases as re-ceptor expression is low.
- Intraoperative ultrasonography is markedly superior to all other methods.

Treatment Approach

- Enucleation of small tu-mors
- Resection of multiple or malignant tumors
- Diazoxide and slowly ab-sorbed carbohydrates to reduce the tendency to hypoglycemia

- Cure only through a surgical procedure
- Benign tumors in the majority of cases, so enucleation sufficient
- Resecting procedures also with multiple tumors (e.g., distal pancreatectomy or duodenum-preserving resection of the head of the pancreas)
- Malignant insulinoma: resection with lymphadenectomy
- Tumor debulking can be useful for symptom control in advanced disease.
- The tendency to hypoglycemia can be reduced by diazoxide and frequent small meals with slowly absorbed carbohydrates.
- Somatostatin analogues, effective only with receptor-positive tumors
- Streptozotocin, 5-fluorouracil, and doxorubicin for palliative chemotherapy

Prognosis

- Malignant insulinoma: the 5-year survival rate is 60%.

Duodenum and Pancreas—Gastrinoma (Table 22.5)

Epidemiology

- Incidence: 1–5 per 1 000 000 population per year
- Manifestation between the 3rd and 5th decades

Table 22.5   Neuroendocrine tumors of the pancreas and duodenum

	Nature	Symptoms	Location	MEN I-associated	Treatment
Insulinoma	90% benign	Whipple triad: hypoglycemia, blood glucose < 40 mg/dL, instant improvement after giving glucose	Pancreas	5%–10%	Enucleation
Gastrinoma	60% malignant	Zollinger–Ellison syndrome: recurrent ulcers, diarrhea	Pancreas, duodenum	25%–40%	Surgical resection, somatostatin analogues, palliative chemotherapy, possibly radionuclide therapy if appropriate, proton pump inhibitors
Glucagonoma	> 60% malignant	Diabetes mellitus, necrolytic migratory erythema	Tail of pancreas	3%	Surgical resection, tumor debulking if appropriate, somatostatin analogues effective in 50% of patients, palliative chemotherapy
Somatostatinoma	> 75% malignant	Diabetes mellitus, cholecystolithiasis, steatorrhea	Pancreas, duodenum	7%	Surgical resection, tumor debulking if appropriate, cholecystectomy
Vipoma	40–60% malignant	Verner–Morrison syndrome (WDHH): watery diarrhea, hypokalemia, hypochlorhydria	Pancreas	1%	Surgical resection, tumor debulking if appropriate, somatostatin analogues, palliative chemotherapy, volume and K^+ replacement

22

- The second most common NET of the pancreas, accounting for ca. 10%–20% of cases

Etiology

- Ectopic autonomic gastrin secretion leads to gastric hyperacidity and multiple ulcers.
- Inactivation of digestive enzymes and villous atrophy of the duodenal mucosa due to hyperacidity leads to diarrhea.
- About 40% of sporadic gastrinomas are located in the pancreas or duodenum, 80%–90% of them to the right of the superior mesenteric artery in the so-called gastrinoma triangle (**Fig. 22.1**).
- About 25% of gastrinomas occur as part of MEN I syndrome, often multiple and located almost exclusively in the pancreas.

- Frequently located in the gastrinoma triangle

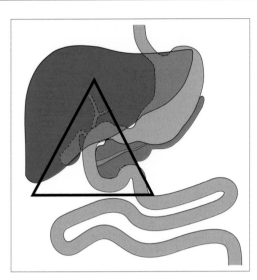

Fig. 22.1 Gastrinoma triangle (head of pancreas–duodenal C–distal common bile duct).

Symptoms

- Treatment-refractory ulcers of the upper gastrointestinal tract

- Treatment-refractory ulcers of the upper gastrointestinal tract due to hyperacidity
- In addition, diarrhea, pain, and vomiting

Diagnostic Approach

- Fasting hypergastrinemia, secretin test
- Chromogranin A usually positive
- Small tumors detected by somatostatin receptor scintigraphy

- Most sensitive screening test: evidence of fasting hypergastrinemia (positive in 90% of patients)
- Suggestive: combination of fasting hypergastrinemia > 1000 pg/mL (475 pmol/L) with intragastric pH < 2.5
- Gastrin level between 150 and 1000 pg/mL confirms the diagnosis by the secretin test (difference between basal and stimulated gastrin concentration > 200 pg/mL after administration of 2 IU secretin/kg body weight IV)
- Chromogranin A elevated in 80%–100% of cases
- Tumor detection by imaging is often difficult in the case of small tumors; lesions located in the duodenum in particular are often less than 1 cm in size.
- Detection of small lesions is possible by somatostatin receptor scintigraphy.

Treatment Approach

- Lifelong proton pump inhibitors
- Somatostatin analogues
- Enucleation or resection with lymphadenectomy

- **Medical:** lifelong acid block with proton pump inhibitors
- Metastases: chemotherapy with 5-fluorouracil, doxorubicin, and streptozotocin, and biotherapy with somatostatin analogues; consider radionuclide treatment if appropriate
- **Surgical removal** by enucleation or resection as attempt at cure
- Lymph node metastases are already present in over 50% of patients, so lymph node dissection is obligatory.
- MEN I-associated gastrinomas must be resected only above a size of 2 cm on account of their low risk of degeneration.

Prognosis

- Slightly aggressive tumor growth in about 75% of patients with a 10-year survival rate of 96%
- Behaves aggressively in 25% of patients with a 10-year survival rate of 30%
- MEN I-associated gastrinomas have a better prognosis than sporadic gastrinomas.

Ileum

Epidemiology

- Incidence: 0.89 per 100 000 population per year (most common site of NET manifestation)
- Main age of manifestation is between the ages of 50 and 60 years.
- About 35% of patients have multiple tumors.

Etiology

- Tumors arise from serotonin-producing enterochromaffin cells.
- They are usually located in the terminal ileum.
- They are usually larger than 2 cm at the time of diagnosis and infiltrating the muscularis propria, so that ca. 35% of patients have lymph node metastases and ca. 20% of patients have liver metastases.
- Besides serotonin, other biogenic amines such as bradykinin and kallikrein also cause carcinoid syndrome.

- Usually located in the terminal ileum
- Malignant, lymph node or liver metastases often already present

Symptoms

- Carcinoid syndrome (ca. 10% of cases) with flushing, diarrhea, and endocardial fibrosis (Hedinger disease) only when liver metastases are present
- In the absence of liver metastasis, complete serotonin degradation in the liver (first-pass effect)
- The endocardial fibrosis leads to right-heart failure due to tricuspid and pulmonary valve insufficiency (most common cause of death)
- Frequent cramplike abdominal pains due to fibrosis in the mesentery (desmoplastic reaction) as a result of autocrine release of tumor products; bowel ischemia in worst case
- Rare symptoms: bleeding, cough, dyspnea, telangiectasias, and hyperpigmentation

- Carcinoid syndrome (flushing, diarrhea, endocardial fibrosis) only with liver metastases
- Right-heart failure as a result of endocardial fibrosis is the most common cause of death.
- Cramplike abdominal pains due to desmoplastic reaction of the mesentery with risk of bowel ischemia

22

Diagnostic Approach

- Lead parameter: 5-HIAA in acidulated 24-hour urine with sensitivity and specificity > 90%
- Serum chromogranin A: sensitive but nonspecific
- Echocardiography to diagnose endocardial fibrosis and its consequences

- Lead parameter: 5-HIAA level in urine
- Serum chromogranin A level
- Echocardiography

Treatment Approach

- **Medical:** somatostatin analogues and interferon-α as biotherapy
- Palliative chemotherapy is possible.

- Somatostatin analogues, interferon-α, palliative chemotherapy

- Radical resection with lymphadenectomy with curative intent

- **Surgical:** Because of the high risk of metastasis, a radical procedure with segmental small bowel resection including locoregional lymphadenectomy is indicated (attempt at cure).
- Second tumors must be ruled out at operation.
- Resection of isolated liver metastases is undertaken with curative intent.
- Advanced disease: tumor debulking is done to control the carcinoid syndrome.

Prognosis

- The 5-year survival rates are 75% with locally limited tumor, 60% with lymph node metastases, and 20%–25% with liver metastases.

Vermiform Appendix

Epidemiology

- Most frequent site of manifestation of gastrointestinal NET

- NET of the appendix is the most common of all gastrointestinal NETs at 30%–45%.
- NETs are found in 3–7 per 1000 appendectomies, usually as an incidental finding.
- Usually, younger patients are affected (in the 3rd or 4th decade).

Etiology

- Usually, serotonin-producing tumors at the appendix tip

- Tumor occurs at the tip of the appendix in ca. 70% of cases.
- It usually produces serotonin.
- When the tumor is < 1 cm, benign behavior can be assumed in over 90% of cases.
- Tumors between 1 and 2 cm in size exhibit uncertain behavior but with a low risk of metastasis, up to 1%.
- Malignant behavior can be expected when the tumor is > 2 cm (risk of metastasis between 20% and 85%).
- Other risk factors for unfavorable behavior: location near the base, lymphatic invasion, infiltration of the serosa or mesoappendix, poor differentiation

22

Symptoms

- Symptoms correspond to acute appendicitis

- Patients are usually operated on for suspected appendicitis.
- Carcinoid syndrome is rare, in < 1% of cases, and is an expression of liver metastasis.

Diagnostic Approach

- Usually an incidental finding, so no preoperative investigations are performed
- Postoperative staging investigations (CT of abdomen, possibly somatostatin receptor scintigraphy) if there is a risk of metastasis

Treatment Approach

- Tumors < 1 cm: appendectomy is sufficient; ileocecal resection is indicated if located close to the base

- Tumors > 2 cm: right hemicolectomy with locoregional lymphadenectomy is necessary
- Tumors between 1 and 2 cm with risk factors (see above): radical operation
- Resection of isolated liver metastases with curative intent
- In advanced stages of tumor, especially with functional activity: operative debulking is performed, or somatostatin analogues or interferon-α is administered systemically to control the hormonal syndrome.

- Appendectomy/ileocecal resection for benign tumors
- Radical resection with lymphadenectomy with curative intent
- Somatostatin analogues, interferon-α, palliative chemotherapy

Prognosis

- The 5-year survival rate is 90%–100% after operative treatment.

Colon

Epidemiology

- Incidence: 0.10–0.31 per 100 000 population per year (very rare)
- Average disease age: ca. 65 years

Etiology

- Located in the right hemicolon in 50% of cases (high density of enterochromaffin cells)
- Usually, poorly differentiated carcinomas with a high potential for metastasis

- Usually, malignant tumors in the right hemicolon

Symptoms

- Nonspecific and similar to those of colon cancer
- Carcinoid syndrome is an exception

- Nonspecific, corresponding to colon cancer

Diagnostic Approach

- Corresponds to the procedure for colon cancer
- When the histology is undifferentiated, always consider the diagnosis of neuroendocrine carcinoma.
- 5-HIAA is found only rarely (especially with highly differentiated NETs of the right hemicolon).

Treatment Approach

- Chemotherapy for poorly differentiated tumors
- Surgical treatment as for colon cancer
- Tumor debulking or treatment with somatostatin analogues or interferon-α for inoperable, highly differentiated and hormonally active tumors

- Resection as for colon cancer

Prognosis

- The 5-year survival rate over all stages is 40%.

22

Rectum

Epidemiology

- Incidence: 0.1–0.14 per 100 000 population per year (very rare)
- Average disease age: between 52 and 59 years

Symptoms

- Usually asymptomatic and an incidental endoscopic finding

- Usually asymptomatic with incidental diagnosis during endoscopic examination
- Rarely, bleeding or constipation
- Never with carcinoid syndrome

Diagnostic Approach

- On endoscopy, firm lesions in submucosal location with a yellowish appearance
- With tumors > 2 cm, staging investigations as for rectal cancer (rate of metastasis between 67% and 100%)

Treatment Approach

- Transanal wedge resection possible for small tumors
- Radical resection for larger lesions without distant metastases

- Tumors < 2 cm, T1/T2, N0 on endosonography: transanal wedge resection
- Tumors > 2 cm, T3/T4 lesion or evidence of locoregional lymph node involvement, provided patient is of M0 status: radical resection
- M1 situation: palliative primary tumor resection, palliative chemotherapy

Prognosis

- The 5-year survival rate is between 80% and 90% for local disease, but only 7%–18% for patients with distant metastases.
- Often diagnosed at an early stage with good overall prognosis

22

■ Gastrointestinal Stromal Tumors

Definition

- Most common mesenchymal tumor of the gastrointestinal tract
- Usually located in the stomach and small bowel

- Most common mesenchymal tumors of the gastrointestinal tract (ca. 1% of all gastrointestinal malignancies)
- Can occur anywhere from esophagus to rectum, and rarely also in the mesentery (stomach 40%–70%, small bowel 20%–35%, colon 10%, esophagus < 5%)
- Nearly always sporadic
- Macroscopically, roundish tumors without a capsule, sharply demarcated from their surroundings
- Soft tumors that rupture easily on manipulation
- Spindle-celled (ca. 70%) and epithelioid (ca. 30%) growth pattern on histology

Epidemiology

- Incidence: ca. 15 per 1 000 000 population per year
- Median age: 55–65 years
- Men affected somewhat more than women.

Etiology

- Cell of origin: Cajal cell located in the muscularis propria of the bowel wall
- Acts as an intestinal pacemaker cell to control bowel motility
- The trigger for development of a gastrointestinal stromal tumor (GIST) is so far unclear.
- The cause is a mutation in the c-KIT gene (80%–85%) or in the PDGFR gene (5%–10%), which code for tyrosine kinases (receptor proteins).
- Through the mutations, uncontrolled sustained activation occurs whereby cell growth is accelerated and apoptosis is inhibited.
- Different mutation sites are known (in c-KIT, exon 9 and exon 11 are affected in particular at 10% and 60%–70%, respectively).
- Assessment of the efficacy of the tyrosine kinase inhibitors when the exact mutation site is known
- GISTs exhibit extremely heterogeneous biological behavior.
- Even small tumors with a low mitosis rate have a potential for metastasis in principle (clear classification into benign and malignant tumors not possible because of the absence of classical histomorphological criteria of malignancy).
- Risk assessment according to tumor size and mitosis rate (**Table 22.6**) and according to the location (GISTs of the stomach has a better prognosis than GISTs of the small or large bowel).

- Cell of origin: Cajal cell in the muscularis propria (pacemaker cell)
- Mutations usually in the c-KIT gene, lead to sustained activation of the corresponding tyrosine kinase
- Very heterogeneous biological behavior
- Risk assessment according to size, mitosis rate, and location

Symptoms

- Uncharacteristic and dependent on location
- In ca. 20% of patients, incidental finding during diagnostic or operative procedures for other indications
- In ca. 40% of patients, gastrointestinal bleeding or abdominal pain, palpable mass in 30% of patients, more rarely dysphagia (esophagus) or obstruction (small bowel)
- In ca. 50% of patients, there are already metastases at the time of the initial diagnosis (frequently the liver [65%] and peritoneum [20%]; lung, bone, and lymph nodes are only affected rarely).

- Uncharacteristic and dependent on the location
- In ca. 50% of patients metastasis already present at the time of initial diagnosis, especially in liver and peritoneum

22

Table 22.6 Assessment of the risk for aggressive behavior with gastrointestinal stromal tumors

Risk behavior	Size (cm)	Mitosis rate (per 50 HPF)	Frequency
Very low	< 2	< 5	12%
Low	2–5	< 5	33%
Intermediate	< 5	6–10	20%
	5–10	< 5	
High	> 5	> 5	23%
	> 10	any	
	any	> 10	

Source: From Fletcher CD, Berman JJ, Corless C, et al. Diagnosis of gastrointestinal stromal tumors: a consensus approach. Int J Surg Pathol 2002;10:81–89.

Diagnostic Approach

- Most important diagnostic investigation is endoscopy with endosonography
- Staging investigations: CT, MRI, abdominal ultrasonography
- FDG-PET: assessment of progress on systemic therapy with imatinib

- Most important diagnostic method is gastrointestinal endoscopy: tumors appear as a hemispherical submucosal bulge covered with intact mucosa; mucosal ulcers and bleeding are possible with large tumors.
- Well-demarcated lesions with a hypoechoic pattern on endosonography
- CT, MRI and abdominal ultrasonography to assess local tumor spread and to detect metastases (liver, peritoneum)
- FDG(Fluordesoxyglucose)-PET provides information about the vitality of the tumor cells, which is important for assessing progress during systemic therapy with imatinib
- By the pathologist: detection of c-KIT (CD 117), determination of the mitosis rate and mutation analysis

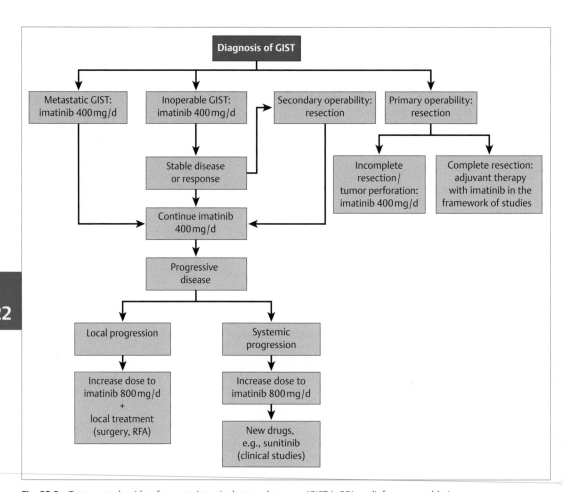

Fig. 22.2 Treatment algorithm for gastrointestinal stromal tumors (GISTs). RFA, radiofrequency ablation.

Treatment Approach (Fig. 22.2)

■ Conservative Treatment

- Conventional radiotherapy or chemotherapy has hardly any effect (response rates < 5%).
- The tyrosine kinase inhibitor imatinib (e.g., Glivec; **Table 22.7**) has been approved since 2002 for systemic therapy.
- Competitive inhibition of c-KIT tyrosine kinase prevents sustained activation of this receptor.
- Currently approved for the treatment of patients with metastatic or unresectable GISTs, after incomplete resection or intraoperative tumor perforation
- Partial remission rates of 66% but no complete remission or cure possible
- With genetic resistance due to secondary mutation, consider treatment with other inhibitors (e.g., sumatinib).

- Systemic therapy with tyrosine kinase inhibitor imatinib for metastatic or unresectable GIST or after R1 resection

Table 22.7 Facts about imatinib

Drug:	Imatinib mesilate
Product name	e.g., Glivec
Mechanism of action	Tyrosine kinase inhibitor
Inhibited enzymes	c-KIT, PDGFR, Bcr-Abl
Approved for	Metastatic, inoperable GISTs
Planned future license	Adjuvant, neoadjuvant therapy, combination therapy if progression
Dosage	400 mg/d p.o.
	800 mg/d p.o. if exon 9 mutation or progression
Side effects	Edema, nausea, diarrhea, muscle cramps, fatigue, bleeding

■ Surgical Treatment

- Surgical R0 resection with a safety margin of ca. 2 cm is the "gold standard."
- Intraoperative tumor perforation must be avoided (**caution:** soft consistency), otherwise an R1 situation may result with high risk for locoregional recurrence.
- Lymph node dissection is not necessary, as lymphatogenous metastasis rates are below 5%, therefore limited resections such as partial stomach wall resection, segmental small bowel resection or transanal wedge resection of the rectum are sufficient oncologically, depending on the tumor size.
- With locally advanced tumors multivisceral R0 resection is indicated.

- R0 resection is the "gold standard."
- Intraoperative tumor perforation must be avoided.

22

Follow-up

- No controlled data available on follow-up
- Structured follow-up is rational after R0 resection of a GIST with intermediate or high risk, because of the high risk of recurrence (recurrence rate up to 54%)
- Physical examination, abdominal ultrasonography, and possibly CT/MRI of the abdomen at 6-month intervals in the first 5 years, then annually
- When the primary tumor organ is accessible, endosonography after 6 months and after 2 and 5 years

Prognosis

- The 5-year survival rate is ca. 50% after R0 resection.
- Median survival time is 19 months with metastatic disease, 12 months with local recurrence.
- The risk of recurrence within the first 5 years after R0 resection is ca. 50%.
- The 3-year survival rate of metastatic GIST has improved to 68% due to the introduction of the tyrosine kinase inhibitor imatinib.

Further Reading

Das Lebenshaus. Im Internet: http://www.lh-gist.org

Füzesi L. Gastrointestinaler Stromatumor: Pathologie. Viszeralchirurgie 2003; 38: 358–362

Grimm O, Dralle H. Chirurgische Therapie neuroendokriner Tumoren von Pankreas, Magen und Duodenum. Onkologe 2004; 10: 1042–1053

Hohenberger P, Wardelmann E. Gastrointestinale Stromatumoren. Chirurg 2006; 77: 33–40

Hohenberger P. GIST – klinische Problemstellungen und offene Fragen. Viszeralchirurgie 2007; 42: 55–60

Klöppel G, Anlauf M, Lüttges J. Klassifikation und Pathologie der neuroendokrinen Tumoren des Magen-Darm-Trakts und Pankreas. Onkologe 2004; 10: 570–579

Plöckinger U, Wiedenmann B. Neuroendokrine Tumoren des Gastrointestinaltrakts. Zeitschrift für Gastroenterologie 2004; 42: 517–526

Source

WHO classification of neuroendocrine tumors of the digestive tract (2000)

23 Soft-Tissue Tumors

H. Brunn

Definition

- Tumors originating in mesenchymal tissue

Epidemiology

- Over 90% of soft-tissue tumors are benign; fibromas and lipomas are the most common.
- Malignant soft-tissue tumors account for about 0.5%–1% of all malignant tumors (but ca. 6%–8% of all childhood malignancies):
  - ► Liposarcoma and leiomyosarcoma are the most common.
  - ► Rhabdomyosarcoma is the most frequent soft-tissue sarcoma in childhood.
- 15% of soft-tissue tumors are located centrally: retroperitoneum, mesentery, mediastinum
- 85% are peripheral soft-tissue tumors: limbs, trunk, head, neck
- The limbs are the most common site.
- Soft-tissue tumors can occur at any age but the incidence increases in older people.

- > 90% of soft-tissue tumors are benign
- Most common site: limbs

Classification

- Tumors can be benign, malignant, and intermediate (biological behavior not assessable with certainty (**Table 23.1**).
- All soft-tissue tumors must be considered malignant until proven otherwise (regardless of site and size).

- Consider all soft-tissue tumors malignant until proven otherwise

Table 23.1 Classification of soft-tissue tumors (examples of the most common tumors)

Tissue of origin	Benign tumors	Malignant tumors
Connective tissue	Fibroma	Fibrosarcoma
Fat tissue	Lipoma	Liposarcoma
Smooth muscle	Leiomyoma	Leiomyosarcoma
Striated muscle	Rhabdomyoma	Rhabdomyosarcoma
Blood vessels	Hemangioma	Angiosarcoma
Lymphatics	Lymphangioma	Lymphangiosarcoma
Peripheral nerve tissue	Schwannoma	Malignant schwannoma
	Neurofibroma	Clear cell sarcoma
Bone and cartilage	Chondroma	Osteosarcoma
		Chondrosarcoma

23

Classification of Malignant Soft-Tissue Tumors
- These are classified both according to UICC stages and according to the TNM system.
- An important distinction is made clinically between
  ► high-grade sarcomas (poorly differentiated, high potential for metastasis), and
  ► low-grade sarcomas (highly differentiated, low potential for metastasis).

Symptoms

Peripheral Soft-Tissue Tumors

- If tumor is not visible externally, diagnosis is often made late because of the uncharacteristic symptoms.

- A painless swelling is the main symptom.
- Pain usually occurs only when neighboring structures (e.g., nerves, vessels, organs) are affected or compressed.

Central Soft-Tissue Tumors
- Uncharacteristic symptoms depending on site and size.

Additional Symptoms
These characteristics make a malignant tumor more likely:
- Rapid growth
- B symptoms (pyrexia, weight loss, night sweats)

Diagnostic Approach

■ Clinical Examination

- Size
- Consistency
- Mobility

■ Diagnostic Imaging

- MRI is method of choice.

- Ultrasonography
- MRI is the method of choice (better contrast between tumor and its surroundings than CT).

Search for Metastases
- Locoregional (e.g., lymph nodes)
- Extraregional (examination of metastasizing organs)
- Systemic (bone scintigraphy, positron emission tomography)

■ Invasive Investigations

Confirmation of Diagnosis by Biopsy
- **Excision biopsy:** Radical removal of tumors < 5 cm with a margin, without injuring functionally important surrounding tissue.
- **Incision biopsy:** Determination of the degree of malignancy and tumor type, biopsy size ca. 2 × 1 cm. **Caution:** incision. Soft-tissue sarcomas have a high tendency to shed tumor cells. Whenever possible, the incision should be within the planned later resection area.

23

Treatment Approach

■ Conservative Treatment

Adjuvant Chemotherapy

- Shrinking of primary tumor, thereby avoiding mutilating operations that interfere with function
- Reduction of distant metastases
- Improvement of prognosis

Indications
- High-grade sarcomas
- Primary radical surgery, not possible

■ Surgical Treatment

Operation Tactics

- Soft-tissue sarcomas are surrounded by a margin infiltrated by tumor (pseudocapsule), which should also be removed, to avoid recurrences.
- Sarcomas spread initially in a longitudinal direction along anatomical planes or within the muscles of a compartment. Transverse spread (e.g., through fascia) occurs relatively late.
- Many tumors can be reduced in size by the use of adjuvant chemoradiotherapy, so that R0 resection or limb-preserving surgery is possible.

Limited Resection (Excision Biopsy)

- Removal of the tumor with a narrow margin of healthy tissue.

Indications
- Benign soft-tissue tumors
- Small peripheral soft-tissue sarcomas
- Central soft-tissue tumors growing in close relation to vital structures, only in conjunction with chemoradiotherapy

Wide Resection (Limited Radical Resection)

- Tumor excision with the greatest possible safety margin taking function into account, removing adjacent structures (fascia, vascular adventitia, perineurium, periosteum) as far as possible. Soft-tissue reconstruction is by local advancement flap and/or split skin graft.

Indications
- Small soft-tissue sarcomas of the limbs; with high-grade sarcomas chemotherapy and/or radiotherapy is necessary
- Low-grade sarcomas

Compartment Resection

- Complete removal of the entire compartment containing the tumor (e.g., muscles, arteries/veins/nerves), followed by reconstruction of the structures (e.g., vessel and nerve replacement, restoration of joint function by muscle transposition). This is therefore a limb-preserving operation.
- **Caution:** The resection is not possible when the sarcoma is in a primary extracompartmental site, for example, in the curve of a joint (e.g., popliteal fossa/groin) or in the distal forearm.

- Not feasible when the sarcoma is in a primary extracompartmental site.

23

Indications
- Soft-tissue sarcomas in the muscle compartments. The affected muscles must always be removed from their origin to their insertion. This removes skip metastases (discontinuous spread of the tumor to connective tissue septa, muscles, or tendons).

Amputation
- The amputation level depends on the affected muscles. All bony origins of the tumor-containing muscle groups must be removed. Amputation does not always signify greater radicality.

Indications
- Large sarcomas of the limbs invading joints or nonreconstructable large nerves (e.g., plexus) and vessels, when compartment resection is not possible.

Supraradical Procedures
- Disarticulation, interscapular thoracic amputation (arm amputation with the shoulder girdle and axillary contents), hemipelvectomy

Indications
- Sarcomas very close to joints and invading the joints

Intralesional Resection
- Palliative tumor debulking
- Resection through the tumor; R0 resection cannot be achieved.

Indications
- Frequently with abdominal sarcomas, chemoradiotherapy is necessary
- Palliative tumor debulking

Prognosis
Unfavorable Prognostic Factors
- Low degree of tumor differentiation
- Tumor size
- Increasing tumor stage
- Deep location
- Located in the trunk or head and neck region
- Advanced patient age

Recurrence Rate
- Wide resection:
  - ► Without adjuvant therapy, 40%–60% risk of local recurrence
  - ► Good local tumor control with adjuvant radiotherapy
- Compartment resection: local recurrence rate 0–10%
- Intralesional resection: local recurrence rate 100%

Further Reading
Feuerbach S, Schreyer A, Schlottmann K. Standards radiologisch bildgesteuerter Biopsien – Indikationsstellung, Technik, Komplikationen. Radiologie up2date 2003; 3: 207–224

Müller J-S, Grote R, Lippert H. Die bildgebende Diagnostik bei Weichteiltumoren. Viszeralchirurgie 2001; 36: 209–221

Prietzel T, Schmidt C, von Salis-Soglio G. Benigne Tumoren der Bewegungsorgane. Orthopädie und Unfallchirurgie up2date 2008; 3: 247–276

23

24 Vascular Surgery

A. Selch

■ Arteries

Anatomy

- The walls of all arteries consist of three layers:
  - ► **Tunica intima** consisting of a layer of endothelial cells and a layer of connective tissue (internal elastic lamina)
  - ► **Tunica media** consisting of circularly arranged elastic membranes (e.g., aorta) or smooth muscle (e.g., limb arteries) to which the external elastic lamina is attached
  - ► **Tunica adventitia,** outer layer with autonomic nerve network and vasa vasorum
- Types:
  - ► **Elastic type:** aorta, initial segments of large arteries; "windkessel" effect due to concentrically arranged elastic membranes
  - ► **Muscular type:** predominates in peripheral arteries; blood flow is regulated by changes in vessel diameter
- Age-related changes: reduction in elastic longitudinal tension, thickening of the tunica intima (**physiosclerosis**), atrophy of the tunica media, and thickening of the tunica adventitia

- Three-layer wall structure

Vessel Replacement

Autologous Veins
- Best results with regard to incorporation, infection risk, and service life of the graft. The disadvantage is the time required for harvesting and preparing the vein. Wound infections and scarring problems in the saphenous vein donor site are described.
- Vein bypass can be performed as reverse or in situ bypass.
  - ► **Reverse bypass:** complete removal of the vein, used in reversed direction
  - ► **In situ bypass:** vein is left in situ and valves are destroyed with a valvulotome

- Best results with regard to incorporation, infection risk, and service life

Synthetic Vessel Replacement
- Replacement of large-lumen vessels (e.g., aorta). Consists of **polyester** or **polytetrafluorethylene (PTFE)**.
- **Dacron grafts** (polyester) vary in their porosity and must be sealed by preclotting prior to anastomosis. Dacron grafts exhibit good tissue compatibility, grow into the tissue and form a neointima. Velour modification of the graft surface can be effected, either on the inside only (**velour graft**), or inside and outside (**double velour graft**).
- A primary seal of Dacron grafts can be achieved by coating the surface, for example, with gelatin, collagen, or albumins, and preclotting can be omitted.
- **PTFE grafts** are nonporous and have a smooth surface, so small diameters (down to 4 mm) are possible, though the occlusion rate increases considerably with decreasing graft diameter. PTFE grafts do not heal into the sur-

24

rounding tissue as well as Dacron grafts (**perigraft reaction**). They are reinforced with rings or spirals when they cross joints or pass through scar tissue.

General Diagnostic Approach

- History, clinical examination, and investigations

■ Diagnostic Imaging

- **Oscillography, rheography, Doppler ultrasonography** and **duplex ultrasonography**. Can be repeated as often as desired; used for screening and follow-up. Baseline for further invasive investigations.

■ Invasive Investigations

- Risk of local or systemic complications
- **Arteriography, digital subtraction angiography, angio-CT,** and **magnetic resonance angiography**. Enable accurate imaging of pathomorphological vessel changes.
- Invasive vessel investigations can cause local or systemic **complications:**
  - ► Local complications occur at the puncture site: these include hematoma, aneurysm of the vessel wall, and arteriovenous fistulas. Vessel stenosis and occlusion are also possible.
  - ► Systemic complications include allergic reactions to the contrast agent, worsening of pre-existing renal failure, or contrast agent-induced hyperthyroidism.

Vascular Injuries

Classification

- A distinction is made between **direct vascular injuries,** in which the vessel wall is penetrated from without inward (laceration, stab wound, gunshot, etc.), and **indirect blunt vascular injuries** or deceleration trauma with injury of the vessel wall from within. Possible consequences are reduced peripheral perfusion or complete vascular occlusion due to intima and media injury with subsequent curling-in and deposition of thrombus on the injured vessel wall.
- Vollmar classification of vascular injuries (**Fig. 24.1**)

Treatment Approach

■ Surgical Treatment

- Restoration of arterial perfusion
- The aim of treatment is restoration of arterial perfusion within the ischemic tolerance period.

24

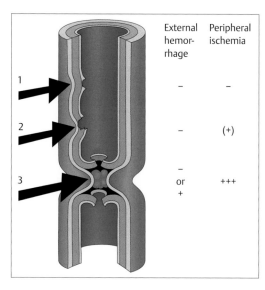

	External hemor-rhage	Peripheral ischemia
1	–	–
2	–	(+)
3	– or +	+++

Fig. 24.1   Classification of vascular injuries according to Vollmar.
Grade 1: circulation not impaired, no bleeding, no peripheral ischemia.
Grade 2: opening of the lumen or injury of the intima and media with bleeding or local thrombus deposition, which may be associated with peripheral ischemia.
Grade 3: division or crushing of the artery with severe bleeding or complete occlusion, peripheral ischemia inevitable.

Operative Technique

- Angio-CT to determine the extent of the vascular injury and to plan the operation
- Exposure of the affected vessels at the site of injury
- Resection of the injured vessel segments
- Primary vascular suture rarely possible, so a graft must nearly always be inserted. Because of the infection risk, the graft should be a vein wherever possible.
- With grade 3 or 4 open fractures, management should ideally be interdisciplinary (traumatologist, vascular surgeon, neurosurgeon). After brief stabilization of the fracture, the veins, arteries, and nerves are repaired, and finally the soft tissues are repaired.
- Subsequent fasciotomy to prevent a compartment syndrome

■ Complications

- Early thrombotic occlusion
- Infection (fatal, particularly when synthetic vascular graft is used)
- Compartment syndrome
- Arteriovenous fistulas
- Suture aneurysms

24

Aneurysms

Definition

- Bulging of the vessel wall where at least one layer of the wall has a defect, in contrast to **ectasia**.
- The causes are arteriosclerosis, inflammation (**mycotic aneurysms**), trauma, and genetic defects (**Marfan syndrome**).

- Bulging of the vessel wall

Classification

- **True aneurysm:** sac or spindle-shaped dilatation of all three layers of the wall
- **Dissecting aneurysm:** tear of the intima leads to dissection of the vessel wall distally with stretching of the outer wall. Distal re-entry of the blood from the dissection space into the original vessel lumen is possible. Occlusion of the originating arterial branches (descending ischemia syndrome) is possible.
- **False aneurysm:** arises as a result of injury of the vessel wall, usually after penetrating injury. This causes a paravasal hematoma to develop, which is limited by a connective tissue capsule following organization.

Location

- Most frequently in the aorta

- The most frequent site of aneurysm is the aorta. About 85% are infrarenal and about 15% occur in the thoracic part of the aorta.
- Thoracoabdominal and suprarenal locations are seldom affected but appear to be increasing in frequency. Peripheral aneurysms are much rarer, mainly in the common and internal iliac arteries, popliteal artery, subclavian artery, and carotid artery.

Symptoms

- **Asymptomatic stage:** Incidental finding during an examination; it does not cause any symptoms. This is by far the most common occurrence.
- **Symptomatic aneurysm:** Symptoms are due to expansion of the aneurysm or pressure on neighboring structures.
- **Ruptured aneurysm:** Rupture is usually retroperitoneal. Classic signs are hemorrhagic shock and severe pain with a sensation of doom. With free rupture into the abdominal cavity, death usually occurs rapidly.
- Symptoms of **acute dissection** are extremely severe, sharp retrosternal pain (differential diagnosis: myocardial infarction, pulmonary embolism, pneumothorax), nausea, vomiting, and acute dyspnea.

Treatment Approach

■ Conservative Treatment

- Strictly speaking, there is no conservative treatment; normalization of the blood pressure (ca. 60% of patients) is desirable.

■ Surgical Treatment

- In the asymptomatic stage, operation is indicated for thoracic and abdominal aneurysms with a transverse diameter > 5 cm. The operation consists of a **tubular** or **bifurcation** interposition graft using the inlay technique. The aneurysm is left in situ and sutured in front of the graft to protect against infection.

Endovascular Transluminal Stent Graft

- Alternative to conventional aortic surgery for infrarenal and thoracic aneurysms.
- Treatment by stent grafts that can be placed endoluminally is possible. With aneurysms of the infrarenal aorta, morphological classification of the aneurysm type is useful as an aid to choosing the procedure. **The Heidelberg–Allenberg classification** has proven useful (**Fig. 24.2**).
  - ► **Type I:** healthy infrarenal aortic segment (proximal aneurysm neck) and healthy aortic segment above the bifurcation.
  - ► **Type II:** preserved proximal aneurysm neck; the aneurysm extends distally as far as the bifurcation in type IIA and beyond the bifurcation in type IIB. Types IIA and B can be treated with a Y-shaped endovascular stent graft. Type IIC extends distally as far as the iliac bifurcation and an endovascular graft is not possible distally without blocking the internal iliac artery. Treatment is surgical in this type.
  - ► **Type III:** no infrarenal neck; fixation of an endovascular graft is not possible.
- Endovascular transluminal stent graft can be used in about 30% of aortic aneurysms that require treatment.

• Morphological classification for selecting procedure

Acute Limb Artery Occlusion

Pathogenesis

- The cause of acute arterial occlusion is either **embolism** due to dislodged thrombotic material or **acute arterial thrombosis** where the arterial wall is already damaged.
- The heart is the main source of arterial embolism (atrial thrombi with absolute arrhythmia, post-infarction embolism with cardiac mural thrombi), more rarely aneurysms (e.g., aorta), or detached atherosclerotic plaques (carotid artery).
- In exceptional cases, an atrial myxoma (obtain embolus histology!) or a so-called paradoxical embolism from a venous thrombus through a patent foramen ovale is the source of embolism.
- Rare causes are trauma or post-traumatic vascular changes or a dissecting aneurysm.

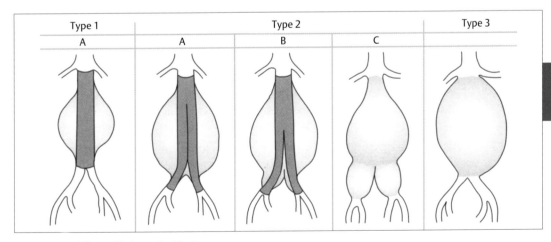

Fig. 24.2 Heidelberg–Allenberg classification

24

Symptoms

• Pratt 6 Ps rule

- **Progressive tissue ischemia** distal to the artery occlusion. Development of typical clinical symptoms depending on the **sensitivity to hypoxia** of the respective tissue (nerves first, muscle second, skin third).
- The characteristic symptoms are the **Pratt 6 Ps**: pain, pulselessness, paralysis, pallor, paresthesia, prostration.
- An abrupt onset of symptoms in a patient with a history of heart disease or with an absolute arrhythmia is typical of arterial embolism. Arterial thrombosis usually has a subacute onset in a patient with pre-existing peripheral arterial disease.

Diagnostic Approach

- In clinically obvious cases, no further diagnostic investigations but immediate treatment.
- Palpation of pulses and physical examination are not sufficiently reliable, so if acute limb ischemia is suspected, **Doppler examination** of the peripheral vessels should always be performed. With acute embolic vascular occlusion there is no Doppler signal over the arteries at the ankle.
- When the clinical evidence is unclear, especially in the presence of incomplete ischemia and known peripheral arterial disease, **angiography** or **angio-CT** is recommended, provided the ischemia tolerance allows this.

Treatment Approach

• Restoration of perfusion by embolectomy

- Acute limb ischemia requires immediate parenteral anticoagulation to avoid apposition thrombosis. Intravenous injection of heparin 5000 IU is indicated.
- The method of choice in complete ischemia syndrome is operative restoration of perfusion by embolectomy using a Fogarty catheter. The success of treatment should be confirmed by intraoperative angiography. Fibrinolytic therapy with rt-PA via local catheter lysis is indicated particularly in the case of occlusion of a bypass graft.
- Local catheter lysis can be combined with percutaneous intervention techniques such as aspiration thromboembolectomy.

Distant Embolectomy Using a Fogarty Catheter

Operative Technique

- Expose the vessels at readily accessible sites (groin, elbow); usually possible under local anesthesia.
- After looping and excluding the vessels, arteriotomy: preferably longitudinal in the leg and transverse in the arm.
- Longitudinal arteriotomy provides a better view of the opened vessel with easier extraction of thrombus or embolus.
- Closure of the arteriotomy by direct suture or with an expansion patch in the event of stenosis (vein, bovine pericardium, or PTFE).

Acute Mesenteric Artery Occlusion

Pathogenesis

- Acute mesenteric artery occlusion usually affects the superior mesenteric artery and is generally caused by an **embolus,** more rarely by arterial thrombosis. The diagnosis is usually suggested by absolute arrhythmia or a history of myocardial infarction.

Symptoms

- **A three-phase course** is typical of acute mesenteric artery occlusion:
  - ► Acute onset of **upper** and **central abdominal pain** with nausea and vomiting, sometimes with bloody diarrhea also.
  - ► After ca. 6 hours: development of **paralytic ileus** with relatively little pain for ca. 6–12 hours.
  - ► Development of **spreading peritonitis** with rapidly progressing deterioration in the patient's general condition and increasing shock symptoms.

• Triphasic course

Diagnostic Approach

- If acute mesenteric infarction is suspected, immediate imaging of the abdominal aorta and its visceral branches by **angiography** or **angio-CT.** If imaging is not possible without losing time, laparotomy should be performed if the condition is suspected clinically.

■ Differential Diagnosis

- All causes of an acute abdomen must be considered in the differential diagnosis:
  - ► Hollow organ perforation
  - ► Obstruction due to adhesions
  - ► Appendicitis
  - ► Pancreatitis
  - ► Myocardial infarction
  - ► Nonocclusive mesenteric ischemia

Treatment Approach

- **Aim:** restoration of bowel perfusion as quickly as possible by **embolectomy** or **thrombectomy** of the superior mesenteric artery or reperfusion by a **bypass procedure.**
- Since untreated acute mesenteric infarction causes death, there are **no contraindications** even in patients of advanced age or with high general risks.

• Restoration of bowel perfusion

24

Operative Technique

- The abdomen is opened through a midline laparotomy.
- Operability is assessed.
- The transverse colon is elevated, the greater omentum is displaced upward and the small bowel to the right.
- Exposure of the superior mesenteric artery at the lower border of the pancreas.

- A loop is placed around the superior mesenteric artery and a longitudinal arteriotomy is made near its origin.
- Embolectomy or thrombectomy is performed using a Fogarty catheter.
- Closure of the arteriotomy by direct suture or with a patch, if possible using a vein.
- Aortomesenteric bypass with a vein is rarely necessary.
- Synthetic material can also be avoided by aortic transposition of the superior mesenteric artery.
- After successful reperfusion, resection of infarcted segments of bowel is performed.
- If the vitality of the bowel cannot be assessed with certainty, a second-look relaparotomy after 24 hours is scheduled.

Chronic Arterial Disease of the Limbs

Pathogenesis

- Due to arteriosclerosis in over 80% of cases

- Chronic arterial disease is due to **arteriosclerosis** in over 80% of cases.
- **Obliterative** and **dilating** forms
- Rare causes are media calcification of Mönckeberg type (stony hard, often bandlike calcium deposits in the vessel wall without intimal thickening and with a patent lumen), diabetic angiopathy (affecting smaller and medium-sized vessels), and inflammatory vascular processes such as endangiitis obliterans or giant cell arteritis. Fibromuscular hyperplasia is rarer.
- **Risk factors** for the development of atherosclerosis are ethnicity, sex, age, smoking, diabetes mellitus, hypertension, dyslipidemia, inflammatory markers, hyperviscosity and hypercoagulability, hyperhomocysteinaemia, and chronic renal failure.

Atherogenesis
- The exact mechanisms of atherogenesis have not yet been clarified in detail. It is still disputed whether **plasma factors** (e.g., elevated low density lipoprotein [LDL] cholesterol) lead directly to atherosclerotic changes in the vessel wall or whether **injury to the vessel wall** is the primary process (response to injury).
- In the "**combined hypothesis**" the two approaches are linked: according to this theory, elevated LDL levels can damage the endothelium and thus trigger the subsequent cascade of platelet aggregation, release of platelet-derived growth factor (PDGF) and proliferation of smooth muscle cells. Factors that can lead to initial endothelial damage are high shear forces, toxic substances (e.g., in cigarette smoke), viruses, or bacteria (*Chlamydia pneumoniae*).
- The most important steps in atherogenesis are as follows:
  - ► **Endothelial damage**
    - Formation of adhesion molecules
    - Adhesion of monocytes to the endothelium
    - Permeability for serum lipids and cellular blood components
  - ► **Formation of fatty streaks**
    - Lipid accumulation in the intima
    - Transmigration of monocytes into the intima and transformation to macrophages
    - Phagocytosis and oxidation of lipids by macrophages

- ► **Formation of a neointima**
  - – Immigration of vascular muscle cells
  - – Plaque growth through proliferation of muscle cells and macrophages
  - – Formation of an extracellular connective tissue matrix
- ► **Vessel occlusion**
  - – Organization and calcification of the plaques
  - – Retraction and plaque rupture
- ► **Deposition of platelets and thrombosis**

Location

- Chronic peripheral arterial disease (PAD) affects the lower limb in 90% of cases and the upper limb in 10% of cases.
- In the lower limb, a distinction is made according to the location of the occlusion between the **pelvic type** (aortoiliac level), **thigh type** (femoropopliteal level), **lower leg type** (crural level) and **multilevel type** when more than one level is affected.

• Lower limbs affected in particular

Classification

- **Fontaine** classification:
  - ► **Stage 1:** arterial occlusion or stenosis without symptoms
  - ► **Stage 2:** pain on exercise (intermittent claudication)
    - – **2a:** walking distance > 100 m
    - – **2b:** walking distance < 100 m
  - ► **Stage 3:** rest pain, especially at night
  - ► **Stage 4:** local tissue destruction (necrosis, gangrene)

Symptoms

- The symptoms depend on the site of occlusion:
  - ► **Aortoiliac occlusion:** pain in the buttocks and thigh, potency disorders
  - ► **Femoropopliteal type:** pain located in the lower leg (calf)
  - ► **Crural type:** pain in the distal lower leg and foot, delayed wound healing

Diagnostic Approach

- The diagnosis is confirmed and treatment is planned by means of **angiography** (digital subtraction angiography), **angio-CT**, or **magnetic resonance angiography.**

Treatment Approach

■ Indications

- The treatment is guided by the clinical stage and site of occlusion. It ranges from conservative measures to eliminate and treat risk factors along with exercise training to percutaneous transluminal angioplasty with and without stents and to complex vessel reconstructions.
- In the TASC-2 classification, the common vessel lesions are divided into four different lesions for both the aortoiliac region and for the femoropopliteal segment, and interventional or operative treatment options are then in accordance with these.

• TASC-2 classification for deciding treatment

24

• Surgical vessel reconstruction

■ **Surgical Treatment**

• **Bypass grafting** with anatomical and extra-anatomical reconstruction using autologous vein or synthetic grafts
• **Thromboendarterectomy** with and without a patch
• **Profunda revascularization**
• A **hybrid procedure** is a combination of surgical vessel reconstruction with intervention in another vessel segment.

■ **Complications**

• Secondary bleeding
• Early occlusion, usually due to poor anastomosis technique or incorrect diagnosis (deficient outflow)
• Delayed wound healing, especially frequent at the groin
• Graft infection, which generally requires removal of the graft
• Ischemic colitis after operations on the infrarenal aorta and inadequate collateralization through the marginal arcade
• Potency disorders with procedures on the distal aorta
• Late bypass occlusion, usually due to deterioration of the inflow or outflow

Subclavian Steal Syndrome

Definition

• Subclavian steal syndrome is due to proximal occlusion or high-grade stenosis of the subclavian artery proximal to the origin of the vertebral artery. The left side is usually affected.
• Reversed flow in the vertebral artery is characteristic.

Pathogenesis

• Rarely congenital, usually develops on the basis of arteriosclerotic changes
• In women, an inflammatory origin is also possible.

Symptoms

• When the arm is exercised, blood is withdrawn from the vertebrobasilar circulation region with neurological symptoms such as **dizziness, ataxia,** or **drop attacks**.
• **Blood pressure** difference between the right and left arm

Diagnostic Approach

• Diagnosis by **duplex ultrasonography:** characteristic reversal of flow in the affected vertebral artery, degree of stenosis in the proximal subclavian artery or occlusion can be demonstrated.
• **Angiography** is employed only when the findings are unclear and to carry out an intervention.

Treatment Approach

• The treatment of choice is **peripheral transluminal angioplasty** (PTA) with and without **stent implantation.**

- Surgical methods such as transposition of the subclavian artery to the common carotid artery or a **carotid-subclavian bypass** are employed in symptomatic patients only after failure of the interventions.

■ Veins

Anatomy

- Veins are thin-walled, wide-lumen vessels with semilunar valves.
- Intact valves reduce the hydrostatic pressure on the vessel wall.
- Three-layer wall structure on histology with **tunica intima, tunica media,** and **tunica adventitia.**
- On the basis of their position, a distinction is made between **deep subfascial veins** and **superficial epifascial veins.**
- There are direct connections between the different vein systems through **communicating veins.**

General Diagnostic Approach

- Clinical inspection and palpation, tests of function such as Trendelenburg or Perthes test
- Simple Doppler ultrasonography, duplex ultrasonography, and phlebography
- Functional conclusions can also be drawn from **venous occlusion plethysmography** and **light reflection rheography.**

Varicose Veins

Definition

- According to the WHO definition, **saclike dilatations** of veins, often with a tortuous course, are designated varicose veins.

Epidemiology

- Most common vascular surgical disorder of veins. About 20% of men and up to 35% of women in Europe are affected.

Classification

- A **pathogenetic** distinction is made between primary and secondary varicose veins. Secondary varicosity is a result of other underlying diseases, usually deep vein thrombosis in the leg or dysplasia.
- A further subdivision is made according to the affected veins into **major veins, side branch veins,** and **perforating veins:**
  - ▸ The major veins are the long and short saphenous veins.
  - ▸ Side branch varicosities affect larger side branches such as the lateral or medial accessory saphenous vein.
  - ▸ Perforating varicosities arise from incompetent perforating veins.
- Varicosities of the long saphenous vein are most common; Hach has divided them into four stages on the basis of Doppler ultrasonographic criteria.

- Hach classification

24

Treatment Approach

■ Indications

• Complications are an indication for surgery

• Surgery is indicated to prevent chronic venous insufficiency or when complications such as **variceal bleeding** or **varicophlebitis** are present.

■ Surgical Treatment

• Precise mapping of the varicose veins by duplex ultrasonography or ascending phlebography in preparation for operation. Confirmation of patency of the deep vein system should be sought.

Operative Technique

• Exposure of the proximal site of incompetence; this is usually at the opening of the long or short saphenous vein
• Exposure and division of all branches of the saphenofemoral junction ("vein star")
• Exposure of the distal site of incompetence and removal by means of a vein stripper from central to peripheral
• Removal of varicose side branches through tiny accessory incisions (miniphlebectomy)
• Search for incompetent perforating veins, subfascial ligature of these

---

■ Complications

• Delayed wound healing, especially in the groin
• Injury of the saphenous nerve
• Lymph fistula
• Recurrent varicose veins

Phlebothrombosis

Definition

• Acute complete or incomplete thrombotic occlusion of the deep veins, predominantly in the lower limb and pelvis and in the veins of the neck and arm. Venous clots tend to grow and embolize to the lung.

Pathogenesis

• Virchow triad

• **Virchow triad:**
  ► Changes in the vessel wall/endothelium: inflammatory, degenerative, traumatic, allergic
  ► Changes in blood flow: immobilization, varicose veins, paralysis, local outflow obstruction, fractures
  ► Changes in the composition of the blood: polycythemia, erythrocytosis, thrombocytosis, hyperfibrinogenemia, thrombophilia, activated protein C resistance (factor V mutation)

24

Symptoms

- Dull, dragging pain in the entire leg, sensation of heaviness, acute edema with visible increase in leg circumference, cyanosis, inflamed veins over the dorsum of the foot (Pratt warning veins)

Diagnostic Approach

- **Clinical signs,** all highly sensitive but accuracy still only ca. 50% (**Table 24.1**)
- Measurement of **D-dimers** allows thrombosis to be ruled out if result is negative.
- **Continuous wave Doppler** is a simple method for looking for proximal thrombosis; **duplex ultrasonography** can replace phlebography in routine investigation. **Phlebography** can be employed if the results are unclear.

Table 24.1   Clinical signs of thrombosis

Sign	Pain
• Payr sign	• Pain on the sole of the foot, e.g., on tapping
• Bisgaard sign	• Retromalleolar pain
• Homans sign	• Calf pain on plantar flexion
• Lowenberg test	• Calf pain produced by blood pressure cuff
• Meyer pressure points	• Tender points over deep veins
• Pratt sign	• Tenderness in the popliteal fossa

Treatment Approach

■ Indications

- **Recent lower leg and femoral thrombosis:**
  - ▶ In ambulant patients **compression therapy** (elastic bandaging or well-fitting compression stocking) and immediate **heparinization** (ideally with low molecular weight heparins)
  - ▶ No immobilization
  - ▶ Early **oral anticoagulation** desirable in the absence of contraindications
- **Massive pelvic vein thrombosis:**
  - ▶ Temporary **immobilization** for 5–7 days
  - ▶ Temporary **cava filter** if there are floating thrombi in central veins and when bilateral pulmonary artery embolism has occurred.
  - ▶ **Fibrinolytic treatment** with streptokinase, urokinase, or rt-PA only in exceptional cases. The same applies for operative thrombectomy (only isolated acute pelvic vein thrombosis).
- **Phlegmasia cerulea dolens** poses a vital threat to the limb. Rapid surgical measures are necessary, such as **thrombectomy** in combination with **fascial splitting** of the thigh and lower leg.

- Treatment predominantly conservative
- With phlegmasia cerulea dolens, rapid thrombectomy and fasciotomy

■ Aftercare

- Both compression and oral anticoagulation are prescribed for 6 months; after pulmonary embolism, oral anticoagulation is continued for at least 1 year.
- Proximal thrombosis or multi-level thrombosis: compression treatment for 2 years is recommended.

- Compression
- Oral anticoagulation

24

- Lifelong oral anticoagulant therapy in congenital protein C, protein S, or antithrombin 3 deficiency states or the homozygous form of activated protein C resistance.
- In patients with contraindications to oral anticoagulation, therapy with low molecular weight heparins is an alternative.

Further Reading

Diehm C, Allenberg J-R, Nimura-Eckert K. Farbatlas der Gefäßkrankheiten. Berlin, Heidelberg, New York: Springer; 1999

Norgren L, Hiatt WR, Dormandy JA, Nehler MR, Harris KA, Fowkes FGR. Konsensuspapier der Fachgesellschaften zur Behandlung der peripheren arteriellen Verschlusskrankheit (TASC 2). gefaessmedizin.net: 2007; 3 (Suppl. 2)

Vollmer J. Rekonstruktive Chirurgie der Arterien. Stuttgart, New York: Thieme; 1996

25 Emergency and Trauma Surgery

M. Fuchs

■ Polytrauma

Definition

- Injuries of different body regions or organ systems occurring at the same time, at least one of which, or a combination of several, is life threatening.

• Life-threatening complex injuries

Scoring Systems, Documentation

- Identification of the injured patient at the accident site as multiply injured, subsequent treatment in a trauma center
  - ► Glasgow Coma Scale (GCS)
  - ► CRAMS scale (Circulation, Respiration, Abdomen, Motor, Speech)
- Scores for injury severity: decision-making aid for operative procedures, intubation and ventilation, primary amputation, validation of quality of care
  - ► Abbreviated injury scale (AIS)
  - ► Injury severity score (ISS) according to Baker et al. 1974
  - ► Hannover Polytraumaschlüssel (PTS)
- DGU [German Society for Trauma Surgery] trauma register form at four specific times: S: basic data, history of accident, A: pre-hospital, B: emergency department, C: intensive care unit, D: conclusion

• Scores record the severity of injury and are used to validate the quality of care.

Management of Polytrauma

This extraordinarily complex medical problem demands time-critical action and great professional competence. There must be close interdisciplinary collaboration among specialists in trauma surgery/surgery, anesthesiology, and intensive care. The team includes other professional disciplines depending on the injury pattern. Procedures in accordance with guidelines improve the quality of care and substantiated documentation is used for quality assurance.

• Close interdisciplinary collaboration

Goals of Acute Treatment

- Restoration/preservation of the circulation (macro- and microcirculation), BP > 80 mmHg
- Oxygen supply at pulmonary and cellular level with O_2 saturation > 90%
- Pain relief
- Avoidance of sepsis

Treatment Principles

- Time-critical action in the acute phase:
  - ► Rational surgical measures
  - ► Hemostasis
  - ► Debridement, fasciotomy

• Time-critical action and observation of whole body reaction

- ► Fracture stabilization, for instance, with an external fixator
- ► Avoidance of stressful operations and long operation times
- Monitoring for trauma reaction, strategies to alleviate the systemic inflammatory response syndrome (SIRS):
  - ► Individualized volume replacement
  - ► Organ support and replacement therapy (ventilation, hemofiltration, dialysis)
- Consistent prophylaxis of septic complications:
  - ► Antibiotic therapy, thrombosis prophylaxis, replacement of coagulation factors
  - ► Parenteral nutrition, early changeover to enteral feeding
  - ► Positioning treatment

Phase-Dependent Diagnostics and Therapy

- Diagnostics and surgical therapy are adapted to the overall severity of the trauma and depend on the phase.

■ Pre-Hospital Phase

- Life-saving measures in the pre-hospital phase

- Brief clinical assessment (vital signs, injury pattern)
- Initial treatment of shock (volume replacement, oxygen)
- Intubation
  - ► Indication: hypoxia, unstable thorax (flail chest), paradoxical respiration, aspiration, bleeding from the oropharynx, GCS < 7, severe shock state
- Chest tube
  - ► Indication: unstable thorax, cutaneous emphysema, high ventilation pressure, respiratory rate < 10 or > 30/min, congested neck veins when tube is in correct position
- Make patient fit for transport

■ Resuscitation Room Phase

- Clinical examination according to ATLS principles, baseline investigations, and urgent essential invasive measures

- Clinical examination from head to toe according to ATLS principles (Advanced Trauma Life Support)
- Technical examinations: radiographs of chest, pelvis, and spine and ultrasonography of abdomen and pleura or CT as "trauma spiral"; radiography of limbs depending on clinical signs
- Insertion of a bladder catheter, urinalysis if bloody urine is noted

■ Emergency Operating Room, Intensive Unit (Table 25.1)

- Immediate operations in emergency OR and day 1 surgery

- Internal fixation of open fractures, surgical "baseline management," operative decompression of compartment syndromes
- Laparotomy (bleeding from parenchymal organs, perforation)
- Stabilization (circulation, gas exchange, laboratory parameters)
- Monitor function of organ systems, recording "tendencies"
- Supplementary radiological investigations, for example, contrast CT and angiography

Table 25.1 Operative (op) treatment according to phase

Op phase 1 Vital indication	Op phase 2 Primary operation	Op phase 3 Second-look operation	Op phase 3 Delayed operation
• Control of massive bleeding • Decompression of: tension hemothorax, epidural hematoma	• Intracranial bleeding • Injury of major vessels • Hollow organ injury • Open fracture • Pelvic and spinal injury • Compartment syndrome • Dislocation • Joint fracture	• **Caution:** high incidence of multiorgan failure	• Reconstruction of soft tissues • Change of procedure (external fixator–medullary nail) • Joint reconstruction • Peripheral ORIF (open reduction internal fixation) • Reconstructions: urology; maxillofacial surgery; neurosurgery)

■ Intensive Unit, Operating Room

• Stabilization (circulation, gas exchange, laboratory parameters)
• Sepsis protection by debridement of extensive areas of necrosis and evacuation of large hematomas (in scheduled second-look operations that are less stressful for the patient)

• Stabilization phase in the intensive unit

■ "Delayed Primary Surgery"

• Operation timing: extensive operations can be planned for when the patient is in a stable condition after 5–6 days (the incidence of multiorgan failure is significantly raised on days 2–4).
• Fracture stabilization by definitive fixation (ORIF: open reduction internal fixation)
• Parameters that influence immunological stress reaction: patient's preoperative status, extent of the operative procedure.
• Laboratory parameters with predictive value:
  ► Platelet count (< 90 000/μL)
  ► PaO_2/FiO_2 (< 200)
  ► 24-hour fluid balance (> 3 L)
  ► Creatinine (> 90 mmol/L)
  ► Bilirubin (> 25 μmol/L)

• Complex surgical reconstructions, supplementary fracture internal fixation, or early change of procedure takes place from day 5 onward.

Prognosis

• The care level of the facility providing primary treatment (basic care, trauma center) influences the overall prognosis.
• Target criteria of scoring systems: injury severity, survival after polytrauma (ISS, AIS, RTS [revised trauma score], TRISS method [trauma injury severity score], PRE chart [preliminary outcome based evaluation]).

■ Head Injury

25

Definition

Direct (blunt, sharp) or indirect (acceleration) application of force to the skull and/or brain and its surroundings, leading to disturbance of its function. There is an association between the primary mechanical damage and the development of secondary brain damage.

• Force acting on the skull, brain, and surroundings with disturbance of function

Classification

- Head injury (Glasgow Coma Scale; Teasdale and Jennett 1974; **Table 25.2**) is classified into three degrees of severity according to the clinical findings (Herrmann 1991): mild (GCS 13–15 points), moderate (GCS 9–12 points) and severe (GCS 3–8 points).

Table 25.2   Classification according to the Glasgow Coma Scale

Reaction	Stimulus	Score (points)
Eye opening	Spontaneous	4
Eye opening	To command	3
Eye opening	To painful stimulus	2
No eye opening	Despite painful stimulus	1
Purposeful motor response	To command	6
Localized withdrawal	Painful stimulus	5
Withdrawal	Painful stimulus	4
Abnormal flexion	Painful stimulus	3
Extensor response	Painful stimulus	2
None	Painful stimulus	1
Oriented	Verbal response	5
Confused	Verbal response	4
Inappropriate words	Verbal response	3
Incomprehensible sounds	Verbal response	2
No reaction	Verbal response	1

Diagnostic Approach

- Diagnosis by clinical examination and contrast CT

- Clinical examination: local findings, level of consciousness, vital parameters
- Radiological investigations: standard x-ray of skull and lateral cervical spine; higher-grade head injury: contrast CT and CT of cervical spine; repeat CT after 12–24 hours

Treatment Approach

- Conservative treatment measures consist of reduction of external stimuli and intensive therapy, operation for severe head injury

Pre-Hospital Care
- Ensure vital functions
- Moderate hyperventilation
- Sedation

Intensive Therapy
- Ventilation
- Treatment of cerebral edema
- Correction of electrolytes and coagulation factors
- BP control
- Parenteral and enteral nutrition
- Monitoring of intracranial and cerebral perfusion pressure

Surgical Measures
- Decompression of depressed fractures
- Dural closure: frontobasal fractures (risk of infection), compound fractures

- Hematoma evacuation: osteoclastic trepanation for space-occupying bleeding
- Removal of larger perforating foreign bodies

■ Complications

- Circumscribed or extensive functional deficit culminating in brain death
- Posttraumatic epilepsy
- Cranial nerve injury with functional deficit
- Carotid artery–cavernous sinus fistula

■ Fractures

Definition

Direct or indirect application of force that exceeds the elasticity of bone. Periosteum, endosteum, cortex, and nutritive vessels are divided. Neighboring structures such as vessels, nerves, muscles, tendons and skin can be injured.

- Great variability in clinical and radiological severity

Classification (Tables 25.3, 25.4, 25.5, 25.6)

- Fracture classification is used for clear fracture description and forms the basis for standardized treatment.

Table 25.3 Basic principles of AO fracture classification

Step 1: coding of bone and segment	1 = humerus
	2 = forearm
	3 = femur
	4 = lower leg
	5 = spine
	6 = pelvis
	7 = hand
	8 = foot
	Position within the region:
	1 = proximal
	2 = shaft
	3 = distal
Step 2: fracture typing	**Shaft fracture:**
	A = simple (contact > 90%)
	B = wedge (little contact)
	C = complex (no fragment contact)
	Joint fracture:
	A = extra-articular
	B = partial joint fracture
Step 3: classification according to difficulty and prognosis	1 = easy
	2 = difficult
	3 = very difficult
Steps 4 and 5: subgroups (n = 27) and qualifications (n = 9)	

25

Table 25.4 Classification of compound fractures

Grade I	Skin wound < 1 cm, insignificant contamination, penetration from within, simple fracture form such as transverse or oblique fracture
Grade II	Skin wound > 1 cm, extensive soft-tissue damage, slight to moderate muscle crushing, flap formation or detachment, simple transverse or oblique fracture with a small area of comminution
Grade III	Extensive soft-tissue destruction (skin, muscle, vessels, nerves), heavy wound contamination, extensive bone comminution **IIIa:** adequate bone cover, part break **IIIb:** periosteal stripping, bone lies free, massive contamination **IIIc:** vessel injury requiring reconstruction
Grade IV	"Subtotal" (incomplete) amputation injury, with less than one quarter of the soft-tissue cover intact and extensive injuries of nerves and blood vessels

Source: From Gustilo RB, Anderson JT. Prevention of infection in the treatment of one thousand and twenty-five open fractures of long bones: retrospective and prospective analyses. J Bone Joint Surg Am 1976; 58: 453–458.

Table 25.5 Classification of soft-tissue damage with closed fractures

Grade 0	Absent or insignificant soft-tissue injury, indirect force, simple fracture form
Grade I	Superficial abrasion, contusion with fragment pressure, simple moderately severe fracture form
Grade II	Deep contaminated abrasion, skin and muscle contusion due to direct force, potential compartment syndrome, moderate to severe fracture form
Grade III	Extensive skin contusion or crushing, subcutaneous detachment, overt compartment syndrome, blood vessel injury, severe fracture form

Source: From Tscherne H, Oestern H-J. Die Klassifizierung des Weichteilschadens bei offenen und geschlossenen Frakturen. Unfallheilkunde 1982; 85: 111.

Fracture Forms
- Shaft fractures
- Joint fractures
- Fractures of small and flat bones
- Childhood fractures

Special Forms of Fracture
- Fissure: not all of the bone structure is divided
- Pathological fracture (spontaneous fracture): minor or no trauma; causes are bone tumor, cyst, metastasis, osteoporosis
- Transitional fractures: in the transitional age between adolescents and adults when the epiphyses are partially fused (two-plane and three-plane fracture)
- Greenstick fracture in children: periosteal tube intact or only partially damaged

Table 25.6   Classification of childhood fractures

Salter–Harris	Aitken	Description	Illustration
I	0	Slipped epiphysis	
II	I	Slipped epiphysis and meta-physeal wedge	
III	II	Epiphyseal fracture + epiphyseal wedge (joint fracture)	
IV	III	Epiphyseal fracture: epi- and metaphyseal wedge (joint fracture)	
V	–	Crush injury of the growth plate	

Diagnostic Approach

■ Clinical Examination

- Definite signs of fracture:
  - ► Crepitation
  - ► Visible bone fragment in the case of a compound fracture
  - ► Abnormal position/mobility apparent with shaft fractures
- Nondefinite signs of fracture:
  - ► Pain
  - ► Impaired function
  - ► Swelling
  - ► Deformity with fracture in the region of a joint

■ Diagnostic Imaging

- Radiograph examination in two planes (showing the neighboring joints)
- Additional oblique or targeted views; stress views, if necessary
- CT examination (if necessary with 2D and 3D reconstruction)

- Most important diagnostic measures are definite clinical signs of fracture and x-ray photos in two planes along with CT.
- Problem: assessment of the severity of the individual injury, injury pattern, and impairment of the patient's overall status

25

Classification

- Traumatic
- Chronic recurrent
- Habitual
- Congenital

Symptoms

- Definite signs
  - ▸ Resilient fixation due to tension of capsule, ligaments, and muscles
  - ▸ Deformity
  - ▸ Palpable empty socket
  - ▸ Abnormal position of the joint head
- Nondefinite signs
  - ▸ Pain
  - ▸ Swelling
  - ▸ Hematoma

Diagnostic Approach

• Clinical examination is always supplemented by diagnostic imaging

- Radiographs in two planes before and after reduction
- Stress views: to find out the direction and extent of any instability
- MRI: concomitant injury of cartilage, capsule, ligaments, menisci, limbus, muscles
- Doppler ultrasonography, angiography: if vessel injury is suspected

Treatment Approach

• Closed reduction is the acute treatment of choice. Concomitant injuries that cause persistent instability undergo post-primary reconstruction.

Closed
- Shoulder dislocation: Hippocrates, Arlt, or Kocher method
- Reduction by traction and countertraction in the direction opposite to the movement that caused injury
- As soon as possible under analgesia or regional or general anesthesia to avoid further pressure injury

Open
- If there is an obstacle to reduction due to interposition of ligaments, tendons, or bone fragments (fracture dislocation)
- Open dislocation: immediate operation because of the infection risk
- Concomitant vascular injury for the purpose of vascular reconstruction

After reduction (open/closed) immobilization depends on the affected joint, instability, and treatment measure employed.

■ Complications

- Concomitant injuries (blood vessels, nerves, cartilage, menisci, ligaments, tendons, muscles, bones). The concomitant injuries often require post-primary reconstruction to avoid recurrent dislocation.
- Late damage (osteoarthritis, recurrent dislocation, unstable joint, impaired range of motion)

■ Soft-Tissue Injuries

The trauma management of soft-tissue injury is based on knowledge of all the relevant parameters influencing the injury and determines the sequence of diagnostic and therapeutic measures in the form of an individually optimized "master plan" (**Tables 25.7, 25.8**).

Classification

Table 25.7 Classification of soft-tissue injuries according to the level of the acting energy

Open soft-tissue injuries	Incised, stab and bite wound	Low energy injury
	Abrasion, tear, impalement, gunshot wound	Low to high energy injury
	Avulsion or explosive wound, traumatic amputation	High energy injury
Closed soft-tissue injury	Contusion, crushing, abrasion, detachment, avulsion	Low to high energy injury

• The multi-facetted soft-tissue injuries make classification necessary as a basis for a multi-stage treatment plan

Table 25.8 AO classification of soft-tissue injury

IC = integument closed	IO = integument open	MT = muscle-tendon injury	NV = neurovascular injury
IC 1 = skin intact	IO 1 = skin penetration from within	MT 1 = no muscle or tendon injury	NV 1 = no neurovascular injury
IC 2 = contusion	IO 2 = skin opening from without < 5 cm	MT 2 = circumscribed loss of one muscle group	NV 2 = isolated nerve injury
IC 3 = circumscribed detachment	IO 3 = skin opening from without > 5 cm	MT 3 = injury of two or more muscle groups	NV 3 = isolated blood vessel injury
IC 4 = extensive detachment	IO 4 = circumscribed detachment with skin loss	MT 4 = division/loss of entire muscle groups	NV 4 = combined neurovascular injury
IC 5 = contusion necrosis	IO 5 = extensive detachment with skin loss	MT 5 = compartment syndrome	NV 5 = subtotal/total amputation

Diagnostic Approach

• Visible skin damage
• Degree of wound contamination
• Contact surface of the traumatizing object
• Direct/indirect force
• Direction of the acting force
• Affected body region
• General condition of the injured person

• Soft-tissue injury should be understood as a multifactorial event.

A local shock state of variable severity develops as a result of injury, and this determines the prognosis of the injury.

25

The clinical picture and nature of the injury allow conclusions to be drawn about the causal kinetic energy and the true extent of the trauma. This classification is easier with open injuries than with closed injuries.

Treatment Approach

First Aid at the Accident Site
- Sterile wound cover (left in place until operation)
- Fracture reduction
- Immobilization by splinting
- Hemostasis by local compression (tourniquet only in exceptional cases)

Clinical Treatment (Fig. 25.1)
- Reduction of dislocations and fractures
- Systemic antibiotic therapy, tetanus prophylaxis
- Radical surgical debridement (scheduled review after 24–48 hours if appropriate)
- Neurovascular reconstruction with suture/interposition graft (nerves can also undergo secondary reconstruction)
- Immobilization by splinting

- Surgical debridement in conjunction with an external fixator is the basic treatment in severe, open soft-tissue injuries

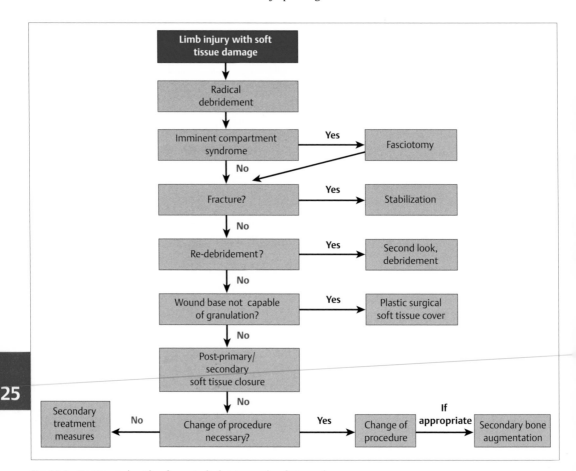

Fig. 25.1 Treatment algorithm for acute limb injury with soft-tissue damage.

- Soft-tissue relief by transfixation of neighboring joints with an external fixator
- Fracture fixation (external fixation, undrilled interlocking nail), with subsequent change of procedure if appropriate
- Wound drainage, local antiseptic wound dressing if appropriate
- Open wound treatment of bite wounds to ensure drainage of secretion

Soft-Tissue Closure
- Temporary with synthetic skin substitute
- Primary or secondary suture, dynamic wound closure (banding)
- Soft-tissue distraction
- Local or free flap cover
- Secondary healing
- Split-skin or full-thickness skin graft after wound conditioning

■ Complications

Complications are possible depending on the severity of injury. They must always be considered when planning treatment.
- Seroma, hematoma
- Necrosis
- Infection
- Compartment syndrome
- Secondary injury of vessels, nerves, tendons, and ligaments

• Infection is a feared complication.

Late Complications
- Loss of function and impaired range of joint motion
- Poor cosmetic result

■ Bone Infection

Definition

- Infection of the bone (osteitis, osteomyelitis) with clinical and laboratory signs of inflammation and finding of microorganisms.

Etiology

- Nonspecific form: *Staphylococcus aureus*, and also *Escherichia coli*, *Pseudomonas aeruginosa*, *Staphylococcus epidermidis*, Proteus spp., streptococci
- Specific bone infection by the causative organisms of tuberculosis, syphilis, typhus

• Commonly *Staphylococcus aureus* infection

Route of Spread (Fig. 25.2)
- Hematogenous: for example, staphylococci in hematogenous osteomyelitis
- Direct: after open fracture or by continuity if there is infection in the surroundings
- Postoperative: after internal fixation, joint aspiration, joint prosthesis, osteotomy

25

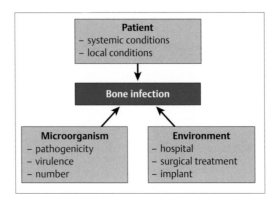

Fig. 25.2 Factors influencing bone infection.

Classification

• Acute and chronic forms

The course of the infection and the clinical picture are determined by the virulence of the pathogens on the one hand, and on the other hand by the strength of the immune forces.

The possible manifestation forms are:
• Highly acute form with a septic course
• Acute osteitis/osteomyelitis
• Chronic osteitis/osteomyelitis
• Brodie abscess
• Chronic sclerosing form

Diagnostic Approach

• Bacterial detection is always desirable

• Clinical symptoms: local signs of inflammation, fistula
• General symptoms: fever, malaise
• Pathogen detection (aspiration, blood culture)
• Laboratory inflammatory parameters (leukocytes, C-reactive protein, erythrocyte sedimentation rate)
• Imaging methods:
  ► MRI with contrast enhancement
  ► Triple-phase scintigraphy, leukocyte scintigraphy
  ► Conventional radiographs in two planes
  ► Ultrasonography
  ► Fistula filling

Treatment Approach

• Eradicate basis of infection by removal of avascular tissue due to bone and soft-tissue destruction along with antimicrobial treatment

■ Conservative Treatment

• Start treatment as soon as possible.
• Acute hematogenous osteomyelitis in children is treated conservatively with consistent immobilization.
• High-dose systemic antibiotics are administered.

■ Surgical Treatment

• Treatment is focused on local surgical measures and antibiotic therapy

• Radical surgical debridement of:
  ► Nonvital bone, sequestrum, opening of medullary cavity
  ► Adjacent infected, necrotic soft tissues, fistula track

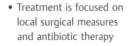

- Copious wound irrigation, jet lavage
- Local application of antibiotic vehicles (beads, fleece, spacer) according to antibiotic sensitivity
- Defect management:
  - ► Avoid formation of a cavity, drainage.
  - ► Cover with skin/muscle flap.
  - ► Autologous cancellous bone graft.
  - ► Wound management can be open, semi-open, or closed
- Plan scheduled review operation
- Stabilization:
  - ► After internal fixation: if implant site is vital, leave implant (e.g., plate) in place initially, otherwise switch to external fixator
  - ► External fixator: when free from infection change later to internal fixation
  - ► Arthrodesis
- Antibiotics: empirical initially, according to sensitivity after bacterial identification
- Hyperbaric oxygen therapy as an additional measure
- Infected arthroplasty prosthesis:
  - ► Early infection with preservation of the prosthesis: local surgical treatment, local and systemic antibiotics
  - ► One- or two-stage prosthesis revision
  - ► Resection arthroplasty (e.g., Girdlestone hip)
- Secondary bone reconstruction (callus distraction, bone grafts)
- Amputation

■ Complications

- Persistent infection with transition to chronic or chronic recurrent form:
  - ► Sepsis
  - ► Abscess formation, fistulation
  - ► Pseudarthrosis
  - ► Pathological fracture
  - ► Recurrence
  - ► Chronic course
- Growth disorder in children due to involvement of the growth plate

- Transition to the chronic form is feared.

■ Nerve Injury

Classification (Table 25.9)

- Direct (laceration, stab wound) or indirect damage (contusion, traction, deceleration)

- Direct or indirect trauma
- Degrees of severity: neurapraxia, axonotmesis, and neurotmesis

25

Table 25.9 Classification of injuries of peripheral nerves

Neurapraxia (I)	Temporary dysfunction (nerve contusion) without interruption of continuity, no peripheral degeneration, reversible
Axonotmesis (II)	Destruction of the axons and myelin sheaths, peripheral degeneration, little connective-tissue proliferation, regeneration complete
Neurotmesis (III)	Total/subtotal division of nerve fibers and enveloping structures, peripheral degeneration, regeneration highly impaired to impossible, indication for surgery

Source: From Seddon HJ. Three types of nerve injury. Brain 1943; 66: 237.

Diagnostic Approach

- Meticulous clinical examination: which nerve, where injured, degree of severity
- Nerve conduction speeds, electromyography: objective measure of clinical findings and for follow-up observation

Treatment Approach

- Conservative treatment for neurapraxia and axonotmesis
- Neurotmesis: reconstruction of the nerve using microsurgical technique

Conservative (Stages I and II)
- Physiotherapy, passive joint exercises, avoidance of contractures
- Electrostimulation

Surgical (Stage III)
- Operation timing: primary, post-primary (< 2 weeks), secondary (> 6 weeks)
- Reconstruction of the nerve using microsurgical technique
- Suture technique: epineural, perineural, interfascicular interposition grafts

■ Late Sequelae

- Motor deficit, muscle atrophy
- Sensory deficit with trophic disturbances
- Joint contractures
- Development of neuroma with neuroma pain

■ Tendon Rupture

Etiology

- The cause is often inappropriate loading or previous damage.

- Rare: exceeding the physiological tear strength of a healthy tendon
- Common: inappropriate loading or previous damage of the tendon texture

Mechanism of Injury
- Uncoordinated rapid force that exceeds tear strength
- Direct trauma (blow, impact, kick)
- Sudden stress on a previously damaged tendon (degeneration, steroids, systemic disease)

Symptoms

- Functional deficit of the affected muscle (e.g., with displaced muscle belly)
- Deformity of involved joints
- Nonspecific local symptoms (pain, swelling, hematoma, palpable gap)

Diagnostic Approach

- Clinical examination, ultrasonography

- Specific tests positive (e.g., Thompson test for Achilles tendon rupture)
- Imaging (ultrasonography, MRI)
- Radiographs (bony avulsion, joint deformity as indirect sign)

Treatment Approach

■ Indications

- Conservative, functional, surgical—depending on the tendon, anatomical region, and cause
- Treatment is more likely to be surgical when there are fewer possibilities for compensation in the movement segment and conservative/functional treatment measures are less established.

• Operation indicated for dehiscence, functionally significant deficit, and old rupture

Indication for Conservative Treatment
- Partial tendon rupture with preserved function
- Tendon rupture of a muscle with more than one belly with compensation by intact parts
- Elderly patients with reduced functional demand and with risk factors
- The results are similar compared with surgical treatment (Achilles tendon)

Indications for Surgical Treatment
- Complete tendon tear with dehiscence
- Functional deficit without possibility for compensation
- Open tendon injury
- Old rupture with clinically relevant functional deficit
- Injury with a defect (reconstruction: tenoplasty, interposition graft)

■ Conservative Treatment

- Functional bracing or special splint limits range of motion and ensures contact of the tendon ends
- Isometric exercises under physiotherapist instruction

■ Surgical Treatment

- Atraumatic exposure of the tendon ends
- Sparing the gliding layers and vascular supply (peritendineum, annular ligaments, retinacula, etc.)
- Atraumatic approximation, adapting the instruments and suture material to the size of the tendon

■ Postoperative Care

- Functional therapy (passive supportive treatment initially, later active) to improve histomorphological healing and functionality
- Dynamic fixation (e.g., Kleinert method for finger flexor suture)
- Protection of the rupture zone against major axial traction (splints, ortheses)
- Limited range of motion (splints, special shoe for Achilles tendon)
- Physiotherapy of agonist and antagonist muscles and neighboring joints

25

Further Reading

Baker SP, O'Neill B, Haddon W, Long WB. The Injury Severity Score: a method for describing patients with multiple injuries and evaluating energency care. J Trauma 1974; 14: 187

Debrunner AM. Orthopädie, Orthopädische Chirurgie. Bern: Hans Huber; 2002

Dittel K-K, Weise K. Komplikationsmanagement in der Traumatologie. Stuttgart: Thieme; 2003

Ewerbeck V, Wentzensen A. Standardverfahren in der operativen Orthopädie und Unfallchirurgie. Stuttgart: Thieme; 2006

Herrmann HD. Neurotraumatologie. Weinheim: Edition Medizin VCH; 1991

von Laer L, Kraus R, Linhart WE. Frakturen und Luxationen im Wachstumsalter. 5. Aufl. Stuttgart: Thieme; 2007

Mutschler W, Haas N. Praxis der Unfallchirurgie 2. Aufl. Stuttgart: Thieme; 2004

Stürmer KM. Leitlinien Unfallchirurgie. Stuttgart: Thieme; 2001

Teasdale G, Jennett B. Assessment of coma and impaired consciousness. A practical scale. Lancet 1974; 2: 81

Wirth CJ, Kohn D. Gelenkchirurgie. Stuttgart: Thieme; 1999

Illustration Credits

Fig. 2.1 from Thieme Atlas of Anatomy, Neck and Internal Organs. © Thieme 2006. Illustration by Karl Wesker.

Figs. 2.2, 2.3, 2.6 from Frilling A, Weber F. Endokrine Chirurgie. Schilddrüsenkarzinom. Allgemeine u. Viszeralchirurgie up2date 2007;1:73–88.

Figs. 6.1, 8.1, 17.2, 18.1 from Thieme Atlas of Anatomy, Neck and Internal Organs. © Thieme 2006. Illustrations by Marcus Voll.

Figs. 7.3–7.5 from Schumpelick V. Hernien. 4th ed. © Thieme 2005.

Fig. 11.2 from Schmidt G. Sonographie des Gastrointestinaltraktes. In: Schmidt G, ed. Kursbuch Ultraschall. 4th ed. © Thieme 2003.

Fig. 14.8 from Seegenschmiedt MH, Betzler M. Moderne Behandlungskonzepte beim Analkarzinom. Viszeralchirurgie. 2001;36:119–125.

Index

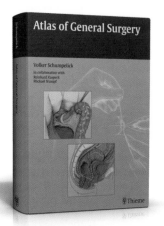
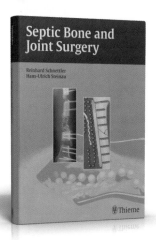
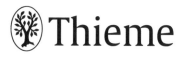

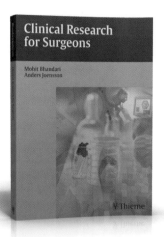
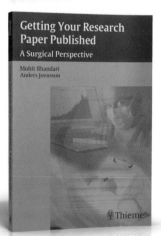
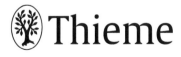